HOW MUCH RISK?

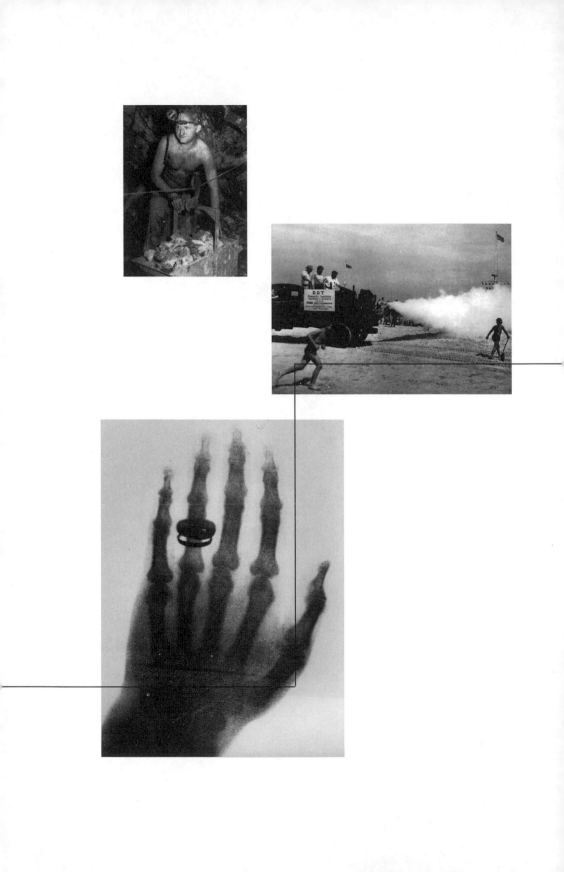

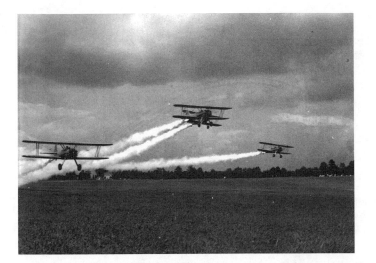

HOW MUCH RISK?

A GUIDE TO UNDERSTANDING
ENVIRONMENTAL HEALTH HAZARDS

Inge F. Goldstein
Martin Goldstein

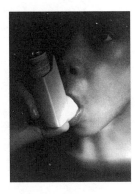

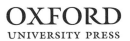

OXFORD
UNIVERSITY PRESS

2002

OXFORD
UNIVERSITY PRESS

Oxford   New York
Athens   Auckland   Bangkok   Bogotá   Buenos Aires   Cape Town
Chennai   Dar es Salaam   Delhi   Florence   Hong Kong   Istanbul   Karachi
Kolkata   Kuala Lumpur   Madrid   Melbourne   Mexico City   Mumbai   Nairobi
Paris   Sao Paolo   Singapore   Taipei   Tokyo   Toronto   Warsaw

and associated companies in
Berlin   Ibadan

Library of Congress Cataloging-in-Publication Data
Goldstein, Inge F.
How much risk? : a guide to understanding environmental
health hazards / by Inge F. Goldstein, Martin Goldstein.
p.   cm.
Includes index.
ISBN 0-19-513994-1
1. Environmental health. 2. Risk assessment.
I. Title: Guide to environmental health hazards.
II. Goldstein, Martin, 1919 Nov. 18–   III. Title.
RA566.27.G65 2001
615.9'02—dc21   2001021985

9 8 7 6 5 4 3 2 1

Printed in the United States of America
on acid-free paper

To our children's children, in the inverse order of their arrival:
Eyal (Didi), Ari, Avital and Teddy.

The human understanding when it has once adopted an opinion (either as being the received opinion or as being agreeable to itself) draws all things else to support and agree with it. And though there be a greater number and weight of instances to be found on the other side, yet these it either neglects and despises, or else by some distinction sets aside and rejects; in order that by this great and pernicious predetermination the authority of its former conclusions may remain inviolate. And therefore it was a good answer that was made by one who when they showed him hanging in a temple a picture of those who had paid their vows as having escaped shipwreck, and would have him say whether he did not now acknowledge the power of the gods,—"Aye," asked he again, "but where are they painted that were drowned after their vows?"

FRANCIS BACON, *NOVUM ORGANUM*

PREFACE

In March of 2001, Christine Todd Whitman, appointed as administrator of the Environmental Protection Agency some months previously by the incoming President Bush, announced that the EPA was rescinding a decision made during the Clinton presidency to lower the acceptable level of a known carcinogen, arsenic, in drinking water. The present standard, 50 parts per billion, has been in force since 1942; the rescinded level would have been 10 parts per billion, the maximum level permitted in European countries. Ms Whitman justified the decision by stating that there was not a sufficient scientific basis for the 10 parts per billion standard. In her words, "When we make a decision on arsenic, it will be based on sound science and solid analysis."

According to the *New York Times*, a factor in the decision was a claim by the mining industry, and by municipalities with high levels of arsenic in their drinking water, that reaching the 10 part per billion level would cost too much. Within the United States the problem appears most severe in New Mexico and other western states, but is even more severe in some other countries around the world. Whitman's decision has been both harshly criticized and warmly defended.

We wrote this book to explain to the concerned reader how science evaluates the health hazards of environmental pollutants: what constitutes "sound science and solid analysis." We use a "case-history" approach, describing in some depth a number of examples of the investigation of specific health hazards about which there has been controversy. They include radiation from radon in homes and from nearby nuclear facilities, toxic waste dumps, air pollution, pesticides, electromagnetic fields, and arsenic in drinking water; hazards blamed by some for causing cancers of various kinds including breast, lung, and skin cancer and childhood leukemia, as well as asthma and other respiratory diseases.

Our goal is to help the concerned reader understand better the issues involved in such evaluations. We are well aware that not all the scientific concepts relevant to environmental health are easy to explain in lay language but we think it is important to make the attempt. Ignorance of them is responsible for exaggerated fear among some, and apathy in the face of real dangers among others.

We make no exaggerated claims for what science can do; we deal as much with the limitations of science as with its successes. The basic scientific principles we describe apply equally well to establishing the health risks of arsenic in drinking water as they do to other currently recognized hazards not discussed in this book, and to those that may arise in the future.

We have done our best to present in an unbiased way the controversies over whether and to what extent specific suspected hazards do harm. We expect that both environmental activists who believe the environment is dangerously polluted to the point that human health is threatened and industrialists who believe that panic about the environment is leading to economically disastrous overregulation will find things to criticize and things to welcome in this book. Perhaps it will help them recognize that there are things on which they may agree.

Science provides a basis for standards to protect human health. Setting such standards, however, is not a purely scientific process: it involves questions of values also, of political and economic choices. These questions are not covered in this book for three reasons. First, such questions lie outside our area of competence: we have opinions about them but only as concerned ordinary citizens, not as "experts." Second, there are many other books that deal with them. Third, explaining the science alone easily fills a book.

All of us, experts or not, have to make informed choices about issues of environmental health, both policy choices and the ordinary choices of daily life. We need to ask what should be regulated, what the benefits of regulation are, what it will cost, and if it is worth it. We also need to know whether to eat an apple that mght have been sprayed with a pesticide, or to warm ourselves at night with an electric blanket, or to install an exhaust fan in the basement. If we understand how science answers the questions we put to it, and, as important, what questions it cannot answer, we can make more sensible choices, and work for more realistic goals.

ACKNOWLEDGMENTS

We are deeply grateful to the Alfred P. Sloan Foundation for a generous grant that made writing this book possible, and to the Rockefeller Foundation for the award to us of a joint residency in September 1998 in the intellectually stimulating, humanly warm, physically beautiful, and gastronomically challenging atmosphere of the Villa Serbelloni, Bellagio, Italy.

We want to thank a number of busy fellow scientists, who were never too busy to read, comment on, and criticize various chapters in this book, or otherwise give us the benefit of their advice or opinions. Many are from our home institution, Columbia University, and include Habibul Ahsan, David Brenner, Patricia Cohen, Victor Gann, Reba Goodman, Tom K. Hei, Judith Jacobson, Andrew Rundle, Regina Santella, Sam Shapiro, and Mary Beth Terry; David Brenner and Tom K. Hei in particular were generous of their time in explaining their own research and providing access to material prior to publication. Others to whom we owe heartfelt thanks include Ethel Gilbert and Michael Alavanja of the National Institutes of Health, Meir Stampfer of Harvard University, Jonathan Samet of Johns Hopkins University, Carol Bodian, Susan Teitelbaum, and Mary Wolff of Mt. Sinai School of Medicine, Susan Klitzman of Hunter College of the City University of New York, Judy Klotz of the New Jersey Department of Health and Senior Services, Anne Aschengrau of Boston University, Julia Brody and Ruthann Rudel of the Silent Spring Institute, Ted Litovitz of Catholic University, Kevin Costas of the Massachusetts Department of Health, Wayne Ott of Stanford University, Leeka Kheifetz of the Electric Power Research Institute, Mel Greaves of the Institute of Cancer Research, London, and Joachim Heinrich and Irene Brueske-Hohlfeld of the G.S.F. (Environmental Research Institute), Munich, Germany.

None of them are responsible for any mistakes we may have made.

Special thanks go to members of our own family, who read chapters and made sure we knew when they had trouble understanding them, Harold, Eric, Michael, and Aviva Goldstein and Richard Miller, and to Michael for drawing the picture of the Texas sharpshooter.

CONTENTS

1 Introduction: What We Hope to Do, 3

2 Atomic Bombs, Nuclear Fallout, and Dental X-Rays, 13

3 Radon in Your Basement, 59

4 Childhood Leukemia Near Nuclear Plants, 101

5 Breast Cancer, Part 1: The Rise of Activism and the Pesticide Hypothesis, 135

6 Breast Cancer, Part 2: Testing the Pesticide Hypothesis, 171

7 Power Lines, Magnetic Fields, and Cancer, 199

8 Cancer from the Landfill? 235

9 Asthma, Allergy, and Air Pollution, 269

10 Summary: Lessons from a Disaster, 303

Bibliography, 317

Index, 325

HOW MUCH RISK?

1

INTRODUCTION: WHAT WE HOPE TO DO

IN THE MOVIES

The movie *Erin Brockovitch*, starring Julia Roberts, opened in the spring of 2000 to excellent reviews and immediate popular success. Advertised as being "based on a true story," it describes how an uneducated but feisty young woman discovers a cluster of diseases in a small California town, including uterine and breast cancer, Hodgkin's disease, brain cancer, colon cancer, asthma, heart disease, and disorders of the immune system, which she attributes to contamination of the town's drinking water with chromium, a toxic metal, due to negligent waste disposal practices of a large corporation. She then initiates a class-action lawsuit on behalf of the victims, which is settled for $333 million, the largest sum yet won in such a suit. The true story on which the case was based involved the Pacific Gas and Electric Corporation, which really did settle the lawsuit by paying out $333 million. Whether the willingness of the corporation to settle for this amount proves that the chromium did cause all the diseases claimed is an interesting question, which this book may shed some light on, but not directly answer.

The movie is one of a number of recent films reflecting a widespread fear that the environment is being polluted by hazardous chemicals and harmful radiation that cause cancer and other diseases, and a need to identify and seek restitution from whoever is responsible.

3

CIVILIZATION AND ITS MALCONTENTS

People living in the advanced industrialized countries of the world suffer from mixed feelings about their high standard of living. They are fully aware of its advantages, both for health and for the quality of life generally: greater freedom from infectious diseases, better medical care, longer life span, a higher standard of living, more choice in work and play. But there is a sense of disadvantages as well: concerns about a loss of community and of cultural diversity, about an obsession with material possessions, about pollution and destruction of the environment. In this book we will open only one of these Pandora's boxes: the problem of environmental pollution and human health.

People of the advanced countries live longer, healthier lives than their preindustrial ancestors and their contemporaries in the less-developed world. But they wonder if pollution of the environment by chemicals or radioactivity, by-products of their modern industrialized society, has replaced some threats to health with others: replaced smallpox and malaria with cancer and asthma. In this book we describe how scientists have investigated a number of specific threats to human health—from high energy radiation, from electromagnetic fields, from chemical hazards like pesticides or toxic waste dumps, from air pollution—what kind of evidence they need, what they have concluded about the risks these hazards pose, and what still remains to be done.

This book is written to be understood by lay readers and has two goals. The first is to present the current scientific picture on these hazards. The second is a more general one: to describe just how environmental health hazards are studied scientifically, as an example of how science in general functions, how it succeeds, and how and why it often fails.

TOXIC CHEMICALS FROM A DUMP SITE

The following stories are something like that told in the film *Erin Brockovitch*, except that there are no happy endings. Sadly, they are much more typical of what happens in such episodes.

Pelham Bay Park, a good-sized public park, is located in the Bronx, one of the five boroughs that make up New York City. The park is adjacent to Pelham Bay, an arm of the Atlantic Ocean. In 1963 a portion of the park was turned over by the New York City Parks Department to the city's Sanitation Department, for the construction of a euphemistically named sanitary landfill, a dumping ground for domestic garbage, street sweepings, and construction and other commercial waste. People from residential neighborhoods adjacent to the park objected to the construction of the landfill, but were unable to stop the dumping until 1978, after enduring some fifteen years of foul smells, heavy traffic of dumping vehicles, and the general ugliness of the site.

A few years after dumping was stopped, the U.S. Senate Committee on Crime heard testimony from a driver for an oil-refining company to the effect that toxic substances had been illegally dumped at the landfill. In 1986 a five-year-old girl we will call Ellen living in the neighborhood of the site became ill with leukemia. Her mother, bringing her in to a local clinic for treatment each week, was struck by the fact that she was meeting many of her neighbors there, also bringing in children for treatment of leukemia. She and other concerned parents began to compile a list of the cases in the neighborhood and found twelve cases, a number that seemed unreasonably large to her and her neighbors.

Could the chemicals illegally dumped in the landfill be causing the leukemia? Although the full extent of toxic substance dumping could no longer be determined, benzene and other toxic chemicals could be detected in the air, in ground water near the dump, in the water of Long Island Sound just offshore, and in the fish and shellfish there. Benzene in particular is a known cause of leukemia.

As by this time health and the environment had become a politically important issue, the Pelham Bay community was able to force an investigation by the New York City Health Department and the New York City Department of Environmental Protection. To answer the concerns of the community, the Department of Health did a study to determine if the rates of leukemia in particular and cancer in general were high in the vicinity of the dump site. The main conclusion was that although leukemia rates were higher than normal, the increases were not "statistically significant" and were attributed to "chance."

This conclusion, so contrary to the impressions of concerned members of the community, was greatly disturbing to them. Although the Health Department had attempted to explain their methods and results in lay language, there was a considerable use of technical terms, and of graphs and tables difficult for a nonspecialist to make sense of.

One of the authors of this book, who was a member of a scientific advisory committee to the community and who had had some experience in writing about science for nonscientists, was asked to write an explanation of the Health Department reports in language a lay reader could better understand. This book grew out of that experience.

CANCER CLUSTERS, WOBURN AND ELSEWHERE

The story of the Pelham Bay landfill and the cases of childhood leukemia in its vicinity is unfortunately a common one. It is one of thousands of episodes, in the United States and elsewhere, in which someone becomes aware that there are many more cases of some disease in her neighborhood than seems reasonable, and wants to know why. The community as a whole becomes concerned and demands that health authorities investigate the problem. Such a local excess of disease is called a cluster, and clusters of cancer have lately attracted considerable attention.

The cluster of childhood leukemia cases in Woburn, Massachusetts, is among the best known, having inspired the best-selling book *A Civil Action* and later a film. The story, similar to that of Pelham Bay, began with the suspicions of a concerned mother of a child with leukemia, who organized a voluntary survey within the community that turned up an unexpectedly large number of cases of childhood leukemia. This led to a Massachusetts Department of Public Health investigation and a dramatic lawsuit. In Woburn as in Pelham Bay there was a plausible source of contamination: chemical wastes dumped or otherwise carelessly handled. In Woburn they entered the water table from which one part of the town, where many of the leukemia cases had occurred, drew its drinking water. In spite of years of study by several groups of scientists, there as yet is no agreed-on explanation of the cluster. The parents there know their children have suffered and died, but have not as yet received a clear answer. Why is it taking so long? (fig. 1-1).

In the town of Toms River, in southern New Jersey, still another concerned mother whose child developed a rare form of central nervous system cancer sparked the collection of data on childhood cancer that showed high rates in the community, and again an investigation of the cluster by the New Jersey Department of Health was begun, which is still going on. The department issued a preliminary report in 1997, which concluded that in the years 1979 to 1995 the rate of childhood cancers in Toms River was four times the average in the rest of the state. There were excesses both of leukemia and of brain and nervous system cancers. Again, as in Woburn,

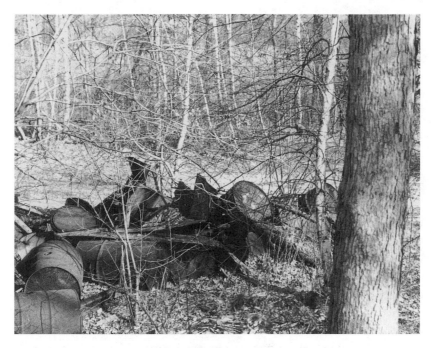

FIGURE 1-1 Abandoned drums of chemicals rusting away in the woods around Woburn, Massachusetts. Courtesy of the U.S. Environmental Protection Agency, New England office, Boston, MA.

a source of contamination of the water supply by industrial chemical wastes was known, and is now under study. Will the investigation come up with an answer that will satisfy the people of Toms River?

WHO IS TO BLAME?

One cannot ask for a Hollywood ending to all these episodes; but one might hope for closure: first of all for a definitive answer to the question, what caused the cancers? then for an assurance that the source of contamination has been eliminated, and finally for some sort of restitution to be made to the families of the victims. It does not usually happen that way, contrary to the impression *Erin Brockovitch* may give. Some of the contaminated sites have been cleaned up, but in neither Pelham Bay, Woburn, nor Toms River have clear causes of the cancers yet been established, in turn making it harder to win suits for wrongful injury. The anguish of the parents who believe that their children sickened or died as a direct result of gross carelessness and irresponsibility can be imagined. Their attitudes toward health authorities and scientists, who have failed to establish any clear cause or dismissed the clusters as merely chance occurrences, have ranged from impatience to fury, and who can blame them? Do not diseases have causes? Can not science find them? How can a high rate of cancer next door to a toxic waste dump be caused by chance?

THE ATOMIC BOMB

High-energy radiation is a well-established cause of leukemia, as was confirmed by a study of survivors of the atomic bombing of Hiroshima and Nagasaki. We begin the book with this tragic episode because it is a model for studies of other environmental health hazards. It required a laborious effort to reconstruct the dose of radiation each survivor received, which has enabled us to make good estimates of just how many cancers of each kind the radiation from the bombs in Japan caused, to set safety standards for radiation exposure, and to predict the consequences of other exposures, from nuclear plant accidents like Chernobyl down to dental X-rays.

Some clusters of childhood leukemia or other cancers have been attributed to fallout from nuclear bomb tests and nuclear plant accidents, or careless disposal of radioactive waste. For example, fallout from U.S. weapons tests in the 1950s and 1960s exposed areas of the state of Utah, and excess cases of childhood leukemia were reported in some of the small towns in its path. The U.S. Atomic Energy Commission denied at the time that the fallout was any significant health threat, no more so than getting a few medical X-rays. Were these cases of leukemia caused by the radiation?

RADON IN HOMES

Not all exposure to high-energy radiation takes place as a result of the development and use of nuclear energy or from medical X-rays; there are natural sources of radiation exposure—for example, radon in our homes. What is radon and how does it get into our homes? How do we know it is there? How much harm does it do? Some scientists have claimed that it is responsible for about 10% of lung cancer in the United States, but others think that this figure is far too high. Who is right?

THE NUCLEAR PLANT NEXT DOOR

In a small town adjacent to a nuclear fuels reprocessing facility in England there was a cluster of childhood leukemia cases: the rate during a fifteen-year period was about ten times the average in England generally. The facility was subsequently revealed to have emitted more radioactivity as a result of a major fire and a number of smaller accidents than authorities had ever acknowledged. Was the radioactivity responsible?

BREAST CANCER AND PESTICIDES

Breast cancer has apparently been increasing over the last fifty years in Western industrialized countries, and industrialization has been blamed for the increase. Excess rates of breast cancer among women have been reported in some areas of the United States. It is particularly high in the northeastern urban belt, from Philadelphia to Boston, and also in the San Francisco area in California. Women living on Long Island, New York, on Cape Cod, Massachusetts, and in San Francisco, concerned about the high rates in their areas, have organized activist groups to demand scientific studies to explain them. In response, studies have been funded to investigate the role of pesticides, toxic waste dumping, and electromagnetic fields in some of these areas. What have these studies found? What is known about the causes of breast cancer?

The techniques of molecular biology have been used to show that a small proportion of women have a genetic predisposition to breast cancer that gives them a very high risk of the disease. Are there genetic sensitivities to chemicals in the environment that play a role in breast cancer? What is known about the molecular biology of cancer in general and breast cancer in particular?

POWER LINES, ELECTRIC BLANKETS, AND CANCER

High-energy radiation, from radioactive substances or from X-ray machines, is invisible and odorless: we may not know that we have been exposed until we become ill, unless we use devices like radiation counters or film badges to warn us. Electromagnetic fields, from electric currents flowing either in power lines, in the wiring in our homes, or in appliances used close to the body such as electric blankets, hair dryers, or the now ubiquitous cellular phones, are also invisible and odorless. Are they a threat to health? On one hand, a number of scientists have reported excess childhood leukemia, brain and breast cancers, birth defects, and psychological problems in people living close to power lines or otherwise exposed to such fields. On the other hand, other scientists have found no such excesses. Some physicists have claimed that it would violate the laws of physics for weak fields coming from electric currents in the home to have any health effects at all. If scientists disagree, how do ordinary citizens decide what to do? Such electromagnetic fields are all around us in the modern world; we are all exposed. Just how serious a hazard are they? Is it true that the laws of physics guarantee that these fields are harmless?

ASTHMA: A DISEASE OF CIVILIZATION?

Cancer is not the only disease attributed to exposure to environmental hazards. Asthma, a disease characterized by acute attacks of breathing difficulty on exposure to various airborne agents, has been increasing dramatically, mostly in industrialized countries. Is this increase caused by air pollution? Is it caused by some other consequences of industrialization? There is something paradoxical about who suffers most from asthma: in the United States poor minority populations in the inner cities have the highest rates, while in most other countries, there is more asthma among people in the higher social classes. Why is this so?

HOW DANGEROUS IS ARSENIC?

We use the as yet unresolved question of how much harm results from arsenic in drinking water, a matter of serious concern in the United States and even more serious concern in other countries around the world, to summarize the main points we want to make about evaluating health hazards. They include the importance of knowing precisely which people were exposed and how much, the problem of estimating the harm done by low exposures from studies of high exposures, the need for coherence among the different scientific disciplines before conclusions can be drawn, the particular and growing importance of molecular biology in health studies, and last but not least the limitations of science.

THE MANY ENVIRONMENTAL SCIENCES

There is no cut-and-dried procedure for answering the questions we have asked, no one kind of scientist called an "environmental scientist" to turn to. If there is such a thing as "environmental science," it is the combined activity of different scientists from various disciplines, using different approaches and different techniques, hopefully coming up with a coherent answer, but sometimes with conflicting conclusions. Obviously harmony among them is more convincing than discord.

There is one discipline of special importance to environmental health controversies because it is of special importance to the questions of health and disease in general, and will play an ever-increasing role in the future. Molecular biology is concerned with understanding on the basis of the behavior of individual molecules how genetic predispositions and environmental factors act together—as they must in all kinds of diseases. This field, which has greatly illuminated the causes and progression of cancer and other diseases, is in the process of rapid change and development. It will give us not only a more fundamental understanding of disease but also quite practical knowledge: an increasing ability to tell which environmental exposures caused specific cases of disease, how to find out which individuals are genetically susceptible to specific environmental agents or genetically resistant to them, and much else. For example, it is now possible to detect by simple blood tests which women have a certain genetic predisposition to breast cancer that puts them at very high risk. The complete genetic makeup of all human beings, the "human genome," has just been deciphered, and the impact on research into human diseases is incalculable.

ENVIRONMENT, GENES, AND LIFESTYLE

The word "environment" unfortunately is used in two not-quite-overlapping senses, and in this book we will need both of them. When we contrast the relative influences of heredity and "environment," we are using it in one sense, to refer to all influences on the development and functioning of an organism other than those determined by that organism's genes. High-energy radiation, chemical toxins, deciding to delay pregnancy, getting too little exercise are in this sense all environmental factors, as contrasted with inherited ones. In the second sense, we contrast "environment" with "lifestyle." As an example, smoke from one's own cigarette is a lifestyle choice, and smoke from somebody else's an environmental hazard, which is why smoking in many public places is banned. Pesticides in food is an environmental hazard, eating a diet high in fats a lifestyle one. When personal choice is involved, we speak of lifestyle; the things we are exposed to whether we want them or not form the environment.

We also use the term "lifestyle" to describe differences between one society and another. Here personal choice is less important; in highly industrialized societies we are exposed to higher electromagnetic fields, get more medical X-rays, eat richer diets, have few children, and so on. The line between environment and lifestyle is sometimes hard to draw, but the distinction is useful. As we said earlier, we will have to use the word "environment" in both senses, and hope the context will make clear which sense is implied.

WHAT WE TRY TO DO HERE

In this book we will try to answer the questions we have asked here, and others like them, about some current environmental health concerns. Many will not have answers yet, and some may get answers only as new scientific techniques are developed. We want to explain not only what scientific research has found about the health effects of certain specific environmental exposures but also the way scientists in general approach such questions. The particular controversies we describe were chosen to meet two criteria: they are of current concern, and they illustrate some basic principles of science and the methods used to resolve them. Our intention is to give the reader some sense of how the scientists that deal with these issues go about their mission: how causes of disease are discovered, what kind of evidence is needed to show causation, how that evidence is obtained, and how it is used. We hope it will help the reader understand other environmental problems, those we have left out and those that will arise in the future, to which the same basic principles will apply.

Most of what we read or hear about environmental issues is not based on science. Some of it is the expression of self-interest or ideology, and some is the expression of ignorance and fear. Science is the only antidote to ignorance and fear, and the best answer to the distortions and omissions of those engaged in advocacy for a cause.

2

ATOMIC BOMBS, NUCLEAR FALLOUT,
AND DENTAL X-RAYS

THE DISCOVERY OF HIGH-ENERGY RADIATION

One of the first pictures made with X-rays by Wilhelm Roentgen, when he discovered them in 1895, was of the hand of a colleague of his, a Dr. von Koelliker (fig. 2-1). The bones of his hand and a ring he was wearing stand out clearly; the flesh appears as a faint halo around the bones. A glance at the photograph makes it obvious why the medical possibilities of X-rays were almost immediately recognized. X-rays were used first for diagnosis, and later for treatment of disease as well, but they were the first form of radiation shown also to cause disease. In the early years of radiology, radiologists used to hold the X-ray film in place close to the patient's body, thus receiving intense exposures of their hands. There were unexpected difficulties in arranging for a celebratory dinner for the Society of Radiologists in Philadelphia on the twenty-fifth anniversary of the discovery of X-rays: so many of the members had lost fingers or hands that they found it too awkward to eat in public.

The discovery of X-rays led in 1896 to the discovery of radioactivity by Henri Becquerel, who observed, almost by accident, that compounds of the metallic element uranium emitted a kind of radiation that like X-rays passed through the black paper photographic film was wrapped in and darkened the film. Marie and Pierre Curie, following up his work,

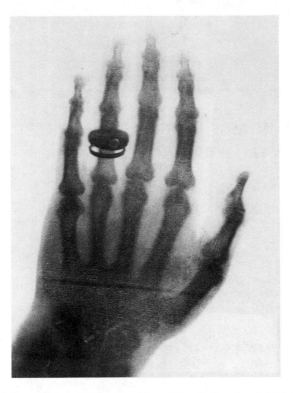

FIGURE 2-1   X-ray of hand with ring. One of the first pictures made by Roentgen in 1898. Copyright Bettman-Corbis.

found that the strongest sources of the radioactivity were impurities in the uranium compounds and were able to extract small quantities of other much more radioactive elements from them, including polonium and radium. Becquerel and the Curies were awarded the Nobel Prize in physics in 1903.

At first, the energy given out steadily by radioactive substances could not be explained, and some scientists proposed that they might provide unlimited sources of energy. It was soon shown that radioactive substances, like any other fuel, are used up as energy is given out: the radioactive atoms are undergoing disintegration into other, different kinds of atoms. When an atom of uranium-238 emits alpha radiation, it changes at the same time into an atom of a rare element called thorium, also radioactive. After a series of other radioactive decays the process ends with nonradioactive lead (see fig. 3-5, page 65).

Marie Curie died of a blood disease, probably leukemia, in 1934. Her daughter Irene Joliot-Curie, who also devoted her research career to radioactivity, died of leukemia in 1956. Their deaths were probably caused by their exposure to radioactive substances, making Marie one of the first casualties of the era she pioneered. There were many others, even before nuclear bombs were dropped on Hiroshima and Nagasaki. In the 1920s a number of women employed to paint the numbers on the dials of luminous watches with compounds of radium were found to have suffered deterioration of the jawbones. They had ingested radium by licking the paint brushes to produce a fine point at the tip. Many eventually died of bone cancer and anemia.

Before the hazards of high-energy radiation were fully recognized, radioactive substances were advertised as good for health. Mineral waters with dissolved radon or radium were widely advertised, and a toothpaste containing radon was marketed before World War II. There are some who still believe in its benefits today. There are abandoned mines in Montana equipped with benches on which people wishing to inhale radon may sit. There is a health resort in the republic of Georgia (formerly part of the Soviet Union) where people may have enemas or vaginal douches using water solutions of radon. The authors of this book, on a visit to Carlsbad (now Karlovy Vary) in the Czech Republic, were offered bottles of mineral water at dinner, drawn from natural springs in the area, with the quantity of radioactivity listed conspicuously on the label. We were told that people come from all over the world to Carlsbad to drink this water (fig. 2-2).

Just how harmful is high-energy radiation? How large a dose will cause leukemia? Is it possible that low doses are beneficial? In this chapter and the next two we describe how such questions are answered.

THE BOMB

What It Was Like

The nuclear bomb dropped on Hiroshima on August 6, 1945, killed about one hundred thousand people almost immediately, the majority by the force of the explosion, the subsequent collapse of buildings, and the resulting fires. It is estimated that about thirty thousand were killed directly by radiation, and thousands more died of acute radiation sickness within a few weeks. Almost as many died in the bombing of Nagasaki three days

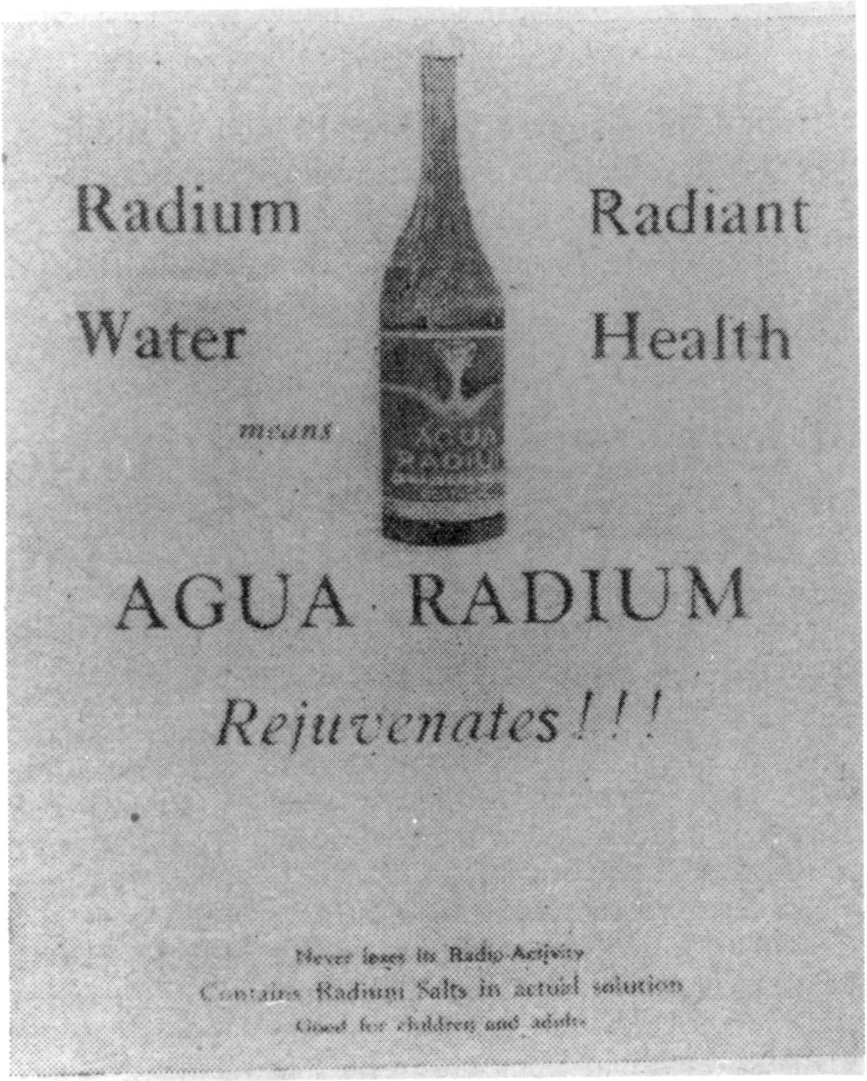

FIGURE 2-2 Advertisement for "Agua Radium," sold to the public during the 1920s and 1930s, to be mixed with milk to make it "more digestive for all children and invalids." Reproduced from an article by A. M. Jelliffe and F. S. Stewart, "Radium Vita Emanator—An Unusual Potential Radiation Hazard," in the *British Medical Journal*, v. 2, pp. 305–306 (1969). Reproduced with permission of the BMJ Publishing Group.

later, the causes of the deaths in about the same proportion. Still thousands more in both cities, less strongly exposed, suffered from acute radiation sickness but recovered.

These dry statistics do not give any sense of the horror of the experience. For that we must turn to the testimony of some of the survivors. Here are brief passages from a memoir by a Japanese physician, Michihiko Hachiya, who was working in a hospital in Hiroshima the day of the bombing. Dr. Hachiya was injured in the bombing and immediately hospitalized, but reports graphic observations by friends and colleagues.

Dr. Tabuchi:

> Hundreds of injured people who were trying to escape to the hills passed our house. The sight of them was almost unbearable. Their faces and hands were burnt and swollen: and great sheets of skin had peeled away from their tissues to hang down like rags on a scarecrow. They moved like a line of ants. All through the night, they went past our house, but this morning they had stopped. I found them lying on both sides of the road so thick that it was impossible to pass without stepping on them.

Mr. Katsutani:

> The sight of the soldiers, though, was more dreadful than the dead people floating down the river. I came onto I don't know how many, burned from the hips up; and where the skin has peeled, their flesh was wet and mushy. They must have been wearing their military caps because the black hair on top of their heads was not burned. It made them look like they were wearing black lacquer bowls.
>
> And they had no faces! Their eyes, noses and mouths had been burned away, and it looked like their ears had melted off. It was hard to tell front from back.

Dr. Hanaoka:

> Between the Red Cross Hospital and the center of the city I saw nothing that wasn't burned to a crisp. Streetcars were standing at Kawaya-cho and Kamiya-cho and inside were dozens of bodies, blackened beyond recognition. I saw fire reservoirs filled to the brim with dead people who looked as

though they had been boiled alive. In one reservoir I saw a man, horribly burned, crouching beside another man who was dead. He was drinking blood-stained water out of the reservoir. Even if I had tried to stop him, it wouldn't have done any good; he was completely out of his head. . . .

. . . [T]hat pool wasn't big enough to accommodate everybody who tried to get in it. You could tell that by looking around the sides. I don't know how many were caught by death with their heads hanging over the edge. In one pool I saw some people who were still alive, sitting in the water with dead all around them. They were too weak to get out. People were trying to help them, but I am sure they must have died. (figs. 2-3, 2-4)

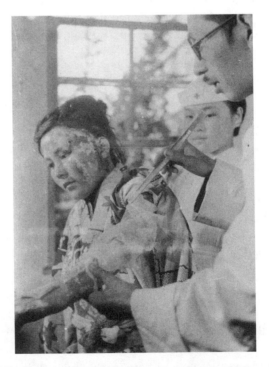

FIGURE 2-3 Treating a burned survivor of the atomic bombing of Japan. Courtesy of the Atomic Bomb Casualty Commission Archives, Houston Academy of Medicine—Texas Medical Center Library.

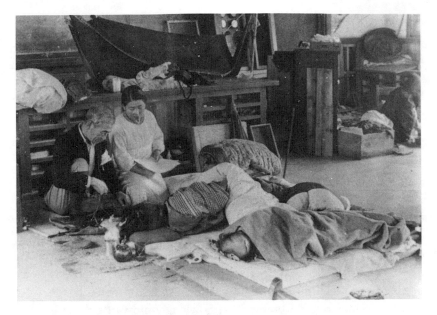

FIGURE 2-4 A family member and nurse comforting survivors in a Hiroshima first-aid station. Courtesy of the Atomic Bomb Casualty Commission Archives, Houston Academy of Medicine—Texas Medical Center Library.

Neither Dr. Hachiya nor anyone else in Japan, including Japanese physicists, had any idea the United States was working on a nuclear bomb. Dr. Hachiya's first guess, on observing that many of the survivors were suffering nausea and diarrhea, was that they were suffering from dysentery from bacteria contained in the bomb: the United States was engaging in biological warfare. However, on August 8, a Japanese nuclear physicist examining the city concluded that a nuclear bomb had been used. Japanese physicians and biologists began studying the effects of the radiation almost from the first day, and after the Japanese surrender they were joined by American scientists, who arrived in Hiroshima on September 8.

The two groups joined efforts on a study of how much harm human beings suffer from exposure to high-energy radiation. The research effort is still continuing today, more than fifty years after the event. What questions had it sought to answer? More specifically, we expect that the more exposure a person has received, the greater that person's risk of harm: of leukemia, of breast cancer, of giving birth to a retarded child. Just what is the relation between the amount of exposure and the risk of each of these outcomes? Can this tell us the risk from a chest X-ray? From fallout from nuclear weapons testing? From living near the Three Mile Island nuclear power plant at the time of the accident there? The study of the survivors of the Hiroshima and Nagasaki bombs is our best single source of knowledge for answering such questions.

A New Age

The first response to the atomic bombing of Japan, at least in the United States and among its allies in World War II, was euphoria at the sudden, painless (for them), victorious peace that followed. But doubts and concern began almost immediately, first among scientists who had worked on the bomb and understood its dangers; many became active in support of civilian control of atomic energy, bans on nuclear testing, and nuclear disarmament. Public concern increased at first gradually, and then accelerated after the disclosure of a number of episodes in which people were exposed to radiation without their knowledge, most often accidentally as the result of carelessly conducted nuclear weapons tests, but in some cases quite deliberately in experiments unpleasantly reminiscent of those done by German physicians on concentration camp inmates during the Nazi era.

There are features of radiation that makes it particularly frightening: it is not detectable by the senses: it is invisible, odorless, tasteless. Exposure to fatal or near-fatal doses can take place without the victim being aware of it at the moment. This combination of undetectability and official obfuscation, together with the horrors of the nuclear bombing of Japan, have fueled public fears of nuclear energy. There is fear of accidents at nuclear plants. There is concern about disposal of nuclear wastes that remain radioactive for thousands of years. There has been intense scrutiny of the dangers to health of working in or living near nuclear facilities, particularly after reports of increased rates of leukemia and other cancers in their vicinity.

This increasing public awareness of the risks of exposure to high-energy radiation was one major reason for the rise of the environmental movement, another being the London "smog" episodes of 1952 in which four thousand people died in just a few days from exposure to high levels of air pollution (discussed in chapter 9), and still another the publication in 1963 of the book *Silent Spring*, by Rachel Carson, describing the effects of pesticides on wildlife (discussed in chapter 5).

FALLOUT FROM NUCLEAR TESTS AND
NUCLEAR ACCIDENTS

Fallout and Disinformation

In 1951 the U. S. government began above-ground tests of nuclear weapons at a site in southern Nevada. The site was selected because it was not near any major population centers and because the expected zone of fallout, determined by prevailing wind direction and amount of rainfall, was sparsely populated. Unfortunately, "sparsely populated" does not mean empty of people.

It was a difficult time, the beginning of the Cold War. Berlin had been blockaded by Soviet forces in 1948. The Soviet Union exploded its first atomic bomb in 1949, which surprised the U.S. government but not U.S. physicists, who were well aware that once it was known a bomb could be made, it would be easy for any country with a competent scientific base to make one. In 1950 the Korean War began. There was considerable pressure from the military for testing weapons, and the Atomic Energy Commission (AEC), although a civilian agency, had the responsibility for running the program.

When the agency planned the tests, some thought had been given to possible exposure of nearby populations, but the sense of urgency overrode such concerns. The problem was treated as one of public relations, rather than of protecting people. The system for monitoring fallout was primitive and far from adequate; better methods were available but not used. There were only a few monitoring stations, and only one was located in southern Utah, where the known wind patterns would have suggested that the fallout would be greatest. No search for possible contamination of the food chain, particularly of milk, was done until the test series was almost over, in spite of the fact that the danger to children from radioactive iodine in milk was well recognized at the time.

About 100 bombs were exploded at the Nevada site during the years from 1953 to 1958, the total energy (equivalent to about one million tons of TNT) being more than fifty times that of the bomb dropped on Hiroshima. Amateur prospectors who used Geiger counters to search for uranium deposits reported that at times the counters would give off-scale readings. There were many deaths of sheep pastured in areas suspected to have suffered high local fallout. Within a year or two people living in the area began to report symptoms such as skin burns, and illnesses and deaths, particularly from cancer, which many of them attributed to radiation. In some of the small towns in southwestern Utah, where the fallout was assumed to be heaviest, clusters of childhood leukemia were reported subsequent to the tests. The numbers of cases was not large, but childhood leukemia is a rare disease in any event. In two nearby small towns in Utah, Parowan and Paragonah, with a combined population of about a thousand and where everyone knows everyone else, four cases within a few years when childhood leukemia had hardly ever been seen before were alarming.

The response of the AEC was not to acknowledge responsibility or improve its inadequate monitoring system but rather to deny that the tests could have caused any of the illnesses or animal deaths, to ignore or dismiss the Geiger counter readings, to suppress reports written by their own scientists that suggested harm from the fallout, and to falsify some of the data on fallout they had collected to make it seem that safety guidelines were being met. When the AEC was sued by ranchers whose sheep had died, the commission concealed from the court what their own scientists had concluded: the deaths had been caused by radiation, probably ingested when the sheep grazed on grass coated with radioactive dust. The court judgment went against the ranchers, but when the dishonesty of the AEC was revealed in the 1970s through the use of the Freedom of Information Act, the ranchers reopened the case, and this time the same judge decided in their favor. The judgment was overturned on appeal, and the Supreme Court declined to hear the case.

What Harm Was Done?

It has been hard to tell in retrospect whether people in Utah were really harmed by the fallout. Why? A portion of the radioactive substances emitted by a nuclear device exploded above ground goes up into the stratosphere, and is circulated all around the world before it is eventually deposited on the earth. Much of the radioactivity will have decayed by the time this has taken place. Another portion, in the dust cloud caused by the explosion, is carried by winds to nearby areas and reaches the ground either when the dust settles, or more rapidly if rain or snow brings it down. How much radioactive dust is deposited depends therefore on highly local weather conditions and local topography: winds die down or suddenly blow harder, a rainstorm may drench one small area and miss an adjacent one a half-mile away. The result is that even in an area in which the average level of fallout is low, there can be local "hot spots" of high radiation. If the AEC had used many more monitoring devices, and there is no good reason why there should not have been one in every small town in the area, more would have been known about the exposures of individuals living there.

So there is no answer yet to the question: was there really as much excess childhood leukemia in the immediate path of the fallout as the people of Utah believe? Thanks to the decision by the AEC to deal with safety issues in the irresponsible way they did, it remains open. Was this the only course the AEC could have followed at the time, even considering the needs of national security, and under the pressure of the Soviet nuclear bomb program? The people of Utah, patriotic and politically conservative, initially supported the necessity of testing. If the AEC had been more honest in warning them that there was some risk from fallout, had set up an adequate monitoring network to warn local communities when needed, and advised what measures to take to minimize the risk, there would have been less suspicion of government, less anger, and, just possibly, less cancer.

This sad story has a moral that applies to any study of environmental health hazards, not just radiation: if we do not know what people were exposed to and how much, we can conclude very little. The better we know exposures the more confidence we can have in the conclusions we draw.

In the United States there have been attempts to estimate retrospectively the exposures from nuclear weapons tests using other data, to see if they have caused increases in leukemia and thyroid cancer. We will describe them later in the chapter.

THE STUDY OF THE BOMB SURVIVORS

Why We Need to Know Exposure

Our knowledge of the harm radiation, and for that matter any environmental hazard, can do to human beings comes first and most significantly from epidemiological studies: the comparison of rates of disease in exposed and unexposed human populations. Specifically what we need is what is called a dose-response relation: how much a person's risk of cancer is increased by a particular dose of radiation exposure. Obviously, if we do not know who has been exposed and to how much, we cannot proceed, as is amply borne out by the history of the U.S. nuclear bomb tests. The exposure of each individual in the study of the Japanese survivors of the nuclear bombings in World War II could be estimated in ways we will describe, which is what makes this study so valuable.

Finding out how much disease rates have increased is harder than it sounds: the diseases caused by radiation are not different in kind from diseases that occur in its absence: cancers, birth defects, blood abnormalities all occur anyway. Radiation only increases their rates. As of this writing there is no way to distinguish a cancer caused by radiation exposure from a cancer of the same kind that occurs spontaneously, though study of the genetic makeup of the cancerous cells may yet make it possible. (See "How Is the Harm Done?" [p. 56] and discussion of the molecular biology of cancer in chapter 6.)

The Life Span Study

Over the course of the Japanese study, approximately 85,000 survivors were identified and have received careful medical surveillance from then on, still continuing today. About half of them are still alive, almost fifty-five years after the bombing, and are still showing new effects of their exposure, so the book is not yet closed on what is now known as the Life Span Study.

While the Life Span Study is our best single source of information about the health hazards of high-energy radiation from sources outside the body, radiation emitted from radioactive elements selectively absorbed by organs of the body requires separate study. Both kinds of exposure occur from fallout. In this and the next chapter we will discuss examples of internal sources in some detail: thyroid cancer from radioactive iodine in fallout and lung cancer caused by deposition in lung tissue of radioactive elements formed from the decay of radon.

What Is Radiation?

The bomb victims were exposed to high-energy radiation, sometimes called ionizing radiation. Such radiation has enough energy to directly break the chemical bonds that hold molecules together. There are two different kinds of ionizing radiation. X-rays and gamma rays are forms of electromagnetic radiation and travel at the speed of light. Alpha rays and beta rays are composed of particles of matter travelling at high speeds but less than the speed of light. Neutrons, uncharged particles found in the nuclei of atoms, can travel at high enough speeds to constitute ionizing radiation (see "What Is Ionizing Radiation?" [p. 49] for more details on ionizing radiation and how it is measured). Both particle and electromagnetic radiation are emitted when atoms undergo radioactive decay, either naturally or in a nuclear device, and by particle accelerators commonly used in research laboratories. In addition, radiation of both the particle and electromagnetic kind are produced in stars and in the course of other astrophysical processes, though we are shielded from much of such radiation by the earth's atmosphere.

The bombs dropped on Hiroshima and Nagasaki emitted most of their ionizing radiation in the form of neutrons and gamma rays, though the relative proportions of each were different in the two bombs.

How Radiation Harms

If the chemical bonds broken by ionizing radiation are those of the molecules of DNA in the nuclei of cells, mutations may result, and sometimes this starts a process that ends in cancer. "DNA" is an abbreviation for the molecule that carries the genetic information that determines the functioning of a cell. These molecules are duplicated and passed on to daughter cells on cell division. Sometimes a mutation, a change in the chemical structure of the DNA molecule, can be passed on to the daughter cells and their descendants. Some mutations are harmful, so that the cell that bears them functions less well, dies earlier, and has fewer offspring. Certain mutations, however, confer a reproductive advantage on the cell and its descendants. Further mutations may eventually give rise to cells that can reproduce out of control, leading to cancer (figs. 2-5, 2-6).

It is important to realize that the same diseases that result from radiation exposure occur also in its absence. Radiation does not produce unheard-of monsters, the two-headed children of science fiction. Instead it adds to the number of cancers, other illnesses, birth defects, and mutations that occur for other reasons.

Living beings are exposed to some radiation from radioactive elements in the natural environment and cosmic rays from outer space, and have been from the dawn of life. In addition to natural sources of radiation, all of us are exposed to a number of man-made sources: we get medical X-rays, and are subject to fallout from nuclear tests, nuclear accidents, and the normal operating emissions of nuclear power plants. Most of the time and in most places, these man-made sources add only a little to the natural background.

The evidence we have from studies on both humans and animals shows that natural radiation accounts for several percent of mutations and

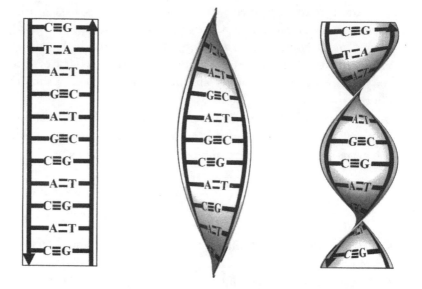

FIGURE 2-5   DNA. The figure shows the "double-helix" structure, which can be visualized by twisting a ribbon about its long axis. One DNA molecule lies along each edge of the twisted ribbon. DNA molecules can be thought of as having a "head" end and a "tail" end; the two molecules face in opposite directions. The base-pairing that holds the two molecules together is also shown: A (adenine) with T (thymine) and G (guanine) with C (cytosine). Figure prepared by Professor Andrew Rundle, Columbia University, and used with his permission.

cancer. Mutations also occur spontaneously; there is enough energy in the form of heat in living tissue to cause them. Certain chemicals are also known to be mutagenic, but it is not known what fraction of mutations might be due to such chemicals in the environment.

Cancers in the Nonexposed

Since the cancers and genetic defects caused by radiation do not differ in kind or in severity from illnesses that occur in its absence, we must compare the rates in groups exposed to different levels of radiation to the rates of these various illnesses in the absence of radiation exposure. Of the roughly 85,000 survivors whose dose of radiation could be estimated, about 35,000 received so low a dose they could be regarded as not exposed. The rest received doses that varied from low up to near-fatal levels.

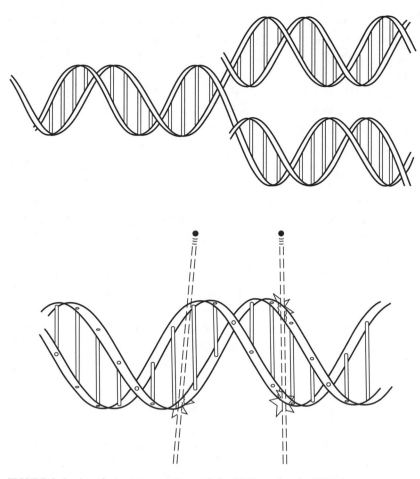

FIGURE 2-6 Another representation of the DNA molecule. This figure illustrates how the two DNA molecules separate during replication, each molecule acting as a template for forming a new molecule (above), and the breaking of the DNA molecule by alpha particles (below). One alpha particle is shown breaking one of the two DNA strands, and another breaking both at once. Reproduced from David J. Brenner, *Radon: Risk and Remedy,* W.H. Freeman and Co., New York, 1989, and used by courtesy of Professor Brenner.

How Much Radiation Did They Get?

We have used the term "dose" of radiation: it is necessary to define it.

The dose for gamma rays or X-rays is the total energy of the radiation absorbed by an individual person, corrected for that person's size. Obviously a given amount of radiation energy absorbed by a large person will do less harm than the same amount absorbed by a smaller person.

The dose is therefore defined as the energy absorbed per kilogram of the person's mass. Energy here is measured in joules. How much energy is a joule? A 100-watt electric bulb uses 100 joules each second, so a joule may seem like a very small amount of energy, at least in terms of ordinary experience. As will be seen, a total dose of X-rays or gamma rays of 5 joules per kilogram over the whole body is usually fatal. Why so little energy can do so much harm will be explained later.

Unfortunately, the dose alone is not enough to predict damage: equal doses of different kinds of radiation are not equally harmful. A given dose of neutrons, for example, is roughly ten to twenty times more biologically damaging than the same dose of X-rays or gamma rays. The current standard unit of "equivalent" dose corrects for this relative degree of harmfulness. It is called the sievert and is described in more detail in "What Is Ionizing Radation?" X-rays are used as a reference: the sievert for X-rays is defined as 1 joule per kilogram of body mass, and the sievert for neutrons, assuming neutrons are ten times more damaging, is 0.1 joule per kilogram of body mass.

A whole-body equivalent dose of 5 sieverts is usually fatal to a human being; when we express equivalent doses in sieverts in later discussion, it will be helpful to think in terms of what fraction of a fatal dose the number of sieverts correspond to (table 2-1).

What Did the Bombs Emit?

One of the greatest challenges in determining the health effects of radiation among the bomb survivors has been estimating what equivalent dose of radiation each individual in Hiroshima or Nagasaki actually received. While today workers in nuclear plants or those otherwise exposed to radiation on their jobs wear badges that record their exposures, the bomb victims in Japan obviously did not. It was therefore necessary to divide

TABLE 2-1   Exposures to Various Doses of Radiation

	Total Dose
Fatal whole body dose	5 sieverts
Increase of total cancer deaths by 0.8%	0.1 sieverts
Medical X-rays: barium enema	0.004 sieverts = 4 millisieverts
Medical X-rays: chest	0.0001 sievert = 0.1 millisieverts
One year's exposure to natural background radiation	0.003 sieverts = 3 millisieverts

the problem into two parts to determine, first, how much ionizing radiation the bombs emitted, and, second, how much of that radiation reached each survivor.

Although it was known very precisely how much uranium was used in the Hiroshima bomb and how much plutonium in the Nagasaki one, it was not known so precisely how much of the fuel in either bomb actually underwent fission. The result was that the actual energies released have had to be estimated in a variety of indirect ways, including observing knocked-over telephone poles and crushed oil drums, and physical and chemical changes produced by radiation in such structural materials as roof tiles and steel girders, and in crystals of quartz and other substances in the soil, at various distances from the point over the city where the bomb exploded (the epicenter). In the period before nuclear testing was banned, the AEC exploded bombs made up to closely resemble the bomb actually used on Nagasaki, and measured their radiation outputs. However, no corresponding experiment was done for the Hiroshima bomb.

The primary radiation from the bombs consisted of a mixture of gamma rays and neutrons, the Nagasaki bomb having a lower proportion of neutrons than the Hiroshima bomb. As noted, neutron doses do more biological damage than gamma ray doses. However, even the ratio of neutrons to gamma rays was not precisely known for either bomb, and estimates of these ratios have changed many times over the years as more information became available. One current view is that the neutron proportion of the radiation in both cities was relatively minor, so that the effects on health were primarily due to the gamma rays, but even now this is still a matter of dispute. The estimates of radiation from the two bombs have undergone several revisions in the past, and the question is clearly not yet settled.

The Radiation Dose to the Victims

The uncertainties over how much and what kinds of radiation the bombs gave out are not so great as the uncertainties over what dose each survivor received. The thirty-five thousand most heavily exposed individuals in the study were asked where they were at the time of the explosions so that their distance from the epicenter could be determined, whether they were indoors or out, whether they were standing or sitting and which way they were facing, what clothes they were wearing, what kind of building they were in at the time—concrete structure, wooden house with tile roof, and so forth—and even whether the building collapsed immediately or survived the first five seconds after the explosion, thus giving them protection from secondary radiation (from radioactivity produced by the neutrons and gamma rays of the initial explosion, most of which dies away in a few seconds). Using such information, the dose to each person could be estimated. By and large the estimates were consistent with the duration and severity of the acute radiation sickness or other symptoms the individuals suffered. Yet for more than a hundred people this method of estimation did not seem to fit: the doses calculated from the information they provided should have been fatal, yet obviously were not. Was this because these individuals for some reason were unusually resistant to radiation, or because they misremembered the details of their exposure at the time of the blast? The answers will probably never be known.

WHAT THE SURVIVORS SUFFERED

Putting It All Together

The goal of the study was to calculate the health risk of radiation exposure for people in general from the specific experience of the Hiroshima and Nagasaki survivors. What are the chances that a person will suffer some particular health consequence—leukemia, lung cancer, breast cancer—from a given dose of radiation? To do this a complete dossier was made for each individual in the study, including age at the time of exposure, the dose estimated from the information she provided about where she was at the moment the bomb went off and how well shielded by clothing or buildings, and her subsequent health history, up to the present time. Did she die of breast cancer in 1978 or in an auto accident in 1973, or is she, at least at this moment, alive and well? As time goes on, and more of the survivors and controls become ill or die, the information is added to the dossiers. This will continue until all subjects in the Life Span Study have died.

Solid Tumor Cancers

The rates of solid tumor cancers, such as those of the breast and lung, did not begin to increase noticeably among the survivors until fifteen or more years after the bombing, and are still increasing today, so the estimate of the total number caused by the bombing is preliminary, and we will not have a complete picture until all the survivors have died.

In the period from 1950 to 1990 there were 7,578 deaths from forms of cancer other than leukemia among the survivors. From the known rate of cancer deaths in Japan it was concluded that about 330 of the deaths can be attributed to radiation, not quite a 5% increase. This is a smaller relative increase in deaths from solid tumor cancers than from leukemia, which increased about 50%, but because leukemia is a rare form of cancer, the actual number of deaths from solid tumor cancers is larger. Not all kinds of solid tumor cancers have increased to the same extent. Breast cancer rates are about 50% higher; colon, lung, and ovarian cancers have increased also, but some other forms, such as cancers of the esophagus and bladder, have increased only marginally so far. The risk of breast cancer and some of the other cancers was found to be greater the younger the victim was at the time of exposure. As we noted, in the aging group of still-living survivors of the bombing there will be many more deaths from cancer, and probably the number of cancers attributable to radiation will turn out to be a higher proportion than has been seen so far (table 2-2).

A Dose-Response Relation: The More Radiation, the More Risk

Table 2-2 shows clearly that the risk of solid tumor cancers increases with the dose of radiation. For example the percentage of the total cancer deaths that resulted from radiation was about 3% for doses between 0.005 and 0.1 sieverts, about 12% for doses between 0.2 and 0.5 sieverts, and almost 50% for doses over 2 sieverts. This unmistakable dependence of risk on dose is

TABLE 2-2   Radiation and Solid Tumor Cancers: A Dose-Response Relationship

Dose Range, Sieverts	Total Cancer Deaths Expected[a]	Deaths in Excess of Number Expected	Percentage of Deaths Due to Radiation
0.005–0.1	2,710	85	3.0
0.1–0.2	486	18	3.6
0.2–0.5	555	77	12.2
0.5–1.0	263	73	21.7
1.0–2.0	131	84	39.1
>2.0	44	39	47.1

Note: The large number of deaths in the group with lowest dose reflects only that there were many more people in this dose category: about 33,000, compared to only 700 exposed to more than 2 sieverts.

[a]Expected number of cancer deaths in the absence of radiation.

an example of what is called a "dose-response relationship." It says more than "Radiation causes cancer"; it tells us that the more radiation a person is exposed to, the greater his risk. It makes sense that this should be so, and the fact that it is so clear-cut adds to the confidence we have that radiation exposure causes cancer. It also makes it simpler to estimate the effects of low doses, which, as we will see, cannot easily be measured directly (fig. 2-7).

Leukemia

The leukemias, forms of cancer affecting the blood-cell-producing system of the body, are unusual in that the time period between exposure and disease is much shorter than for most other cancers, which usually take

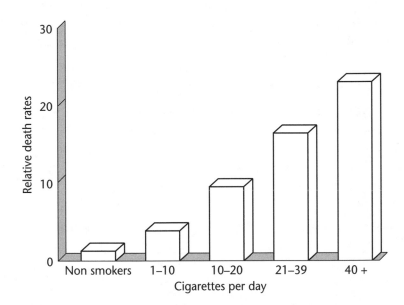

FIGURE 2-7 The classic dose-response relationship: number of cigarettes smoked and death rate for lung cancer. The "relative death rate" is the ratio of the death rates for smokers of various numbers of cigarettes to the death rate of nonsmokers. For nonsmokers, therefore, the relative death rate is 1.00. For smokers of more than 40 cigarettes a day, the relative death rate is over 20. Reproduced from David J. Brenner, *Radon: Risk and Remedy,* W. H. Freeman and Co., New York, 1989, and used by courtesy of Professor Brenner. The figure was prepared from data in an article, "Smoking and Cause of Death among U.S. Veterans: Sixteen Years of Observation," by E. L. Rogot and J. L. Murray, published in *Public Health Reports,* v. 95, pp. 213–22 (1980).

twenty or more years to develop after exposure to radiation or to toxic chemicals. An increased rate of leukemia among the survivors of the bombing reached a peak between five and seven years after the bombing, and then began to decline, so that it is now possible to estimate the total number of cases of leukemia caused by the bombing. Leukemia is a relatively rare disease even among people exposed to radiation, so the number of additional cases is small. Between 1950 and 1990 there were 249 deaths from leukemia in the 85,000 survivors while only 162 would have been expected, so that there is an excess of 87 cases attributed to the radiation exposure, an increase of over 50%.

The solid tumor cancers not only showed a clear dose-response relation, but also the relation is one of simple proportionality: if you double the dose, you double the cancer risk. The leukemias showed a dose-response relation also, but a more complicated one: doubling the dose increased the risk of leukemia by more than double (fig. 2-8). This made the analysis of the relation between leukemia and dose more complex, and predicting the effect of low doses on the leukemia risk less reliable. Also the small number of cases of leukemia makes precise statistical analysis harder. (See discussion of "power" in chapter 8.)

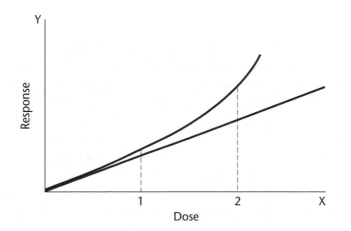

FIGURE 2-8   The figure shows schematically the difference between a linear and a quadratic dose-response relation. In a linear relationship, doubling the dose (going from point marked 1 to point marked 2) produces double the response. The particular quadratic relation shown corresponds to the dose-response relation found for leukemia in the Life Span Study: doubling the dose produces more than double the response.

Most of the excess leukemia deaths occurred among the small number of more heavily exposed survivors. Those receiving doses greater than 2 sieverts suffered leukemia at almost fifteen times the expected rate.

Severe Retardation and Other Effects

There were harmful effects other than cancer. One of the most tragic was a severe mental retardation among some children exposed prenatally. There were about 500 live births among women who were pregnant at the time of the bombing. Twenty-one of the children suffered this extreme mental retardation, while only four or five would have occurred in such a group in the absence of the radiation from the bomb. The mothers of these children were exposed between their eighth and fifteenth weeks of pregnancy, a time of rapid development of the fetal nervous system and brain.

There were also less severe consequences observed. Children exposed at an early age were found to be smaller and to have a greater frequency of muscular and skeletal defects than the control group of unexposed children. The blood-cell-producing system of the bone marrow, which is depressed in radiation sickness, has recovered among the survivors, but usually not quite back to the normal level.

The Missing Genetic Defects

On the other hand, genetic effects that could produce disease and suffering in later generations have not been detected so far. Since the bombing there have been about 70,000 live births in which at least one of the parents suffered significant exposure in the bombings. No evidence of an increased rate of mutations have been found in children conceived after the bombing by these heavily exposed parents: no significant increase in leukemia, Down's syndrome, or any other condition suggesting genetic damage. Estimates of how many mutations the radiation exposure could have caused can be made from studies on irradiated mice and their offspring: the estimated number for the first generation of children of the survivors is actually quite small, so that there is no real contradiction between the results on mice and the experience in Japan. In the first generation, mutations in a single gene are the only kinds that are expected. In later generations, more complex genetic defects, resulting from the inheritance of more than one mutated gene from different forebears, are likely to occur, but might be harder to detect and identify.

OTHER EVIDENCE

Why We Need More Information

We have described the health consequences for the bomb survivors as found so far from the Life Span Study, in particular the striking rise in solid tumor cancers among the most highly exposed survivors almost fifty years later. Can we apply the results of that study generally? There was, after all, considerable uncertainty about each survivor's dose. Also the dose in Japan was received all at once, and the more common situations we would want to apply the results to are when the dose is spread out in time, as in exposure to medical X-rays over a lifetime.

Still another question is whether they apply without qualification to non-Japanese peoples, who are genetically different from the Japanese. Should such differences matter? There is no obvious reason to expect Japanese to react differently to radiation from other people; their biology and biochemistry are much the same as everyone else's. It is true that their rates of various cancers are different from those in Western industrial nations: for example, they have much more stomach cancer and much less breast cancer. The reasons are not fully understood, but are probably related to lifestyle differences rather than basic biology.

For all these reasons it is useful to compare the results of the Life Span Study to studies on people exposed to high doses of medical X-rays and gamma rays, and with what we find from experiments on laboratory animals, to see if the dose-response relationships for various cancers and for genetic defects are in accord with those from the Life Span Study. Both kinds of studies have one great advantage over the bomb survivor studies: the doses of radiation are known more precisely. Each has drawbacks. The medical X-ray studies usually involved lower doses of radiation and smaller numbers of people in each study than the study of the bomb survivors. There are uncertainties involved in applying results on animals to human beings.

Medical Exposures

In studies of medical X-rays and gamma rays the doses of radiation received are known or can be closely estimated. One important difference between medical applications of X-rays and exposure to an atomic bomb blast is that with X-rays the doses, even when large, have consisted of smaller doses repeated a number of times. The studies suggest that larger total doses of X-rays and gamma rays can be tolerated when repeated small doses are given than when the same dose of radiation is received all at once. The estimate is that one concentrated dose gives about twice the risk of repeated small doses.

The carcinogenic effects of radiation on breast tissue was determined from the medical records of women with tuberculosis, who had been given many fluoroscopic examinations of the chest, sometimes more than a hundred, and have had a high incidence of breast cancer. In a fluoroscopic examination a screen that emits light when struck by X-rays is held next to the patient, instead of photographic film. The screen may be moved from place to place by the examining physician, who may wish to observe the organs as they move (lungs, heart), or may wish to apply pressure by hand to the patient's body to see how an organ responds. Fluoroscopy involves greater doses and longer exposures than ordinary X-rays.

Examples of therapeutic use of X-rays include a treatment of a disease called ankylosing spondylitis, a very painful arthritic condition of the spine, by irradiation of the lower back. Those treated were found later to have an elevated risk of leukemia. Ankylosing spondylitis is so painful and debilitating a disease that it can be argued that the benefits of radiation outweigh the risks. Unfortunately X-rays have been used to treat far less serious conditions: many children who immigrated to Israel from North African countries suffered from ringworm of the scalp, a parasitic infection common among children in the less-developed world. These children were (successfully) treated by irradiation of the scalp with X-rays. It was later found that their rates of leukemia and thyroid cancer were elevated. The total doses applied could be estimated retrospectively, and the relation between dose and risk determined. Treatments with X-rays for conditions that are not life-threatening or otherwise unbearable are, for obvious reasons, no longer used.

Animal Experiments: The Science of Toxicology

It is morally wrong to do experiments on human beings that we know will harm them and that do not provide compensating benefits for the harm, or to do experiments on them without their informed consent. The humans we can study are either victims of war or of nuclear accidents, or people irradiated for medical treatment. There are limited numbers of such people, and the doses they received are not always accurately known.

In studying the effects on health of any agent whatever, not just ionizing radiation, it is highly desirable to compare the health effects of different levels of exposure, to see if they show a dose-response relation. In the use of X-rays for treatment of disease, the range of doses used may not be large; each patient may receive nearly the same dose, so it may not be possible to see if the harmful effects of the X-rays obey such a relation.

The various groups should be identical in all relevant factors—age, sex, general health, ethnicity, diet, occupation, and so on—a condition not easy to achieve with human beings.

These particular drawbacks can be avoided in toxicological studies by conducting laboratory experiments on animals. Very large numbers of animals can be studied (one study at the Oak Ridge National Laboratory used 7 million mice), the doses can be known with great accuracy, and doses can be so large that clear-cut effects occur. The various exposed groups of animals live under identical conditions—cages of the same size, with the same numbers of animals per cage, identical diet, identical environmental conditions. Laboratory animals are much more genetically homogeneous than human populations. Further, the life span of a laboratory mouse is a year or two, so the full effects of exposure can be followed over the lifetime of the animal in a much shorter period than the lifetime of the scientist doing the study. In addition, biological surveillance and testing can be done in ways that cannot be ethically justified on human subjects.

There are also drawbacks. There is always some uncertainty about applying results from experiments on mice to men and women, even if the small size of a mouse is taken into account. Different species of mice show different sensitivities to radiation, and mice may be more or less sensitive than humans, or worse, may be simultaneously more *and* less sensitive, depending on the type of cancer or on the specific mutation. As a result, animal experiments are used to supplement, rather than replace, what we can learn from observations on human beings exposed to radiation.

Informative experiments have been done on human cell lines cultivated outside of the body. Changes in the chromosomes of the cell or in its biochemical functioning caused by radiation can be observed. When we know more about how mutations and other changes in the cell resulting from radiation cause a subsequent cancer—and we are learning fast—such experiments will be even more informative.

HOW MUCH HARM DO SMALL DOSES DO?

Is There a Safe Dose of Radiation?

The Life Span Study, together with studies of the therapeutic use of X-rays and experiments on laboratory animals, enables us today to estimate what levels of radiation are clearly harmful and to set safety standards for external exposure.

We have good reason to fear the terrible consequences of nuclear war and major nuclear accidents. But wars and nearby major accidents are far less common events than exposures to lower levels in occupational settings, minor nuclear accidents, leakage or improper waste disposal from nuclear plants, fallout from distant tests or accidents, the use of X-rays for ordinary diagnostic purposes, radon in our basements, and so on. What are the risks of these more common but lower exposures?

Is there a dose below which no harm at all is done—a threshold—or does any dose, no matter how small, do some damage, and if so, how much? Even if the risk of cancer from a low dose is small, when that small risk is multiplied by a very large number of people exposed, the net effect may be a lot of cases of cancer. The central problem in predicting the health consequences of low doses is that we have no direct experimental data on them. Why is this so, and what can we do to compensate for it?

Extrapolating from High Doses to Low

The studies of bomb survivors, of people treated with X-rays, and animal experiments have told us just how much harm relatively high doses of ionizing radiation from external sources cause. One might think that the same methods should be able to tell us how much harm low doses do. There are after all many more people exposed to low than to high doses: enormous numbers of people get dental X-rays every year, many times more than lived in Hiroshima or Nagasaki. Why not study them: are not the doses better known than in the Japanese study? Unfortunately, it is not so simple; as we have said, people get cancer even without exposure to ionizing radiation. The low doses typically used in dental X-rays would increase the rates of various cancers by such a small amount we would not be able to detect the increases over the background of the much larger numbers of cancers not caused by radiation. Such a study would not have the "power" to detect any health effects (see discussion of power in chapter 8). In brief, the question of how harmful low doses are cannot be easily answered by direct studies, precisely because the effects are expected to be small. Instead, in the absence of evidence to the contrary, it is usually assumed that the dangers from low doses are simply proportional to the dose. In brief, if exposure to a gamma-ray dose of 0.1 sievert per person is found to cause 100 extra cases of leukemia in a group of 100,000 people, then we assume a dose of one hundredth sievert per person would produce 10 cases in a group of the same size, and a dose of a thousandth of a sievert per person would produce 1 case. This assumption is called the "linear no-threshold assumption."

It is a simple assumption to make, and it is the one most commonly used so far, but it has been questioned. It was made originally as a reasonable first guess, not based on direct studies of the health effects of low doses. Increasing understanding of the molecular and cellular events that occur between exposure and the clinical appearance of a cancer has provided a rationale. At least at low doses, when only a small proportion of cells are actually "hit" by a photon or particle of ionizing radiation, it is plausible that the number of mutations produced in the DNA molecules is proportional to the number of photons or particles passing through the organism as a whole, that is, the dose of radiation received.

In any event, this is the current rationale for assuming a simple proportionality between dose and health effects. It is not accepted by everyone. There are some who argue that there is likely to be no harm at all at very low levels; organisms having been exposed to low levels of radiation over the whole course of evolution may have developed some defenses against it. This argument implies a threshold level of dose, below which no harm at all is done. There are others who argue exactly the opposite position; there may be a kind of law of diminishing returns in radiation, so that doubling the dose may produce less than double the number of mutations. If this were so, then assuming a relation of simple proportionality between dose and harm would underestimate the risks of very low levels. Some recent developments in radiation biology have raised new questions about the linear no-threshold assumption, and will be described in chapter 3.

The Natural Background Radiation and Safety Standards

If radiation had no beneficial uses, there would be no reason to allow any exposure at all. Because there are some benefits, a small level is considered acceptable, but of course this is a value judgment, not a scientific conclusion.

The linear no-threshold assumption, together with the results from high exposures, permits us to estimate how many of the cancers that occur naturally could be due to the natural background radiation. It has been concluded that only a few percent of them are (discussed in a later section). An additional exposure comparable to the natural background level has been proposed as acceptable for the population as a whole. For selected groups, such as workers in nuclear plants, uranium miners, medical radiologists and the patients they serve, somewhat greater exposures are accepted. Having a well-paying job—well paying precisely because of the increased risk—is one benefit a worker in the nuclear industry may choose to accept. Similar considerations apply to being a radiologist, to say nothing of the intrinsic satisfactions of such a profession. For the patient, the benefits of prompt and accurate diagnosis are usually clear. There are, however, borderline situations, such as mammographic screening of young women for breast cancer, where it has been argued that the risks of radiation are of the same magnitude or exceed the benefits of early detection.

WHAT IS THE RISK?

Quantitative Risk Estimates

The Life Span Study on the bomb survivors, augmented by what we have learned from studies of exposures to medical X-rays and from animal experiments, and accepting the linear no-threshold assumption (that harm is proportional to dose), permits us to determine a dose-response relation between the health risks of whole body exposure and the dose of ionizing radiation.

For simplicity, we will express the cancer results in terms of the lifetime risk of dying from a radiation-induced cancer due to a single dose of X-rays or gamma rays of 0.1 sievert. We note that a whole-body dose of about 5 sieverts is usually fatal, so the 0.1 sievert dose is about one-fiftieth of the fatal dose. The average dose received by the exposed individuals in the Life Span Study was 0.25 sievert, and at the other extreme, one chest X-ray involves a dose of 0.1 millisieverts, one-fifty-thousandth of the fatal dose (see table 2-1 on page 28). The effect on the lifetime risk of death from cancer for a dose other than 0.1 sieverts can be obtained by simple multiplication or division.

The figures we give were calculated in the Fifth Report of the Committee on the Biological Effects of Ionizing Radiation (BEIR V: see bibliographical notes for this chapter). The committee expressed the results in terms of a lifetime risk of death from different cancers. Since the death rates from various forms of cancer change as new treatments are developed, the figures represent the lifetime risk of getting forms of cancer that would have been fatal during the time period of the study. One source of error is that the Life Span Study is still continuing and will continue until all the survivors have died, and the indications are that the estimated risk of cancer from the bombing will continue to increase as the survivors age.

The lifetime risk of death is calculated per 100,000 people with the age distribution and known death rates from cancer for the United States. The U.S. population is about 280 million, and can be thought of as composed of approximately 2,800 groups of 100,000 people. In a group of 100,000 people, studied for a lifetime, there will of course be 100,000 deaths. Of these, according to present rates, about 20,000 will be from various cancers.

The conclusion of the Japanese study is that if a sudden single dose of whole body radiation of 0.1 sieverts were given to a group of 100,000 people, the number of cancer deaths would be increased 0.8%. In numbers, 160—0.8% of 20,000—would die of radiation-induced cancers that would eventually have died from other causes, including, of course, cancer. Although they would have died anyway, as we all must, they would on average have lived sixteen to eighteen years longer if not exposed to that extra 0.1 sievert of radiation. Of these 160 deaths, about 20 will be from leukemia, and about 140 from solid tumor cancers. Although the excess deaths from specific kinds of cancer differ between men and women, the overall excess death rate is about the same for both.

The Effect of Lower Doses

One chest X-ray, with a dose of 0.1 millisieverts, given to 100,000 people, would eventually cause one-thousandth as many deaths: 0.16, or a little less than one-fifth of a death. This of course means that in a group of 1 million people given one chest X-ray each, there would have been about two extra deaths. If everybody in the United States were given one chest X-ray, there would eventually be 500 deaths attributable to the exposure. This may be compared with the 50 million out of the total U.S. population of 270 million who will die of cancer.

X-ray examinations using barium enemas, which can detect potentially life-threatening intestinal obstructions, involve whole-body doses of about 4 millisieverts, and if given to 100,000 people would lead to about 16 deaths. In 1980, about 5,000 such procedures were performed, corresponding to one death among the 5,000 patients. It is not easy to estimate the number of deaths prevented by the procedure, but people with the kind of symptoms that lead a physician to recommend a barium enema study are, on the average, not in the best of health, and the number that would die in the near future if not given proper medical treatment would surely exceed 16 per 100,000.

How Much Cancer Is Caused by Natural Background Radiation?

The whole-body dose from natural background radiation has been estimated as 3 millisieverts per year (fig. 2-9). One year's accumulated dose of 3 millisieverts would be responsible for 24 deaths in 100,000 people, equivalent to about 0.1% of total cancer deaths in the U.S. population. However, we are all exposed not for one year but for our whole lives. Over a lifetime of exposure to natural background radiation, we might expect, say, fifty or sixty times the number of deaths caused by one year's exposure, implying 6% of all cancer deaths. However in contrast to the acute one-time dose in the nuclear bombing of Japan, the lifetime dose is accumulated at a very low rate. It can be estimated from the studies of medical X-rays that only half as many deaths will result. Therefore we conclude that natural background radiation contributes about 3% to the death rate from cancer.

Have We Underestimated the Risk?

In the next chapter we will discuss some recent evidence that low doses may be more harmful than the linear no-threshold assumption suggests. If this proves to be correct, the share of cancer attributed to natural background radiation will be larger, and so of course will all the estimates of the risks from low doses derived from the Life Span Study.

Radiation Concentrated on Tumors

We have so far discussed the risks from whole-body radiation from external sources only. Not all external exposure to radiation is of this kind: when a patient is X-rayed, it is invariably a specific organ that is exposed,

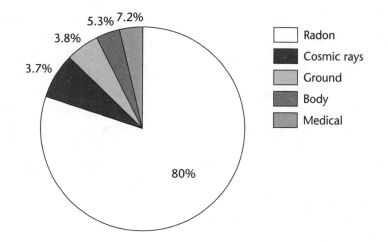

3.7%

3.8%

5.3% 7.2%

Radon

Cosmic rays

Ground

Body

Medical

80%

FIGURE 2-9   Relative amounts of radiation from various sources to which an average person in the United States is exposed. "Ground" refers to radiation received from radioactive elements in various minerals in the ground; "body" refers to radiation from radioactive isotopes in the body, for example from potassium-40, a radioactive isotope of the nutritionally necessary element potassium. Reproduced from David J. Brenner, *Radon: Risk and Remedy*, W.H. Freeman and Co., New York, 1989, and used by courtesy of Professor Brenner. The figure was prepared by him from data in Report No. 93, published in 1987 by the National Council on Radiation Protection and Measurements and in a chapter by A. C. James in *Radon and Its Decay Products in Indoor Air*, ed. by W. W. Nazaroff and A. V. Nero, Jr., John Wiley and Sons, New York, 1988, and used with the permission of the National Council and of John Wiley and Sons.

and the professionals taking the X-rays take precautions to protect the rest of the patient's body. When cancer is treated by radiation, doses higher than a fatal dose of whole body radiation can be focused on the area of a tumor without causing more than temporary radiation sickness, which can be acutely uncomfortable, but is almost never fatal.

Absorption of Radioactive Elements

Radioactive elements, either from the natural background or found there as a result of nuclear tests or accidents in nuclear plants, can be also absorbed selectively by different organs of the body, depending on their chemical nature. Radium and the radioactive form of strontium (strontium-90), being chemically similar to calcium, are absorbed by the bones, radioactive iodine (iodine-131), chemically identical to ordinary iodine, by the thyroid gland. Once there, the atoms of the radioactive elements emit their radiation to the surrounding tissue. Alpha and beta particles do not travel far in flesh, and coming from sources outside the body do not penetrate beneath the skin. When iodine-131 in the thyroid gland decays, it emits beta particles, electrons, that reach the cells in their immediate vicinity, and cancer of the thyroid gland may result.

Polonium formed by the decay of radon, a radioactive gas given out by uranium-bearing minerals, can become attached to dust particles and lodge in the lung tissues. The alpha particles that polonium emits on decay reach the cells nearby and can ultimately cause lung cancer.

ILLNESS FROM NUCLEAR WEAPONS TESTS OR NUCLEAR ACCIDENTS

Fallout and Leukemia in the Whole United States

We now return to the question of how much illness has resulted from the fallout from nuclear weapons tests and from nuclear accidents. It will become painfully obvious why good estimates cannot be made without good knowledge of exposure.

Childhood leukemia is a rare disease, and a cluster of cases in a small community is still only a small number of cases. It is always difficult to identify firmly what caused them, or to rule out chance variation alone as responsible (see discussion of cancer clusters in chapter 4). It is unusual to find situations where a large population has been exposed, and the number of cases of leukemia is correspondingly large enough to rule out chance. However, there was a large exposed population: the whole United States was exposed to fallout from all above-ground nuclear weapons tests conducted by both the United States and the Soviet Union during the 1950s and 1960s.

One study, by V. Archer, of the effect of this fallout on the rate of childhood leukemia in the United States estimated the exposure in each state of the United States from whatever fallout measurements from the time of the tests were available, together with measurements of radioactive strontium in the milk supply and in bones of deceased children. During the period of weapons testing, there were particular time intervals when either the United States or the Soviet Union exploded a lot of weapons, leading to corresponding peaks in fallout. The author noted peaks in the U.S. leukemia rate that followed each of the peaks in fallout by several years.

The total number of childhood leukemia cases in the United States during the period of testing was about 28,000, of which about 2,700, almost 10%, were attributed by Archer to the fallout.

Nuclear Tests, Thyroid Cancer, and Radioactive Iodine

The thyroid gland needs iodine to function, and it absorbs iodine from food. The radioactive form of iodine, iodine-131, is chemically identical to the common nonradioactive form, iodine-127; hence, it is metabolized the same way, and thus is also absorbed by the thyroid. In certain nuclear accidents, such as the Windscale fire in Great Britain (see chapter 4) and Chernobyl, and in the testing of nuclear bombs, iodine-131 was released to the environment and entered the food chain in the milk of cows that had eaten grass contaminated by fallout. Children, who drink more milk than adults, were therefore more at risk. After the Windscale accident, milk from herds in the neighborhood was discarded for a period of several weeks (radioactive iodine-131 has a half-life of eight days). In the aftermath of Chernobyl, exposed inhabitants of the Ukraine were given tablets of potassium iodide as a prophylactic. This increases the proportion of nonradioactive iodine consumed, so that the radioactive form is now a smaller proportion of the total iodine ingested, and therefore a smaller proportion of the iodine absorbed by the thyroid.

There was extensive fallout of iodine-131 from the nuclear weapons tests in Nevada in the period 1950–1956 (fig. 2-10). The National Cancer Institute recently made a retrospective calculation of the total iodine-131 deposited in the United States from the tests, how much of it got into people's thyroid glands, and the likely number of thyroid cancer cases that would result. The calculation was based primarily on scanty data collected by the AEC at 100 locations in the continental United States, supplemented by some recently declassified data on fallout. As the number of locations monitored during the tests averaged two per state of the United States, mathematical modeling and information about rainfall was necessary to make a detailed county-by-county estimate of total iodine-131 deposited. Having estimated local fallout throughout the United States it was then necessary to estimate how much of this landed on grass, was eaten by cows, and found its way into the milk, to be drunk mainly by

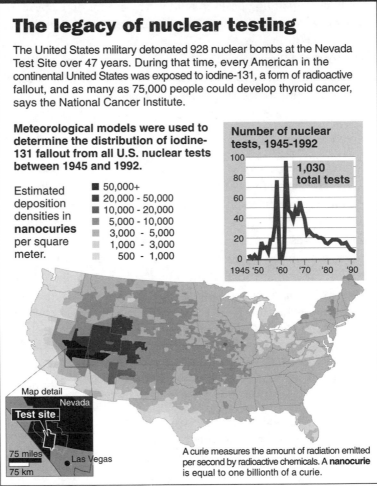

The legacy of nuclear testing

The United States military detonated 928 nuclear bombs at the Nevada Test Site over 47 years. During that time, every American in the continental United States was exposed to iodine-131, a form of radioactive fallout, and as many as 75,000 people could develop thyroid cancer, says the National Cancer Institute.

Meteorological models were used to determine the distribution of iodine-131 fallout from all U.S. nuclear tests between 1945 and 1992.

Estimated deposition densities in **nanocuries** per square meter.

- ■ 50,000+
- ■ 20,000 - 50,000
- ■ 10,000 - 20,000
- ■ 5,000 - 10,000
- ■ 3,000 - 5,000
- ■ 1,000 - 3,000
- ■ 500 - 1,000

Number of nuclear tests, 1945-1992

1,030 total tests

100
80
60
40
20
0
1945 '50 '60 '70 '80 '90

Map detail

Nevada

Test site

75 miles
75 km

Las Vegas

A curie measures the amount of radiation emitted per second by radioactive chemicals. A **nanocurie** is equal to one billionth of a curie.

Source: National Cancer Institute; Department of Energy   **AP**/Wm. J. Castello

FIGURE 2-10   Iodine-131 fallout from nuclear weapons testing in the United States in the 1950s. The map was prepared by the Associated Press from data published by the National Cancer Institute, and is reproduced with permission of the Associated Press.

children. The analysis suggests that 50,000 cases of thyroid cancer have occurred or will occur in the United States among those exposed as children during the testing. The uncertainties in the estimate is so great that the actual numbers might be anything from (approximately) 10,000 to 200,000. This very large range is "the 95% confidence interval" for the figure of 50,000; the probability that the true value lies within this range is 95% (see discussion of confidence interval in chapter 8). The background rate of thyroid cancer in the United States is such that during the lifetime of the generation of children exposed, about 1 million cases of thyroid cancer would occur in the absence of radioactive iodine fallout. So the estimated excess number of thyroid cancer cases caused by the fallout will be either an almost undetectable 10,000 (1% increase) or a quite noticeable 200,000 (20% increase). There has not yet been enough time to tell if there has indeed been an increased rate of this fortunately easily treatable cancer. Among the reasons for this great range of uncertainty are that the estimate of thyroid cancer risk per unit dose of radiation, from the Japanese and medical X-ray studies, is only roughly known; the distribution of the fallout was highly nonuniform, depending on rain, wind, and other local weather conditions; it is uncertain how much grass the cows ate, how much radioactive iodine found its way into the milk, and how much milk the children drank; and last but not least, the quality of monitoring done during the tests was poor.

After Chernobyl

There have been reports of a dramatic rise of thyroid cancer among the children of the Ukraine, but some observers have questioned whether some or most of this rise is not a result of increased medical surveillance since the accident. A study of the exposed population of the Ukraine and Belarus, similar in design to the Japanese survivor study, has begun. Fortunately, there is important information available on individual exposures that was not available in the aftermath of American nuclear weapons tests: measurements of radioactive iodine in the thyroid glands of some 65,000 children, made by Soviet scientists some months after the accident. Studies of leukemia and lymphoma among the workers who cleaned up the nuclear facilities after the accident will also be made. As in Japan, the health effects in people living in the vicinity of Chernobyl will be followed for decades.

SUMMARY

We have described how scientists have used the results of the Japanese bomb survivor studies, combined with studies of people given medical X-ray treatments and animal studies, to estimate the risks of whole-body radiation exposure. The word "estimate" is used advisedly. We have shown that for a number of reasons there is considerable uncertainty in the estimates.

First of all, radiation causes diseases that also occur in the absence of radiation, and we are as yet unable to distinguish cancers or birth defects caused by radiation from those that occur for other reasons. The result is that unless the excess of cancer or other diseases in an exposed group is appreciable compared to the rate in the absence of external radiation, it is impossible to show that radiation has caused any increase. For example, any genetic damage to the children of the bomb survivors, if it occurred, was too small to detect.

A further difficulty was the uncertainty about the dose to each individual, partly from not knowing exactly how much radiation was emitted by the Hiroshima and Nagasaki bombs, but mainly from not knowing enough about the location of each individual exposed, and the extent to which that individual was shielded by clothing or buildings.

Although animal experiments do not share these drawbacks, they have drawbacks of their own. Different species of animals do show different sensitivities than humans to radiation, and the greater genetic and lifestyle diversity of human populations make the extrapolation even more uncertain.

As the estimated risks are often applied to people exposed to much lower doses of radiation than in any of the studies, we rely on the linear no-threshold assumption, not directly tested experimentally but considered plausible, that risk is proportional to dose even at very low doses.

Finally, the results of these studies refer to whole-body radiation. Earlier we have described how radioactive strontium and iodine from nuclear fallout are selectively absorbed by the bones or the thyroid gland, and can cause leukemia in the first case and thyroid cancer in the second. The risk in these cases is not from whole-body radiation and has had to be estimated from other kinds of data. We give one example in the next chapter, on radon in homes.

The uncertainties about our estimates of the harm from radiation may be frustrating. Why can we not have certain answers instead of all this fuzziness? Can science not provide precise answers instead of vague ones with those irritating 95% confidence intervals? Such expectations are natural, but uncertainty is inherent in science. No measurement of anything, whether it is the speed of light, the atomic weight of carbon, or the death rate from lung cancer, is without a range of uncertainty, and awareness of that range of uncertainty is an essential part of the measurement.

In the rest of this book we will describe how other environmental hazards have been studied. Some of them involve high-energy radiation; others are concerned with chemical and biological hazards, or magnetic fields. In all of them the same issues come up time and again: the importance of knowing exposure; distinguishing real health effects of exposure from effects of chance; estimating the harm of low exposures from studies at high exposures; and the need to use all relevant fields of science—molecular biology, the physical sciences, and animal studies. The study of the Japanese survivors of nuclear bombing provides a model for other studies of environmental hazards. Most other studies of environmental hazards we describe here have not come to such firm conclusions.

A CLOSER LOOK: WHAT IS IONIZING RADIATION?

The term "ionizing radiation" unfortunately includes two different kinds of things: electromagnetic waves of short wavelength (X-rays and gamma rays), and atomic or subatomic particles traveling at high speeds, such as neutrons or helium atoms. The reason that two such different things were given the same name is that when radioactivity was discovered, it was first thought that all the radiation given off by radioactive atoms was in the form of electromagnetic waves like X-rays. Although electromagnetic waves and high-speed particles of matter are different kinds of things, they have at least one important feature in common: they may have harmful effects on living organisms.

Bullets and Waves

A fast-moving particle is easy to visualize as like a speeding rifle bullet. Why waves can cause harm to living organisms is less easy to visualize. There are two kinds of motion involved in a wave: ocean waves travel with a definite speed, but the water they move through does not travel with the wave; instead, it undergoes an up-and-down motion. A floating bottle shows the motion of the water; it rises and falls, but does not move in the direction the wave travels. The distance between two wave crests is called the *wavelength*, and the number of times the bottle rises per second is called the *frequency* of the wave (fig. 2-11). Frequency is measured in cycles per second; the scientific term for "cycles per second" is *hertz*; a megahertz is 1 million cycles per second. A sound wave can travel in air, under water, or through solid substances. Sound wave frequencies range from 20 hertz (the lowest sounds the human ear can hear) to 20,000 hertz. Above that it is called "ultrasound," though dogs, bats, and other animals can hear higher frequencies than humans can.

Electromagnetic waves, like ocean waves and sound waves, possess speeds, wavelengths, and frequencies. These three properties are interrelated; the wavelength times the frequency gives the speed. Unlike ocean waves and sound waves, electromagnetic waves can travel in a vacuum, which makes it hard to visualize what it is that is moving. Perhaps this will help: imagine a small, very light compass needle suspended in space above the surface of the earth. When no electromagnetic wave is passing by the needle, it points in a fixed direction, toward the earth's north magnetic pole. As an electromagnetic wave passes by, the needle swings back and forth about its north-pointing direction, just as the bottle floating in the ocean rises and falls.

Electromagnetic waves differ from high-speed particles in a number of ways. First, particles are usually localized at some definite point in space while waves are usually spread out over a considerable region. Second, electromagnetic waves all travel at the same speed in empty space of 186,000 miles per second (300,000 kilometers per second) while ionizing particles travel at different but lower speeds (though sometimes not much less than 186,000 miles per second). Third, when particles are slowed down and brought to rest—for example, when they pass through solid matter—they continue to exist. Electromagnetic waves absorbed by matter cease to exist as waves, and all the energy they carried is converted to other forms of energy, sometimes to extra chemical energy in molecules, sometimes as a heating up of the absorbing matter.

There is a point of confusion, though, about the distinction: according to quantum mechanics, the best theory we have about the properties of matter and energy, under certain circumstances electromagnetic waves can act like particles, and atomic and subatomic particles can act like waves. We will have to pay some attention a little later to the way waves can act like particles when we come to describe how electromagnetic waves can harm living organisms.

Examples of Electromagnetic Radiation

The electromagnetic waves we are most familiar with is the light we see things by, called "visible light." The various colors of visible light correspond to waves

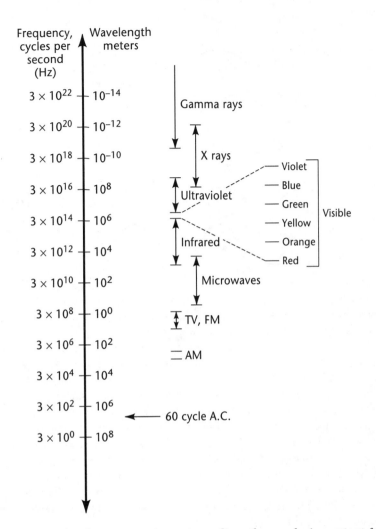

FIGURE 2-12 The electromagnetic spectrum. Since the speed c is constant for all types of electromagnetic waves, and since for all kinds of waves the speed is the product of wavelength and frequency, when the wavelength increases the frequency decreases in proportion. The relation between them is represented on the double-headed arrow in the diagram. Reprinted by permission of the publishers from *The Refrigerator and the Universe,* by Martin Goldstein and Inge F. Goldstein, Harvard University Press, Cambridge, MA, 1993, © 1993 by the President and Fellows of Harvard College.

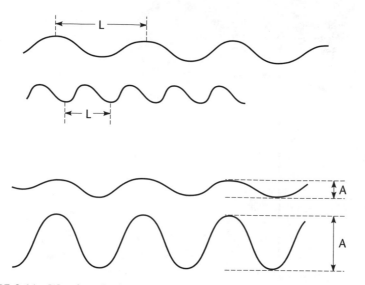

FIGURE 2-11   Wavelength, frequency, speed, and amplitude. A wave is characterized by its wavelength L (the distance between successive crests), frequency f (the number of crests passing a point in space per second), speed v (which can be shown to equal the product of L and f). In a vacuum, the speed of light, and of all other electromagnetic waves as well, is 186,000 miles a second, or 300,000 kilometers a second, and is symbolized by the letter c. Waves also possess an amplitude A, which for sound waves and water waves is related to the total energy in the wave. The energy of electromagnetic waves is carried by individual photons whose energy is proportional to the frequency of the wave. The total energy of any form of electromagnetic radiation is the product of the number of photons in the radiation and the energy of each individual photon. Reprinted by permission of the publishers from *The Refrigerator and the Universe,* by Martin Goldstein and Inge F. Goldstein, Harvard University Press, Cambridge, MA, 1993, © 1993 by the President and Fellows of Harvard College.

of different wavelengths (fig. 2-12). Other kinds of electromagnetic waves include ultraviolet and infrared light, which our eyes cannot directly see, though we can sense either by the warming of our skin. Ultraviolet light has shorter wavelengths than visible light, infrared longer. Microwaves have wavelengths longer than infrared waves, and radio waves longer wavelengths still. The wires that carry 60-hertz electric currents in our houses emit waves with wavelengths of about 5,000 kilometers, about the distance from New York to Paris. X-rays have shorter wavelengths than ultraviolet light, and gamma rays shorter wavelengths than X-rays. Ultraviolet light, X-rays, and gamma rays can affect photographic film just as does visible light.

The different forms of electromagnetic waves differ not only in the lengths of the waves, but also in their frequencies. There is an exact relation between the length of a wave and its frequency: the longer the wave, the lower the frequency. (Their product is the speed of light, 186,000 miles per second in a vacuum for all wavelengths.)

The Energy of Radiation

We know that light sources differ in strengths. A 100-watt bulb emits more light and thus more energy per second than a 40-watt bulb, which in turn emits more than a flashlight. How much energy do the waves carry? Moving particles of matter have more or less energy depending on how fast they are moving and how heavy they are, but if all electromagnetic waves travel at the same speed and do not have weight, how can they differ in energy? The answer given by quantum mechanics is that unlike ocean waves or sound waves in air, electromagnetic waves, even when spread out in space as waves usually are, act as though they carry their energy in little localized particles called "photons," each photon having a fixed amount of energy that depends on the frequency of the wave. This is the sense in which electromagnetic waves can act like particles. The higher the frequency, the greater the energy of the photon. Because higher frequency means shorter wavelength, the individual photons have more energy the shorter their wavelength (fig. 2-12). Thus the energy of one photon of the various forms of electromagnetic waves is smallest for the waves emitted from 60-cycle house current, and increases in the order: radio waves, microwaves, infrared, visible light, ultraviolet light, X-rays, and gamma rays.

The total energy in a beam of radiation, whether electromagnetic wave or particle, is obtained by multiplying the energy of a single photon (or particle) by the number of photons (or particles) in the beam. A 100-watt bulb emits more photons than a 40-watt bulb, but since the color, and therefore the frequencies, of the light emitted by both bulbs is about the same, the average energy of the photons emitted by both bulbs is about the same. Because the 100-watt bulb emits more photons, it emits more energy.

In some situations the total energy of the radiation is what counts, as when a microwave oven is used to reheat a cup of coffee; in others, the energy per photon is what matters. Microwave radiation, when it is at too low a level to heat living tissue appreciably, is not believed to damage the chromosomes of cells directly, but a beam of gamma rays having much less total energy than there is in a microwave oven can do a lot of damage. The damage is done by the individual photons acting as bullets, and a single hit on a single cell may ultimately cause cancer.

Particle Radiation: Alpha and Beta Rays

Examples of the kind of particles that are also called "ionizing radiation" if they are traveling at high enough speeds to ionize atoms include electrons, nuclei of helium atoms or of heavier atoms, protons, and neutrons, all of which can be emitted by radioactive atoms, by nuclear bombs, or by particle accelerators of various kinds. Beams of electrons so emitted were originally called beta rays, beams of helium nuclei alpha rays. The energy carried by each such particle depends both on its mass and on the speed with which it travels. Electrons have very small masses, about one two-thousandth that of a proton or a neutron. A helium nucleus has a mass about four times that of a proton or a neutron (see table A-1).

Ionizing Radiation

We use the term "ionizing radiation" for atomic and subatomic particles only when they have enough energy to "ionize" an electrically neutral atom: that is, to knock one or more electrons out of the atom, leaving it electrically charged, or "ionized." One of the first instruments for detecting the presence of high-energy radiation, the Geiger counter, actually detects the electrons knocked out.

Electromagnetic waves can also ionize atoms if the energy per photon is great enough. The photons of electromagnetic waves of longer wavelength than X-rays, such as ultraviolet, visible, or infrared light, do not have enough energy to ionize atoms, so even a large number of photons from a bright electric light and having a large total energy do not cause ionization.

Ionizing versus Nonionizing Radiation

Ionizing radiation has clear-cut effects on living organisms, usually harmful, though it can be used therapeutically on tumors. It is known to produce

TABLE A-1   Some Atomic and Sub-Atomic Particles

Name of Particle	Mass Relative to Hydrogen Atom (approximate only)	Electric Charge on Particle
Electron	0.0005	−1
Proton	1	+1
Neutron	1	0
Hydrogen atom	1	0
Helium atom (as alpha particle)	4	+2[a]

[a]Helium atoms normally have a charge of zero. The charges given are those they have as an alpha particle ejected from the nucleus of a radioactive atom.

mutations in cells, which in turn can cause cancer and birth defects. Nonionizing radiation can also cause harm if it has enough total energy to cause a rise in temperature: this is why microwave ovens are useful, but why they are designed so that the users are protected from the microwaves.

Measuring Dose and Relative Harm

The dose a person or an animal receives from ionizing radiation of either the electromagnetic wave or the particle variety is defined as the total energy, measured in joules, of the ionizing radiation absorbed *per kilogram* (*2.2 pounds*) *of the organism's mass*. We will see that this is only a crude beginning, and more information will be needed.

The current standard unit of dose is called the *gray*; 1 gray is 1 joule of ionizing radiation absorbed per kilogram. How much energy is a joule? Very little, in fact. A 100-watt electric bulb uses 100 joules of energy in one second. A kilowatt-hour, costing about 5 cents in the Northeastern United States in 2001, is 3,600,000 joules. Why do we use such a small quantity of energy as our standard? The reason is that energy in the form of ionizing radiation is pretty lethal. A dose of 5 grays over the whole body of a 70-kilogram human being (154 pounds) is usually fatal. This is an energy of 350 joules, the amount used by a 100-watt bulb in 3.5 seconds. An earlier unit of absorbed dose, the "rad," still sometimes encountered in the literature, is one-hundredth of a gray. Small fractions of a gray—a milligray (one-thousandth) and a microgray (one-millionth)—are also used.

As we have indicated, the dose absorbed is only a first guess at the amount of harm the person is likely to suffer, as the different forms of ionizing radiation differ in their effects. Neutrons, for example, do more damage than gamma radiation for the same total dose. A unit called the *sievert* is defined so as to take this difference into account. The damage done per gray of X-rays absorbed is taken as a kind of reference, and the damage done by the same absorbed dose (same energy absorbed per kilogram) of some other kind of radiation, say neutrons, compared to it. If the damage is estimated to be twenty times as great, then the number of grays of neutrons is multiplied by 20, a number referred to as the relative biological effectiveness (RBE) for neutrons, to get the "dose equivalent," measured in sieverts.

There are a number of reasons why different kinds of ionizing radiation produces different levels of damage for the same amount of energy. Among them is the fact that some forms lose their energy quickly, often in a single burst, and do not travel far in living tissue, but do a lot of damage in a small region, while others lose it more gradually, and travel long distances, producing many sites of lesser damage along the way. Alpha particles are an example of the first kind, X-rays and gamma rays of the second.

When we estimate "damage," we are dealing with a much less precise quantity than the total absorbed dose. Damage can include death, radiation sickness, cancer, mutations, birth defects, and other outcomes. Obviously, it is a fairly difficult concept to measure numerically, and there is considerable leeway in estimating it. The RBE thus depends on which kind of damage we measure. It also depends in some cases on the rate at which the dose is delivered, a gradual rate of exposure often doing less harm than the same total energy delivered in a sudden burst.

A CLOSER LOOK: HOW IS THE HARM DONE?

The amount of energy in the form of radiation that would constitute a fatal exposure of a human being is actually very little, about the energy needed to warm a teaspoon of cold coffee to a drinkable temperature. How can so little energy kill?

Except at large doses, higher than the minimum fatal dose, radiation harms living beings by its effect on a particular vulnerable part of the cell, the elongated molecules of DNA in the cell nucleus. The DNA molecules contain the genetic information that the cell transmits to the two daughter cells which it forms on cell division, and makes them genetically identical to the parent cell. It was believed until recently that damage to DNA results only from a direct "hit" on the DNA molecule. It has now been discovered that even a hit on the portion of the cell outside of the nucleus, called the cytoplasm, can produce energy-rich molecules called free radicals, which travel into the nucleus and damage the DNA. This discovery has a bearing on the assumption that harm is proportional to dose and is described in more detail in the next chapter.

DNA molecules are constructed in the form of a long chain, composed of millions of smaller molecules linked together. In many synthetic plastics, whose molecules are also constructed in the form of a long chain, there is only one kind of small molecule that makes up the links. In DNA there are four different chemically distinct molecules, and the order in which they appear along the chain determines which protein molecule is synthesized by the cell (see fig. 2-5). The group of links along the DNA chain that carry the instructions for the synthesis of a particular protein molecule is called a "gene"; the total collection of genes, through the proteins they provide instructions for, determines the biological functioning of the individual.

One possible consequence of damage to the DNA molecule is the loss of its ability to reproduce itself during cell division. As cell division is necessary for life to go on, if enough cells are damaged this severely the organism will die. Another possible consequence is that the DNA molecule is chemically altered, but the capacity for cell division is not lost. Instead, however, the two daughter cells will inherit the altered DNA molecule of the parent. Whatever genes have been altered, the corresponding protein is either also chemically altered, or else not produced, or sometimes produced excessively: the cell is said to have undergone a mutation. Most mutations have no effect; some are harmful to the cell, which functions less well, and dies earlier. But sometimes the mutated cell undergoes cell division more rapidly than the normal cell, and its reproductive capacity is not well controlled: the result is often cancer.

Still another outcome is one affecting complex many-celled organisms like us. If there is a mutation in the sperm cells of a man or the ova of a woman, prior to conception, and if that sperm cell or that ovum produces a new individual, all the cells of that individual's body carry the mutated genes. The mutation may, on the one hand, be harmful to the individual, and, on the other, may be passed on to his or her offspring.

Although DNA molecules are very long, they are too narrow by themselves to be visible in the microscope. However, in the cell, two DNA molecules form a composite structure together: each long molecule has the shape of a helix (like the thread of a screw, or a spiral staircase) and the two helices are wrapped around each other to form a "double helix," and surrounded by a protein coat. This structure can be seen under the microscope at certain stages of cell division when stained with suitable dyes. It is called a "chromosome," and human body cells contain forty-six of them (germ cells have half the number). Sometimes radiation causes a break in a chromosome, after which one of the parts may reattach itself to a different chromosome. Such damage can be detected by microscopic examination of the cell. Other mutations involve only a chemical change at one point along the DNA chain. This point mutation cannot be seen with the microscope, but can be detected by the fact that the protein this gene codes for will be chemically altered.

3

RADON IN YOUR BASEMENT

DISCOVERY OF THE PROBLEM

We once saw a science fiction movie in which a monster from outer space is first detected because it sets Geiger counters clicking furiously. We were reminded of that movie by the story of how radon in homes first came to wide public attention. A nuclear power plant was built in a town in Pennsylvania, and like all such plants was equipped with radiation detectors, both to protect the health of employees and to prevent anyone from removing nuclear fuel from the plant. A newly employed engineer at the plant registered a high radioactivity when he walked by the detectors. This was not only alarming but surprising: the plant was not yet operating, and there should not have been any radioactive material around. It was quickly established that the source of the radiation was not the plant but the engineer's house in a nearby suburban community, which had levels of radioactivity almost a thousand times greater than federal standards permit in mines. The radioactivity came from radon gas seeping into the house from the ground.

Cigarette smoking is responsible for about 90% of lung cancers, but 10% of the victims of this disease had never smoked. It was already known that miners exposed to radon gas in uranium mines suffered a high rate of lung cancer, and the question immediately arose: could radon gas in homes be another cause of lung cancer?

Radon in Homes

Radon in homes is not a consequence of the atomic bomb or the building of nuclear power plants; it is one of the major sources of the natural background radiation we are all exposed to. It is present even in outdoor air, and at higher concentrations in homes, castles, peasants' hovels, and caves as long as people have lived in them (fig. 3-1). It is a product of the decay of the element uranium. Uranium is present to some extent in all minerals, so we expect to find more radon in houses built of stone or mineral products like stone, concrete, and gypsum than in houses built of wood, and we expect to find more of it in basements than in attics. Most radon in American homes enters either from the basement or in water that comes from deep wells (fig. 3-2).

Most homes do not have levels of radon anything like what was found in the house of the unfortunate engineer in Pennsylvania, which was built in an area in which the natural radioactive content of the local rock formations happens to be very high. The area is called the "Reading Prong," and is a narrow elongated swath of ground extending through parts of Pennsylvania, New Jersey, and New York (fig. 3-3).

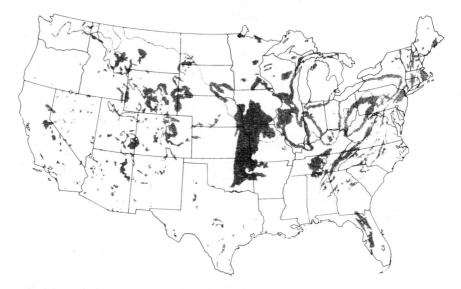

FIGURE 3-1 Areas in the United States where the geological formations are such that radon levels are high. Even within such areas, houses differ greatly in their radon levels, depending on their construction, local geological features, etc. Reproduced from David J. Brenner, *Radon: Risk and Remedy,* W.H. Freeman and Co., New York, 1989, and used by courtesy of Professor Brenner.

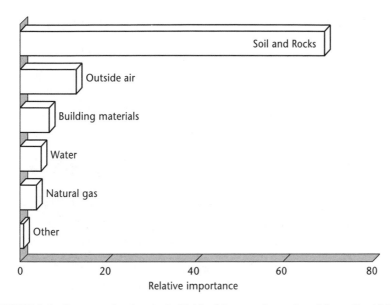

Soil and Rocks

Outside air

Building materials

Water

Natural gas

Other

| 0 | 20 | 40 | 60 | 80 |

Relative importance

FIGURE 3-2   Sources of radon in individual homes. Reproduced from David J. Brenner, *Radon: Risk and Remedy*, W.H. Freeman and Co., New York, 1989, and used by courtesy of Professor Brenner. Adapted by him from *Ionizing Radiation: Sources and Biological Effects*, published in 1982 by the United Nations.

The U.S. Environmental Protection Agency (EPA) has recommended that remedial action to lower radon lovels be taken if the concentration in frequently used rooms of the home exceeds 4 picocuries per liter of air (we will explain what a picocurie is later). About 6% of U.S. homes exceed this standard. High-radon homes are not distributed randomly across the United States., but tend to occur in regions like the Reading Prong, where the minerals in the soil and rocks have high uranium contents.

Figure 3-4 shows the percentage of homes in the United States having given levels of radon, from very low to very high. The EPA action level of 4 picocuries per liter is shown by a dashed line on the figure. What is the risk of lung cancer for the people who live in those homes? Are the people who live in the remaining 94% of homes safe?

External versus Internal Doses

The way radiation affects us depends on whether it comes from sources outside the body or from radioactive elements ingested or breathed in. External sources include X-ray machines and direct exposure to nuclear

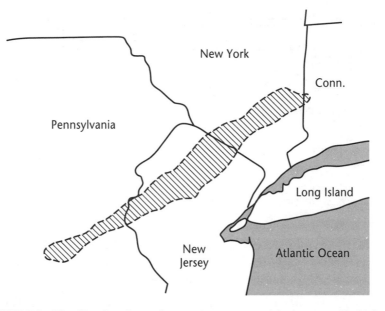

FIGURE 3-3 The "Reading Prong," a contiguous area with an unusually high radon level, lying in the states of Pennsylvania, New Jersey, and New York. Adapted from David J. Brenner, *Radon: Risk and Remedy*, W.H. Freeman and Co., New York, 1989, with permission of Professor Brenner. The map was adapted by him from an article by R. L. Fleisher, "A Possible Association between Lung Cancer and a Geological Outcrop," published in *Health Physics*, v. 50, pp. 823–27 (1986), © by Lippincott Williams and Wilkins and reproduced with their permission.

bombs. Ingested or inhaled radioactive elements are of concern because they are often selectively absorbed by specific organs of the body and produce intense radiation of those organs. Radioactive fallout, from nuclear bomb testing or from nuclear accidents like Chernobyl, involves both kinds of exposure.

Which organ selectively absorbs a radioactive element depends on the chemical properties of that element. Radium and the radioactive form of strontium (strontium-90), being chemically similar to calcium, are absorbed by the bones, radioactive iodine (iodine-131) by the thyroid gland. Embedded there, the radioactive atoms emit their radiation to the surrounding tissue as they decay. Alpha and beta particles have low penetrating power in flesh, and travel only a few thousandths of an inch before coming to rest. But when iodine-131, a beta emitter, is in the thyroid gland,

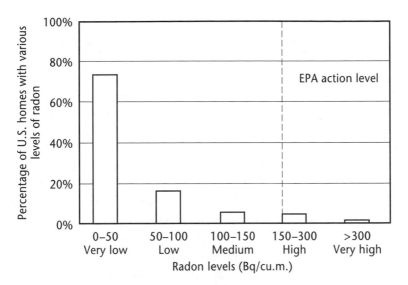

FIGURE 3-4   National surveys of radon levels have been made by sampling representative homes of all kinds, from single family dwellings to apartment buildings. In this figure, the radon levels found are broken up into the following ranges (expressed in bequerels per cubic meter): 0–50 (very low), 50–100 (low), 100–150 (medium), 150–300 (high), and greater than 300 (very high). The EPA remediation level of almost 150 bq/m³ is shown by the vertical dashed line. Over 70% of U.S. homes have radon levels in the very low range. Only 6% exceed the EPA remediation level.

the beta particles can reach the cells in their immediate vicinity, and may cause cancer of the thyroid. Polonium, a solid, formed by the decay of radon, a gas, can become attached to dust particles and when inhaled lodge in the lung tissues. The alpha particles that polonium emits on decay may ultimately cause lung cancer.

Lung Cancer and Radon in Homes

The National Research Council appointed a Committee on Health Risks of Exposure to Radon, composed of specialists in radiation biology and other relevant disciplines, to study the problem of radon in homes. It issued a report in 1999 that critically reviewed over 800 scientific papers on the health effects of radon exposure and concluded that radon in homes in the United States accounts for between 15,400 and 21,800 lung cancer deaths each year.

There are about 157,000 deaths each year in the United States from lung cancer: 95,400 among men and 62,000 among women (the latter figure exceeding the 50,000 annual deaths among women from breast cancer). Ninety to ninety-five percent of the lung cancer deaths are of people who have been smokers. The 15,400 to 21,800 deaths that would not have occurred without radon exposure are thus a significant portion of the total lung cancer deaths, 10% or more. There were 11,000 lung cancer deaths of people who never smoked; of these, the committee estimated that from 1,000 to 3,000 are a result of radon exposure.

It can be seen that radon in homes presents a real health hazard, not so bad as smoking cigarettes but much worse than any yet-demonstrated effect of pesticides, toxic waste dumps, incinerators, or living near nuclear facilities. Further, relatively simple and inexpensive measures—mainly ventilating houses better, particularly their basements—would reduce the risk considerably. It is surprising that so little attention is paid to radon, and so much to hazards that kill or injure far fewer people. Why this is so is a puzzle, which we will return to after we have answered the questions: how were these estimates of lung cancer deaths arrived at, and how controversial are they?

What Is Radon?

Radioactive elements are present in all minerals, sometimes as trace impurities, sometimes as major constituents, as in uranium ores such as pitchblende. Uranium is radioactive, but its rate of decay is very slow, comparable to the age of the earth itself, which is why it can be used for dating rocks that are millions or billions of years old. On decay it forms a long sequence of other radioactive elements that decay in turn, faster than uranium itself. The last element in the sequence is nonradioactive lead.

Figure 3-5 shows the sequence of elements formed when the most common kind of uranium atom, uranium-238, decays. Also shown is the type of radiation emitted when each element decays, and the half-life of the radioactive element, the time it takes for half of any given amount to decay. It may seem strange that some elements repeat themselves as we go down the list; for example, polonium decays to lead, the lead forms bismuth, which in turn decays to form polonium again. The atoms of the second kind of polonium formed, polonium-214, are different from those of the first kind, polonium-218, in the way they decay, although identical in their chemical properties. Why this happens and why two differ-

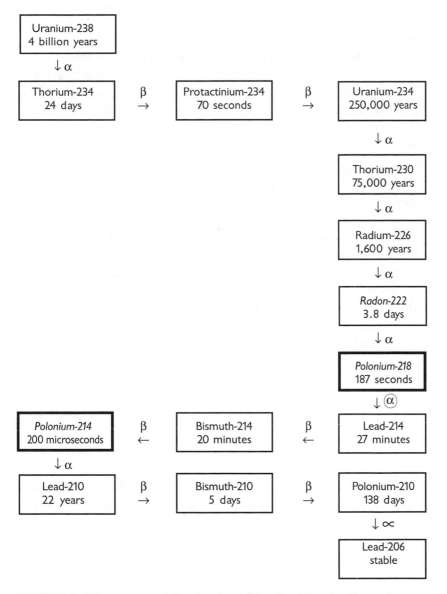

FIGURE 3-5 The sequence of elements formed by the radioactive decay of uranium-238. Radon-222 is one of the elements, which ends with nonradioactive lead-206. The Greek letters alpha (α) and beta (β) show whether the element decays by emission of an alpha or a beta particle. Note also the "half-life" given in each rectangle: 3.8 days for radon-222, 187 seconds for polonium-218, and 200 microseconds for polonium-214. The half-life is the time within which half of the atoms of a radioactive element undergo decay. After two half-lives, one quarter of the atoms of the element have not yet decayed, after three half-lives one eighth, and so on. Reproduced from David J. Brenner, *Radon: Risk and Remedy*, W.H. Freeman and Co., New York, 1989, and used by courtesy of Professor Brenner.

ent kinds of atoms are both "polonium" is explained in "Radioactivity and Isotopes" (p. 97).

One of the elements in this sequence is radon-222, a chemically non-reactive gas, similar to helium and neon. Chemically reactive gases, such as hydrogen or oxygen, can form solids or liquids when chemically combined with other elements. Radon does not combine with anything: it is a gas under all natural conditions, and as such moves around more easily. When it is formed by the decay of radium (itself a decay product of uranium), always present in small amounts in any uranium-bearing mineral, it tends to escape from the rock into the surrounding air, and once there disperses in and moves together with the air. There is such rapid dilution of the radon in air that radon levels outdoors are seldom large enough to pose much of a health threat. The air in enclosed spaces, within homes, is a different matter.

Radon itself decays quickly: in about four days half of it will have undergone conversion to the element polonium, more precisely polonium-218. On further decays eventually polonium-214 is formed. Both forms of polonium, like radon itself, emit alpha particles when they decay, and the danger to health occurs when this happens inside the lungs. The radioactive lead and bismuth atoms in the sequence emit less dangerous beta particles. The elements formed by the decay of radon are sometimes called "radon daughters"; whether this is a sexist designation we leave to the reader. A more neutral term is "radon progeny."

Why Radon Is a Hazard to the Lungs

The concentration of radon in an enclosed space such as the basement of a house comes to a state of balance between radon seeping in from the ground, radon decaying, and radon lost to the outside air through ventilation. The alpha particles emitted by radon gas itself decaying inside the lungs are not particularly harmful because the outer layer of cells in the lung tissue is protected by a layer of mucus, and the particles are mostly stopped in this layer. However, the various kinds of atoms formed from radon decay, including both kinds of polonium, are not chemically inert like radon and immediately attach themselves to particles of dust in the air. These dust particles when breathed in are often trapped in the lung's mucus layer, and once there tend to penetrate through the layer of mucus. Alpha particles from the two kinds of polonium can then reach the outer layer of sensitive lung cells. This is how exposure to radon can cause lung cancer.

Radon: The Main Source of Natural Background Exposure

All of us are exposed to high-energy (ionizing) radiation even in the absence of nuclear plants and atomic bombs. It is part of the natural environment, and includes cosmic rays and X-rays from outer space, and radiation from naturally occurring radioactive substances including radon. Because the atmosphere absorbs cosmic rays, people living at higher altitudes, for example in Denver, Colorado, are more exposed to them. Also because certain geological formations are rich in radioactive elements, there are "hot spots" like the Reading Prong in various places around the world, including localities in Egypt and India, where the natural radiation level is ten times that of the U.S. average. Man-made sources of radiation, such as medical X-rays and fallout from nuclear testing and nuclear accidents, add to our exposure. What is the relative importance of radon, compared to all the other kinds of ionizing radiation? The answer is that about 80% of our exposure to all sources of ionizing radiation combined is ultimately due to radon.

Death in the Mines

One of the great works of Renaissance science is *De Re Metallica*, or "Concerning Metals," by a German engineer who wrote under the Latin name of Georgius Agricola, a translation of his given name of Georg Bauer. This treatise on mining for metals, published in 1556, contains a description of a fatal occupational disease of miners who worked the silver mines in the Erz mountains, on the border region of what is now Germany and the Czech Republic. The disease was known as *Bergkrankheit*, or mountain sickness, and was only identified in this century as lung cancer. At the end of the nineteenth century the region was found to be a source of a uranium ore called pitchblende. Uranium was used before World War II to tint glassware, and after it for other less benevolent purposes. Pitchblende was the ore from which the Curies first extracted polonium and radium, decay products of the uranium.

In the twentieth century the lung cancer of uranium miners was shown to be a result of their radon exposure at work, and measures were taken to improve ventilation in the mines. Unfortunately, many miners working before this was done had already died of lung cancer, and many more who worked at that time are still expected to die of it, as lung cancer does not usually appear until twenty or more years after the initial exposure to cancer-causing agents (fig. 3-6).

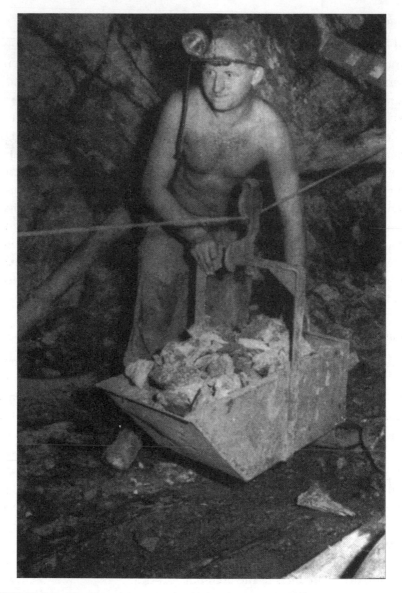

FIGURE 3-6 Uranium miners in the former German Democratic Republic, now
part of the Federal Republic of Germany. Reproduced from photographs in
Seilfahrt. Auf den Spuren des saechsischen Uranerzbergbaus, published by Doris
Bode Verlag, Haltern, Germany, 1991.

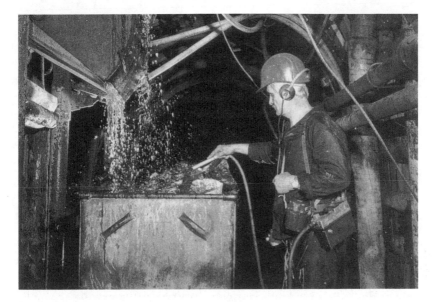

FIGURE 3-6

STUDIES ON HOMES

Lung Cancer and Radon in Homes

Earlier we gave estimates of 15,400 to 21,800 deaths annually in the United States from lung cancer that would not have occurred if there were no radon in homes. One might think that this estimate must have been based on studies of the relation between lung cancer deaths and home radon concentrations. Surely this is the most direct way to answer such a question. Indeed, such studies were begun almost as soon as the risk from radon in the home was recognized. Some have been published and were examined in the report of the Committee on Health Risks of Exposure to Radon, others are still under way. However, most of these studies have not so far helped much in estimating the lung cancer deaths from radon, and we will explain why they have not and why instead we have had to rely on an indirect approach.

The earliest studies did not measure radon in each of the homes in a given area, but only estimated the radon in the homes, in some cases by measuring radon in a few "representative" homes, in others from the general level of natural radiation in the area. The overall lung cancer rate in that area was compared with that in some other area in which the average radon level, similarly determined, was lower. As cigarette smoking is known to be the major cause of the great majority of lung cancer deaths (heavy smokers having ten times the risk of lung cancer of nonsmokers), it is always necessary to take smoking habits into account in any study of that disease. The effect of smoking was estimated in a way similar to the way in which the average radon level in the homes was estimated: an average number of cigarettes smoked was calculated from information about total cigarette sales in the area.

How Much Radon? How Many Cigarettes?

It should be clear that if we use the average exposure to radon of an entire population instead of finding out how much each individual in that population was exposed, and average smoking habits instead of how many cigarettes a day each individual smoked, we will not know whether the individuals who actually got lung cancer really lived in homes with high radon concentrations or how much they smoked. In fact, very few people live in homes with exactly the average radon concentration of their area or smoke exactly the average number of cigarettes, any more than they have exactly the average number (that might be some number such as 2.2) of children.

Studies that use averages over large groups to represent individual exposures are called "ecological" studies by epidemiologists, a use of the term different from its common meaning. Ecological studies are less expensive and time-consuming, and have often been informative, but do not carry much conviction unless confirmed by studies based on exposures determined on individuals. As an example, studies have used the total countrywide consumption of fats as an estimate of the consumption of fats by each individual in that country, and found a relation between high-fat diets and colon and breast cancer. Later studies in the United States that estimated the dietary fat intake of individuals rather than groups have failed to confirm this relation.

The various ecological studies on radon in homes did not show any clear-cut association between radon and lung cancer: some found an association, almost as many found none, and a few found a negative association (as though radon exposure prevents lung cancer).

There were, however, eight nonecological studies that were evaluated by the Committee on Health Risks of Exposure to Radon, in which measurements of radon in the homes of each of the study subjects were made, and their smoking histories determined by questioning them or their families. These, carried out in different countries of North America, Europe, and Asia, were "case-control" studies, in which individuals with lung cancer were identified in a particular area and were then compared to a group of individuals, chosen from the same area, who had not gotten lung cancer, but who otherwise were as much like the cancer victims as possible, particularly with respect to their smoking histories. Then the radon levels in the homes of the cases and the controls were compared to see if the lung cancer cases had been more exposed to radon than the controls.

Fourteen Percent of Lung Cancer Deaths, More or Less

Most of the studies found a statistically significant effect of radon exposure on lung cancer, and there was some evidence that the cancer risk increased with increased exposure—a dose-response relationship. An average over all the studies gave a figure of 14% of lung cancer deaths that could be attributed to home radon concentrations. However, each of the individual studies was subject to statistical uncertainties, and their conclusions differed somewhat. The combined uncertainties (expressed as a 95% confidence interval—see discussion in chapter 8) meant that the annual increase in lung cancer deaths might really be anything from 1% to 30%, a range so wide as to be almost useless. A 1% increase in lung cancer deaths is negligible compared with the risk of smoking a pack of cigarettes a day, which increases the lifetime risk tenfold (in percentage terms, 1000%). On the other hand, a 30% increase, while not as serious a factor as cigarettes, is serious enough.

Why are these studies so uncertain as to be almost useless? Put briefly, they have two kinds of problems. One is the great uncertainty in estimating past exposures to radon, and the second is detecting small increases in the rate of lung cancer, a disease that occurs also in the absence of exposure.

How Much Exposure?

A one-time measurement of radon level in a home, sometimes an average over a period of a month, used in most of these studies, is not likely to represent accurately what the level has been over the thirty or forty years preceding, nor need it represent accurately what radiation dose the lungs of a person living in that home may actually have received. Lung cancer usually occurs 30–40 years after exposure to cigarettes or radiation.

Even people living in the same house get different exposures; some work eight or more hours a day elsewhere, some spend more time in the basement where radon levels are usually highest, some sleep with open windows. Over time, changes in the structure of a home or in the lifestyle of those who live there lead to changes in exposure: adding on rooms, putting a second television set in the basement for the children, installing new windows providing better insulation and therefore less air exchange with the outside air, installing air conditioners so that the windows are closed in the summer.

Old Glass

A remarkable study on radon in homes by M. Alavanja and colleagues at the National Cancer Institute was published subsequent to the publication of the committee report. It used a new method to determine a twenty-five-year average exposure and confirmed the suspicion that a one-time measurement of radon levels in a home gives a poor estimate of that exposure. The researchers examined flat glass in mirrors or windows that had been in place in the home for at least twenty-five years, and exposed to the air of the room in which they were located. When radon in the air near the glass undergoes decay into lead-210 with the emission of an alpha particle, some of the lead atoms undergo enough recoil to be forcibly embedded in the glass. The lead-210 then decays slowly into polonium-210, which in turn can be detected by the alpha particles it emits. By examining "old" glass, an average radon concentration in the vicinity of the glass for the time period the glass has been exposed to the air can be determined. Unsurprisingly, this long-term average did not agree well with current radon measurements in the rooms.

The radon exposures of a group of women in the state of Missouri who had gotten lung cancer were compared to the exposures of a control group, selected to have comparable smoking histories to the lung cancer cases (a "case-control" study). Radon exposures were estimated both by the current air concentration measurements and by the twenty-five-year glass average radon exposure. It was found that the current air measurements had little relation to the risk of lung cancer; on the other hand, the twenty-five-year average determined from the measurements on glass showed a clear statistically significant dose-response relation. The results of this study and another using the same technique will be discussed in more detail in a later section of this chapter.

How Small an Effect Can We Detect?

Another problem in studies of radon in homes is common to many other health studies. No disease or condition caused by one particular environmental hazard is caused exclusively by that hazard. The disease occurs for other reasons anyway, whether or not the hazard is present. The most we expect to find is that the exposure increases the rate of the disease. The "rate" of a disease is defined as the number of cases per thousand or per hundred thousand people per year, usually calculated from data on a very large population—for example, the total population of a large country like the United States. In any health study, what we usually focus on is a small number of cases in a small subgroup of that large population, such as for example one particular county in Pennsylvania located on the Reading Prong. The rate of a disease in a large country does not usually vary much from one year to another, epidemics of contagious diseases being an exception. If, however, we are studying a small subgroup, we invariably find the number of cases will vary appreciably from year to year. While the national rate predicts ten cases per year in a group of the size we are studying, in any one year we may find only seven cases, and the next year eleven. We get ten cases only if we take an average over many years. These annual variations are not "caused" by any factors we can control, but instead appear to occur at random. Because of them, it is often difficult to show that some particular exposure, to radon or to some other hazardous substance, has caused an increase in the number of cases. The reasons that there are random variations are discussed at more length in chapters 4 and 8.

The smaller the number of cases expected in a group being studied, the greater the relative importance of the random variations. Obviously, it is an advantage to study a large group rather than a small one, but it is not always possible: sometimes the number of exposed people is limited, or the cost of studying a large group may be too great.

Detecting Signals over a Noisy Background

This problem is something like the problem of hearing a radio signal over a noisy radio background: signals weaker than the level of noise cannot be distinguished from the noise. The year-to-year random variation is the "noise" background against which we are trying to detect the "signal" of extra cases caused by radon exposure. How great is the range of that random variation? How large must a difference from the expected number of deaths be before we take it seriously? Extensive experience and statistical reasoning have found a very useful rule of thumb for the "noise" level, the range within which the numbers of cases observed in a small group in different years vary randomly about the average number of cases. The square root of the expected average number gives us an estimate of the range of random variation. More precisely, about two-thirds of the time the numbers will lie within that range around the expected average. This may be called "the square root estimate."

The Power of a Study

Suppose we calculate the expected number of lung cancer deaths to be 100 per year, based on the U.S. average rates, in an area where the homes happen to have high radon levels, and in one year we observe 105. Is this alarming, or merely the result of random variation? How many excess deaths must we observe before we take this increase seriously? The square root of 100 is 10, so we should expect to find anything from 90 to 110 deaths in any one year. One third of the years the number of deaths will lie outside this range. We could not possibly detect a 5% increase in the rate, because the five extra deaths would not be noticeable above the "noise." A study in which the expected number of deaths is 100 is said to lack the "power" to detect a 5% increase. On the other hand a 20% increase, leading to twenty extra deaths, is greater than the range of random variation, and could be detected. If we were to study a population 100 times larger, so that the expected number of deaths is now 10,000, the year-to-year variability would be about 100 (the square root of 10,000). The 5% increase in rate now represents 500 deaths, which is larger than the range of random variation and would be easily detectable. Such a large study is said to have the "power" to detect a 5% increase.

We can see that one way to ensure enough power to detect the effects we are looking for is to enlarge the sample. If a study of 1,000 homes does not have the power, study 1,000,000. Unfortunately, if in such a study each home must have its radon levels measured, the cost would be prohibitive.

Another way to increase the power is to select a population for study known to have been heavily exposed, for example, in the workplace or, in the case of radiation, during a nuclear bombing or a nuclear explosion. Then even if the number of people studied is smaller, the number of cases caused by the heavy exposure may be large enough to be detected over the random variations. This approach has problems of its own, but it has been found to be a very informative one in the study of health hazards. (There is further discussion of power in chapter 8).

Real Signals and Real Noise

In the communications industry, two ways have been found to detect signals over a noisy background: one is to transmit the signal many times and take an average, which tends to reinforce the signal and cancel out the noise, and the other is to increase the size of the signal. The first is analogous to using a larger group for the study, the second analogous to studying a more heavily exposed group (fig. 3-7).

STUDIES ON MINERS

Determining Exposure

Not only are workplace exposures to hazardous substances usually greater, but in addition it is often easier to establish what those exposures actually were. In occupational settings the workers often wear exposure detectors, such as radiation badges, now required in mines where there is radon exposure. Often radioactivity or chemicals in the air in a workplace are continuously monitored. The health records of employees may be traceable from employers' records or from health insurance benefits.

Examples of health hazards first discovered by studying occupational groups include asbestos (a cause of both lung cancer and mesothelioma), naphthylamine (a cause of bladder cancer), vinyl chloride (a cause of liver sarcoma), and last but not least, ionizing radiation causing leukemia and melanoma among radiologists and bone cancer in the women who painted the dials of watches with radium-containing paint.

There are several problems with using occupational groups to assess health effects of exposures to environmental agents in the general population.

The "Healthy Worker" Effect

First of all, the employed population does not include children, many elderly people, or people with chronic illnesses or severe physical disabilities. These are groups that will have a different rate of diseases to start

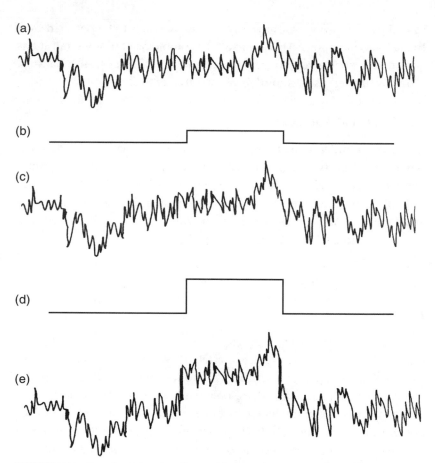

FIGURE 3-7 Signals and noise. Figure (a) is a schematic representation of noise and figure (b) a representation of a signal we desire to detect. The size of the signal is comparable to the ups and downs due to noise, and in the sum of the signal and noise, shown as (c), the signal would be impossible to distinguish from the noise. A larger signal is shown as (d). This signal would be noticeable even when combined with the noise, as shown in (e).

with and may also have a more sensitive response to the exposures under study. Being able to work at all implies that one is healthier than the general population, a factor one must be aware of in making comparisons.

Extrapolation and Its Uncertainties

Second, to apply the results to the less-exposed general population, we must estimate the health effects of low doses by the observations on high ones: the problem of "extrapolation." Often we need to know what will happen in the future, whether because we are investing money in stocks or protecting Earth from a collision with an asteroid. The future is inaccessible to us, and we must make our best guess on the basis of what we know now. The process of using present knowledge to predict future events is one example of extrapolation.

It is not the only example: sometimes it is the past we are ignorant of, and we may still be curious about what it was like. We can still use present knowledge to help us guess. More generally, extrapolation is not only a question of past or future. We have explained why we cannot directly measure how many cancers low doses of radiation cause, yet we need to know to set safety standards. We make the best guess we can from effects at high doses.

In general, when we need to know things that cannot be directly observed, we extrapolate from the knowledge obtained from things we can observe. There is no infallible way to do it, though; it is a question of judgment, and people's judgments differ. Will stock prices continue to rise in the next decade at the same rate they have risen in the last 50 years? Or will the present (mid-2001) signs of weakening in the U.S. economy slow down their rise? Or will war break out unexpectedly in the Middle East and cause a market collapse?

Different people will make different guesses, and if one wants to use a more dignified word than "guess," one can say they use different "models."

Techniques of Extrapolation

The simplest and most obvious model for extrapolation is to assume that whatever happened in the immediate past will continue in the near future. We may visualize this extrapolation by imagining data points, say stock prices, plotted on a graph against the date. So if we have data for the years 2000 and 2001, we imagine drawing a line through the data points and extending this line into the year 2002. Unfortunately, the data points will never lie exactly on one straight line—they will always have some scatter (fig. 3-8)—so we have to choose some "best" straight line going through them, perhaps by placing a ruler so that it comes as close as possible to all of them. Experience shows that different people will place the ruler differently, so this is not a very satisfactory procedure. Fortunately, mathematicians have found an objective procedure for finding this best straight line for us, called "linear regression." There are standard computer pro-

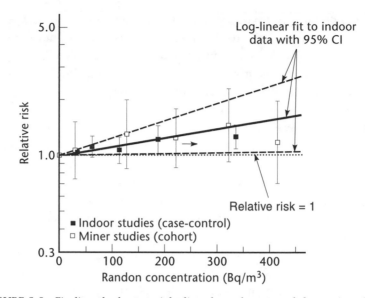

FIGURE 3-8 Finding the best straight line through scattered data points. This is not a schematic representation but a real example. It is an early result in which the "relative risk" of dying of lung cancer found in studies on miners was compared with the "relative risk" found in studies on people living in homes in which radon concentrations had been measured. The ratio of the risk of dying from lung cancer for a person exposed to radon to the risk to an unexposed person of dying from the disease is called the "relative risk." The vertical axis of this figure represents the relative risk, and the horizontal axis the exposure to radon. The results from five studies on miners are shown as white squares; from five studies on homes as black squares. The vertical lines through each square show the 95% confidence interval (CI) of each of the studies. It was assumed that a linear, no-threshold relation holds between relative risk and radon exposure, so that a straight line was drawn through the ten data points which ends at a relative risk of 1.0 for zero radon exposure. A mathematical technique called "linear regression" was used to find the "best" straight line to fit the scattered data points. The technique also enables us to calculate a 95% confidence interval for the best line. The upper and lower limits for this interval are shown as dashed lines. The figure was adapted from a figure in the article, "Studies of Indoor Radon and Lung Cancer Risk," by Jay H. Lubin, in *Implications of New Data on Radiation Cancer Risk*, published by the National Council on Radiation Protection and Measurements, 1997, with the permission of the Council.

grams for doing it, and it is used repeatedly in fitting data to models. Although our extrapolation is not from the past of stock prices to their future, but rather from the cancer risk at high doses to the risk at low ones, the mathematical procedure is the same.

There are more complicated models for the relation of cancer risk to dose than those described by a single straight line. There are models involving curved lines, and even involving two straight lines meeting at one point, one way to represent a threshold for harm. The mathematicians have provided us with procedures and appropriate computer programs for seeing how well these models fit the data, but we will not describe them here.

Miners and Radon

There are a number of major mining areas where miners have been exposed to high levels of radon for a long time. For these miners, reasonably reliable data on lung cancer are available. Many of the mines are uranium mines, such as in Colorado in the United States, in Ontario in Canada, in France, and in the same Erz mountain region described by Georgius Agricola, now divided between Saxony in eastern Germany and the Czech Republic. Radon exposure of miners has also occurred in tin mines in China, which have been in operation for 2,000 years, and iron mines in Sweden. All these mines and the miners who worked in them have been studied extensively for several decades, and like the studies of Japanese nuclear bomb survivors provide us with valuable information about the health effects of radiation exposure.

Measures of Exposure

Radon concentrations in the air either in a mine or a house are still commonly given in picocuries per liter, though this is no longer the unit internationally accepted by scientific societies, which use the becquerel per cubic meter (see "Radon Measures" [p. 96] for more details). A picocurie, originally defined in terms of the rate of decay of radium, is that amount of radium, radon, or any other radioactive material, undergoing 2.2 disintegrations per minute. The U.S. level for radon in homes at which remedial action is advisable is 4 picocuries per liter, corresponding to about 9 disintegrations per minute in each liter of air. A becquerel is that amount of radioactive material undergoing 1 disintegration per second, so that 1 becquerel per cubic meter is the same as 27.3 picocuries.

Working Levels, and Working Level Months

To make matters more confusing, a third unit for the amount of radio-activity, originally applicable to mines, is often used. It is called the Working Level and is defined by the amount of radiation from radon progeny, not radon itself, that was considered "acceptable" in a mine at the time the unit was invented. It is not exactly equal to a definite number of picocuries, but a rough translation from mine to home conditions makes one picocurie per liter of air equivalent to a working level of 0.02.

Exposure: The Product of Radioactive Concentration and Time

All three units, picocurie per liter, becquerel per cubic meter, and Working Level, describe the amount of radioactivity in a particular environment. Obviously the exposure of any individual depends both on the amount of radioactivity and on the time spent there. For miners, exposure is measured by Working Level Months, the product of the Working Level by the number of months the miner was employed in the mine.

The Studies of Miners

The cumulative exposure for each individual miner was assessed from the number of years he was employed in each of the jobs that miners perform, different jobs being associated with different levels of exposure to radon progeny (different Working Levels). The miners more heavily exposed could then be compared with miners of the same age and the same smoking history, who were less exposed because either they worked in mines or sectors in the mines that had much lower concentrations of radon progeny, or else were employed in the mines for shorter periods of time.

As usual, in practice things are always more complicated. Different mines in different countries followed different procedures in measuring radon or radon progeny exposure. At first, after World War II, before the risks were widely recognized and while the pressures of the Cold War were building up, radon in the mines was not always monitored, and monitoring was not as thorough as is required today. As awareness grew, monitoring was done with more care, and in some mines personal monitors were worn by the miners. Also, the working practices in the mines were changed to minimize exposure: for example, ventilation was improved, and wet-drilling used to reduce dust levels. These benefited the miners, but as they were being done at about the time that the accuracy of the monitoring of exposure was being improved, estimates of the heavier exposures of the dirtier past are less precise (fig. 3-9).

Smoking and Radon Exposure: Double Trouble

Since smoking is responsible for 90% of lung cancers in the general population, and miners, unfortunately for them, often smoked more than

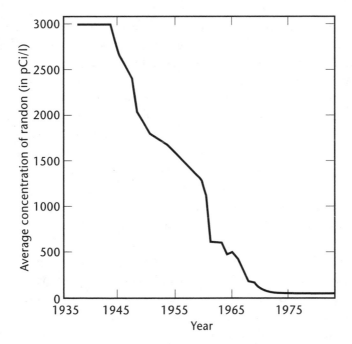

FIGURE 3-9   The decline in average radon concentration in U.S. uranium mines over time, as ventilation and other working conditions in the mines were improved. The radon levels are given in picocuries per liter. Reproduced from David J. Brenner, *Radon: Risk and Remedy,* W.H. Freeman and Co., New York, 1989, and used by courtesy of Professor Brenner. The figure was adapted by Professor Brenner from a figure in a chapter by L. W. Swent in *Radiation Hazards in Mining: Control, Measurements, and Medical Aspects,* ed. by M. Gomez, © 1982 by the Society of Mining Engineers (now the Society for Mining, Metallurgy, and Exploration (SME)), and used with permission of the Society.

men usually do, it is important that we distinguish the risk from radon exposure from the risk due to smoking. Just as the risk to miners from radon was ignored or minimized in the early years of the Cold War, so also was their risk from smoking. At first no records were kept about their smoking habits, and when studies began later, the data on smoking were based on their memories and honesty about their smoking histories, plus some guesswork on the part of the scientists doing the studies. The combination of smoking and radon raises some knotty problems.

Synergism: $3 + 3 = 9$

If in addition to smoking cigarettes one works in a mine with high concentrations of radon progeny how will those two lung cancer-causing agents act together? Is the risk caused by exposure to a certain level of radon progeny just added on to the risks the miners already have from smoking cigarettes? For example, if an exposure to a certain level of radon progeny increases the risk of lung cancer fivefold in non-smokers, and the risk of cancer in smokers not exposed to radon is tenfold, what could be the risk to smoking uranium miners? One possibility is that it is fifteenfold, the sum of five and ten and therefore an additive risk, another is that it is fiftyfold, the product of five and ten and thus a multiplicative risk. If it should come out to be between the two extremes it is called, tautologically, "between additive and multiplicative."

In study after study it was shown that the risk is not the simple sum of the two, but is greater. In other words radon and smoking act in what is called a "synergistic" way: the action of the two together was found in all the studies to be greater than the sum of the effects expected from either alone, but less than the product: it was found to be between additive and multiplicative. The studies did not agree well on exactly how strong the synergistic effect was.

An almost multiplicative risk is found in asbestos workers who smoke. Nonsmoking asbestos workers have a tenfold risk of lung cancer (aside from their special risk of mesothelioma), and heavy cigarette smokers who have not been exposed to asbestos also have a tenfold risk. The asbestos workers who are heavy smokers have, not a twentyfold risk, but rather an almost one-hundred-fold risk (fig. 3-10).

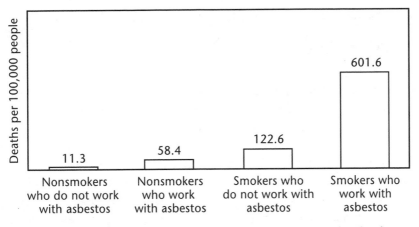

FIGURE 3-10   The death rate from lung cancer per 100,000 people. This figure illustrates "synergism," a combined risk being greater than the sum of the two separate risks acting independently. The combined risk for smoking asbestos workers is approximately the product, not the sum, of the risk to smokers who do not work with asbestos and the risk to nonsmoking asbestos workers.

Other Problems

There were other factors that affected the miners' risk of lung cancer to a lesser extent than smoking that were also taken into account. These included the age of the miner when he was exposed, how far in the past the exposure occurred, and the rate of exposure. A miner exposed for a long time in a mine with a low radon level gets the same total dose as a miner exposed for a short time in a mine with a high level. Are these equally harmful, and if not, which is worse? It appeared that for radon, low exposure rate over a longer period is worse, for reasons not yet fully understood. It is contrary to what was found when the effects of the atomic bombing of Japan were compared with medical treatment with X-rays.

The complete analysis of the miner studies done by the Committee on Health Risks of Exposure to Radon relates the lung cancer risk to the exposure history, the smoking history, and the age of the individual miner. People who are exposed to radon in their homes also have exposure and smoking histories (though their total lifetime exposures are usually less than that of miners), and so from the findings of the miner studies, and the assumption that risk is proportional to dose down to low doses typical of home radon levels, their risk can be calculated.

FROM DANGER IN THE MINES TO DANGER IN HOMES

From the Miners to the Rest of Us

The problem of inferring the health effects of low doses from studies done on high doses comes up repeatedly both in epidemiological studies (on human beings) and laboratory studies on animals, and comes up not only in studies of radiation but of toxic chemicals as well.

The obvious question is why do we not do direct experiments, at least on mice, to determine just what the health effects of low doses are? There is a reason, however, that we often cannot. As we have noted, radiation does not cause diseases or conditions that are unique to radiation. Cancers, mental retardation, birth defects, miscarriages all occur anyway in the absence of radiation; radiation only increases their number. Therefore, if we look for the effects of low doses of radiation, we are necessarily looking for slight increases in the natural rates of various diseases. The lower the dose, the smaller the increase in the rate caused by radiation, and the harder it is to detect above the random variations that always occur. The only way to detect small increases in disease rates is to use a very large number of mice for study. One might think that the question of the safety of low doses is important enough to justify the added cost of studying a large number. However, it is not so simple: a statistical analysis shows that the number needed does not increase simply as the dose decreases, but as the square of the dose. For example, suppose we needed one thousand mice to detect a health effect, say leukemia, with a specific dose of radiation. To see if one-tenth of that dose produces one-tenth the number of cases, we would need not ten times as many mice but one hundred times as many. To show that one-hundredth of that dose produces one-hundredth the number of cases we would need not one hundred times as many mice but ten thousand times as many, in other words, 1 million mice. The reason that we need such large numbers has to do with what we earlier called "the square root law" of random variation (see pp. 73–74), but we will omit the detailed reasoning. Obviously, we cannot go much lower in dose and still detect health effects without enormously large studies, at enormous expense.

The Linear No-Threshold Model

The harmful effects of radiation were first recognized, and can only be directly studied, when the doses are high. Safety standards are necessarily concerned with doses so low that either no harm or acceptable harm would result. What amount of harm is "acceptable" is a value judgment, and we will not attempt to define it here. To determine how low is low enough, one must extrapolate—infer from what we observe with high doses what would happen at low ones. The practice in setting standards is to assume that harm is directly proportional to dose. This implies that there is no dose so small that it does no harm, but also that the lower the dose, the less the harm. At first, there was no strong biological evidence either for or against this assumption, and there was an alternative view that there might be some low dose below which no harm at all was done: a "threshold" dose. Among the arguments for a threshold was that living organisms have been exposed to low doses of radiation from natural sources throughout evolution and may have developed mechanisms to deal with it. The linear no-threshold assumption, that response is directly proportional to dose down to the lowest doses, implies that there is no absolutely safe level of exposure. It seemed a more cautious and prudent one, and in the absence of direct biological evidence to the contrary it was generally adopted.

If there really is a threshold for harm, a dose below which the organism suffers no harm whatever, the linear model would overestimate the risks of low doses. Those who believe in a threshold feel the linear assumption exaggerates the risks, and places unnecessary burdens on beneficial uses of high-energy radiation and nuclear power, burdens of cost and burdens of public anxiety. In particular, critics of the home radon exposure standards set by the Environmental Protection Agency have claimed that homeowners are being panicked into expensive remediation efforts to avoid nonexistent risks. As will be seen shortly, some exciting new experiments on irradiation of single living cells have suggested that the linear no-threshold assumption, justified on the grounds of prudence, may not have been prudent enough. (See figure 3-12 on p. 90.)

Cancer Begins with One Cell

With the advance of molecular biology that began in the 1950s with the discovery of the structure and method of replication of DNA molecules, we understood better how radiation causes cancer: a mutation in a single cell may start that cell and its descendants on a course that ends in cancer many cell generations later, and a mutation can be caused by a single photon or particle of ionizing radiation. If cancer starts with an event in a single cell, it becomes more plausible that no dose, no matter how small, can be harmless, and correspondingly less plausible that there could be a threshold dose. Of course, the more radiation an individual is exposed to, the more mutations are produced, and the more likely cancer will be the outcome.

Determining risks at low exposures from data at high exposures is not only a problem in high-energy radiation, but is a problem shared with other environmental hazards. For example, data from the high exposures of the London Smog Episode were used to estimate health risks from low levels of air pollution (see chapter 9). Standards for known human carcinogens like asbestos and benzene are derived from high exposures in industrial settings. The linear no-threshold model used in the extrapolation from the miners' studies to home radon levels is the simplest model, but might have to be discarded if new biological evidence requires it. This, incidentally, is true of all scientific models: the simplest is best, until it is contradicted by experimental evidence.

A New Discovery, a New Picture

It has recently become possible to observe the consequences of a direct hit by an alpha particle on one individual living cell.

The technique uses a new scientific instrument called a charged-particle microbeam, which can shoot alpha particles at the cell with microscopic precision. The researcher can hit a desired portion of the cell with a specified number of alpha particles: one if the researcher chooses, or three. The particle can be specifically directed to the center of the nucleus, or again, if the researcher chooses, to miss the nucleus and hit instead the part of the cell that surrounds the cell nucleus, called the cytoplasm.

The studies use specially cultivated mammalian cell lines in which mutations can easily be detected. In addition, certain types of mutations, those that involve breaks and rearrangements of the chromosomes, may be observed by microscopic examination. The number of cells killed by different doses of alpha particle irradiation can be determined, and those cells that are not killed may be cultured to see if they have undergone mutation into cancer cells.

Several remarkable discoveries have been made with the microbeam that shed an entirely new light on the question of extrapolation and of the existence of a threshold for damage.

Experiments by T. K. Hei and colleagues at Columbia University have indeed confirmed that a direct hit on the DNA in the cell nucleus by a single alpha particle is enough to produce a potentially carcinogenic mutation. There were, however, a number of unexpected results. It had been previously assumed that a hit on the bulk of the cell outside the nucleus (the cytoplasm) would not cause any mutations. Subsequent experiments by these investigators showed that a hit on the cytoplasm also causes mutations by producing an energy-rich unstable type of molecule called a free radical, which can diffuse into the nucleus and react with the DNA molecule.

Further, the types of mutations produced in the surviving cells depend on whether they are caused by direct hits on the nucleus or on the cytoplasm. Cytoplasmic hits produce what are called "point mutations," changes in one or a few bases in the DNA chain that cause the production of a protein with one or two "wrong" amino acids when the gene is expressed. Nuclear hits produce both point mutations and microscopically observable chromosomal breaks and rearrangements. (See chapter 6 for a more detailed discussion of genes and what they do.)

An additional exciting result is that when the nucleus of a cell is irradiated with an alpha particle, mutations occur in neighboring non-irradiated cells as well. This observation is consistent with previous findings, in which irradiation of 1% of the cells in a colony resulted in mutations in 30% of the unirradiated neighbors. The type of mutations in these "bystander" cells were similar to those in the directly irradiated cell: nuclear irradiation produced visible chromosomal rearrangements in bystanders. It has been shown that the diffusion of energy-rich radicals from one cell to another is not responsible for this "bystander" effect, but instead it involves cell-cell signaling: the emission of certain molecules by cells that influence processes in neighboring cells.

Dose-Response at the Cellular Level?

The mechanism by which irradiation of the nucleus produces mutations in the nuclei of neighboring cells has to do with the ways cells signal to other cells through molecules that can cross the cell membrane. The fact that mutations produced in bystander cells raises a question about the validity of the linear no-threshold model. If hitting 1% of the cells in a colony with an alpha particle causes mutations in 30% of the surrounding cells, it follows that hitting 5% of the cells would cause mutations in essentially all the cells of the colony. Surely it cannot cause mutations in 5x30%, or 150% of them! A kind of "law of diminishing returns" must set in, and there can no longer be a direct proportionality between dose and the number of mutations, except at extremely low doses. The bystander effect implies that doubling the number of cells that are hit by an alpha particle produces less than double the number of mutated cells (fig. 3-11).

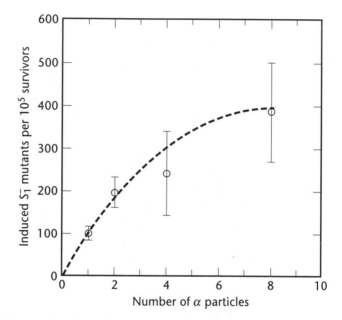

FIGURE 3-11   Why the linear no-threshold assumption may be wrong. Results of an experiment measuring the number of mutants per one hundred thousand surviving cells irradiated with an exact number of alpha particles. The figure shows the numbers of mutants for one, two, four, and eight alpha particles per cell (with 95% confidence intervals). The figure shows clearly a tendency to "saturate," in that eight alpha particles per cell produce less than eight times as many mutants as produced by one alpha particle per cell. In direct studies of health effects on living organisms, whether people or mice, we usually observe health effects at high doses, and are forced to extrapolate to low doses. The linear no-threshold assumption we use for extrapolation would in this case underestimate the effect of the low doses. From an article by T. K. Hei et al., "Mutagenic Effects of a Single and an Exact Number of Alpha Particles in Mammalian Cells," in the *Proceedings of the National Academy of Sciences*, v. 94, pp. 3765–70 (1997). © 1997 by the National Academy of Sciences, U.S.A., and reproduced with its permission.

A further discovery raises still another question about the linear no-threshold model. It applies to somewhat higher doses, when many cells are irradiated by more than one alpha particle. It was found that the number of mutations does not increase in direct proportion to the number of alpha particles passing through a cell. Instead, four alpha particles traversing a cell produce less than double the number of mutations produced by two particles, a further example of diminishing returns. After four or five alpha particles, additional alpha particles cause hardly any additional mutations in cells that survive. Things are complicated even more by the fact that multiple hits kill many cells, and it is only the survivors that can undergo mutations. Another way to put it is that the damage saturates; there is only so much damage possible, and after that point is reached, additional alpha particles do not add much.

It has been shown that at the higher levels of alpha particle radiation that miners were exposed to, the vulnerable cells on the outer surfaces of the lungs, where dust particles containing polonium lodge, actually are traversed by many alpha particles. On the other hand, in the lower exposures more typical of homes, the vulnerable cells are almost never traversed by more than one alpha particle; the majority of cells are not traversed by any.

Prudent, but Not Prudent Enough?

Both the mutations in bystander cells and the complicated effects of multiple hits on a single cell suggest that the linear no-threshold model, extrapolating from the data on miners exposed to relatively high doses, might *underestimate* the harm done by low doses. Putting it another way, the lung cancer risk decreases less rapidly than we would have guessed from the linear model. In contrast, the threshold model predicts a more rapid falloff of risk with decreasing dose than the linear model. Figure 3-12 illustrates the differences among the three models.

From Cells to People

Do these new findings mean we must reject the linear no-threshold model for radon studies? Are low doses of alpha radiation less safe than we thought?

While the microbeam results do suggest that the linear no-threshold model may underestimate the lung cancer risk of low doses of alpha par-

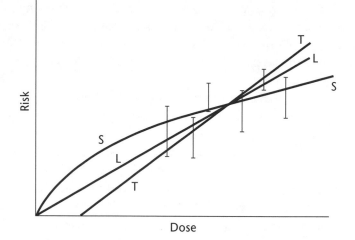

FIGURE 3-12   A schematic representation of three kinds of behavior possible at low doses. The data we obtain from studies is almost always for high doses, and the scatter in the data does not enable us to tell what might happen at the low doses where health effects are too small to measure directly. The relations represented by the letters S, L, and T are three possible models, all of which fit the data points equally well. L is the linear no-threshold assumption, T the threshold assumption (no harm at all below a certain dose), and S a possible model suggested by the data from charged particle microbeam experiments that show saturation at higher doses.

ticles, the word "suggest" is crucial. The microbeam experiments are done on cell cultures, not on living organisms, and they may not apply in a simple way to organisms.

These results are too new; a scientific consensus has not yet formed on their implications for the risks of low-dose radiation of human beings, and the linear no-threshold model is not likely to be rejected until it is. There are many reasons for caution: certainly an experiment showing that a cell has undergone a mutation, or even has been converted into a cancer cell from a precancerous state, does not tell us what will happen in a living organism, man or mouse, composed of billions of interacting cells.

One must hope that the questions of how to extrapolate the high-dose results to low doses raised by these discoveries will be resolved soon. Until it is, the linear no-threshold model will most likely continue to be used.

Fortunately, the lower range of miners' exposures happened to over-lap the higher range of home exposures, so the extrapolation to low doses in homes is not too far from the doses at which we have data on miners. Within the range of miners' exposure, the risk appeared to be proportional to the dose: the linear no-threshold assumption is in accord with the data in this range of doses, although the uncertainties in the data are too great to rule out some alternative models. The true lung cancer risks from home radon exposure are unlikely to be less than those calculated in the committee report, and just possibly they may be greater.

Other Problems

Miners are not the same as the average home-dweller, nor are mines the same as homes. Miners are mostly healthy adult men of working age; home-dwellers include women, children, the elderly, and the ill. Mines are dustier and are ventilated differently from homes. Men who work in mines are doing hard physical labor and breathe harder, inhaling more dust than home-dwellers, who are asleep a large portion of the time they spend at home, and the rest of the time not as physically active. There is no easy way to take these factors into account: the committee considered them, but came to the conclusion that they probably did not affect the relation between exposure and risk by much.

Results: The Lifetime Risk

To summarize, we give the lifetime risk of dying of lung cancer if one lives in a home with a particular level of radon for one's entire life. It should not be forgotten that these risks have been calculated using the linear no-threshold assumption. If there should be a threshold, the calculation overestimates the risks. If the results obtained recently with the alpha particle microbeam are taken at face value, the calculation underestimates the risk.

The calculated risks are different for smokers and nonsmokers, and different for men and for women. The difference in risk between men and women is not because one sex is more susceptible than another, but because in calculating lifetime risks of dying from lung cancer, the life expectancy makes a difference, and women live longer.

Table 3-1 gives the risks for several levels of residential radon concentration that correspond to three possible levels in U.S. homes, a "low"

TABLE 3-1   Lifetime Relative Risk of Dying from Lung Cancer for a Lifetime Indoor Exposure to Radon

Bq/cu.meter (PiC/liter) Exposure	Smokers[a]		Nonsmokers[b]	
	Men	Women	Men	Women
25 (0.7)	1.08	1.09	1.19	1.21
150 (4.1)	1.47	1.52	2.16	2.23
400 (10.8)	2.17	2.23	4.06	4.26

[a]Persons who have ever smoked. [b]Persons who have never smoked.

Note: The relative risk tells us how much our risk is increased by home radon exposure. A relative risk of 1.08, for example, means an 8% increase in risk of death from lung cancer, relative to the risk in the absence of radon. The relative risk of 2.17 for smokers exposed to 400 bq/m^3 is equivalent to an increase of 117% in risk compared to nonsmokers not exposed to radon.

The studies found that while the risk to a miner was primarily determined by his lifetime total dose, the rate at which the dose was received had some effect on the risk. The committee used two different ways of correcting for the rate of exposure. Table 3-1 is based on the correction giving a slightly higher figure.

level of 25 bq/m^3 (about 0.7 picocuries per liter), a "medium" level of 150 bq/m^3 (just about the EPA remediation level of 4 picocuries per liter), and a "high" level of 400 bq/m^3 (10.8 picocuries per liter, more than two-and-one-half times the remediation level). Obviously, the risks of low levels are less, but the proportion of the U.S. homes that have low levels is very large. The result is that there are more deaths from radon-caused lung cancer in homes with levels below the EPA "action" level of 4 picocuries per liter (148 bq/m^3) than in homes above that level.

The numbers listed in the table are not the risks of lung cancer itself, but the "relative risks." Like all diseases or conditions caused by radiation or any other environmental hazard, the disease occurs anyway, in the absence of that hazard. The relative risk for a particular exposure to radon tells us how much the person's risk is increased by the exposure, compared to what it would be without that exposure.

For example, the risk for a male smoker living in a home with a radon level of 150 bq/m^3, about the EPA remediation level, is 1.47 times as great as if he had not been exposed to radon in his home, but still smoked.

Notice that a male nonsmoker living in a home with a 150 bq/m3 radon level has his relative risk of lung cancer increased by a larger factor,

2.16, than a smoker does. This does not imply a greater risk of lung cancer for the nonsmoker, but only a greater relative increase. A heavy smoker already has a tenfold greater risk than a nonsmoker, and the radon exposure increases this to a 14.7-fold risk. The nonsmoker's risk from radon exposure is increased only 2.16-fold, compared to a nonsmoker not exposed to radon. In brief, the proportion of smokers who will die of lung cancer caused by radon will be greater than the proportion of nonsmokers who will die, given the same exposure to radon.

The same reasoning applies to the relative risks of radon exposure to women, which are slightly greater than to men. Since women have a lower rate of lung cancer than men even without considering radon, a higher proportion of men will die (and have died) of lung cancer caused by radon exposure.

Total Deaths from Radon in Homes

The committee also calculated the total number of deaths per year in the United States from lung cancer resulting from residential radon exposure. This required combining the risk for each level of radon exposure with knowledge of how many homes in the United States have that level of radon exposure and how many people of what ages and smoking habits live in them.

Table 3-2 gives the total number of deaths from lung cancer in the year 1993, and the deaths of that total that would presumably not have occurred in the absence of residential radon exposure. Deaths are also categorized by sex and by smoking history. Figure 3-13 gives the percentages of all lung cancer deaths caused by radon associated with the various levels of radon in U.S. homes.

Back to Window Glass

We have mentioned that because it is hard to determine home radon exposures over the lifetimes of the inhabitants reliably, direct studies of lung cancer risks from home exposure have led to estimates with very wide confidence intervals. However we also described one recent study that used alpha particle emissions from flat glass in windows and mirrors that had been in place in the home for at least twenty-five years. Using this more reliable estimate, a significant relation was found between long-term exposure and risk. The relation found actually suggested a greater risk from

TABLE 3-2   Total Deaths from Lung Cancer and the Number Attributable to Radon (United States, 1993)

	Total Deaths	Number of the Total Attributable to Radon
Whole Population	157,400	21,800
Smokers[a]	146,400	18,900
Nonsmokers[b]	11,000	2,900
Men		
Smokers	90,600	11,300
Nonsmokers	4,800	1,200
Women		
Smokers	55,800	7,600
Nonsmokers	6,200	1,700

[a]Persons who have ever smoked. [b]Persons who have never smoked.

Note: The uncertainty in the figures calculated is usefully described by a "95% confidence interval," the range of values within which the true answer is believed to have a 95% probability of lying. (For more detailed discussion of confidence interval, see chap. 8.) For the total radon-caused lung cancer deaths, 21,800, the confidence interval is from 15,600 to 56,700.

home exposure than that extrapolated from the data on miners, but the authors of the paper noted that the 95% confidence interval for the increased risk found in their study was wide enough to overlap the results of the miners' study. They therefore did not claim that the risk from radon in the home was greater than estimated from the miners' risk, and concluded only that more studies on radon in homes and lung cancer should be done using their method of radon dose estimation. A study of this kind done in Iowa has recently been published and gives about the same results.

SUMMARY: HOME RADON LEVELS AND LUNG CANCER

Extrapolation from studies of miners exposed to higher radon levels than those found in homes has provided strong evidence that radon in homes is a significant hazard, accounting for about 14% of lung cancer deaths in the United States. This figure is consistent with the conclusions of the up to now less reliable but direct studies of radon in homes. In turn, lung cancer itself is the leading cause of death from cancer among both men and women. Yet radon has attracted a smaller share of public concern and

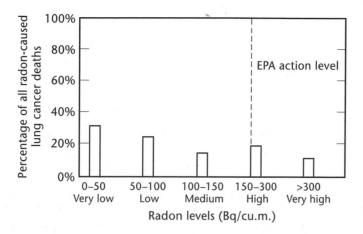

FIGURE 3-13 The percentage of radon-caused lung cancer deaths associated with each range of radon levels in U.S. homes. Data on radon levels in homes (fig. 3-5) was combined with information on what proportion of the general population smokes, and risk of death from lung cancer calculated from the miners' studies. It can be shown that the less than 1% of homes with levels above 400 bq/cu.m. are associated with 6% of the deaths, and the 6% of homes exceeding the EPA remediation level are associated with 30% of the deaths. It is worth noting that 70% of the deaths are associated with radon in homes below the EPA limit. This reflects the very large number of people living in homes with low radon levels: a rather low risk of death affecting a very large number of people still causes a lot of deaths.

the attention of environmental activists than what are often less well established hazards. In other chapters we will discuss some examples of such hazards that may cause much less or even possibly no harm and are much more costly to ameliorate: electric power lines, pesticides, and living near nuclear facilities. In fact, radon in homes is a greater health risk than the fallout from the Chernobyl accident (fig. 3-14).

Measures to reduce radon levels in homes and thereby diminish the risk of lung cancer are not prohibitive in price, costing one or two thousand dollars, yet most homeowners do not bother even to have their radon concentrations measured.

Why has the very real threat posed by home radon levels been mostly ignored? There are a number of factors known to affect how people perceive a risk. One of them whether the risk occurs naturally or as the result of some voluntary choice, or instead is imposed by some impersonal and distant government agency or greedy corporation. This certainly explains

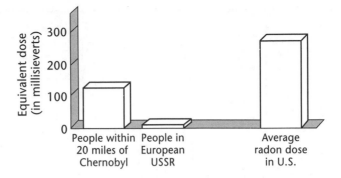

FIGURE 3-14   This sobering figure prepared by Dr. David Brenner compares the average equivalent radiation doses received as a result of the Chernobyl accident with the average dose received from radon in homes in the United States. The doses are given in millisieverts. Three groups are compared: people living within 20 miles of the Chernobyl plant at the time of the accident and who were evacuated, the rest of the population in the European part of the Soviet Union exposed to fallout from the accident, and the entire U.S. population exposed to radon in their homes. Doses from the Three Mile Island accident are too small to be shown on this figure. Reproduced from David J. Brenner, *Radon: Risk and Remedy*, W.H. Freeman and Co., New York, 1989, and used by courtesy of Professor Brenner.

why nuclear processing plants arouse more concern than that most lethal of all known environmental hazards: cigarettes. If it should turn out that the recent studies of single-cell irradiaton with the alpha particle micro-beam leads to a replacement of the linear no-threshold assumption used for extrapolation, and the conclusion that the miners studies under-estimate the risk of home radon exposures, the problem of home radon will surely draw more public attention than it has in the past.

A CLOSER LOOK: RADON MEASURES

By international agreement, the unit currently used for the amount of radio-activity is the bequerel (after the discoverer of radioactivity), which is the amount of any radioactive substance that gives one disintegration per second. One picocurie is exactly 0.037 bequerels. The Environmental Protection Agency, however, still specifies home radon concentrations in picocuries per liter. The internationally preferred unit for concentration is bequerels per cubic meter (bq/m$^{3)}$, a cubic meter being 1,000 liters. The EPA remediation level of 4 picocuries per liter is equal to 148 bq/m^3.

As we have noted above, the health hazards associated with radon actually arise from the radon progeny forms of polonium. A unit of exposure was developed for mines that measures the radon progeny, rather than radon itself, called a Working Level, the term chosen because one Working Level was once considered to be the amount of exposure that should be permitted in a mine.

Unfortunately, the Working Level was defined in such a way that the relationship between picocuries of radon per liter of air in a mine or a basement and the Working Level in that location is not an exact one, and depends on various factors, including ventilation and the amount of dust in the air. An estimate for homes is that 1 picocurie of radon per liter is roughly equivalent to a Working Level of 0.02. The EPA remediation level of 4 picocuries would then correspond to a Working Level of 0.08. Obviously the longer a person is exposed the greater the risk, so the exposure of a particular miner or of a particular home-dweller is the product of the time exposed, multiplied by the Working Level. The exposure of miners is given in Working Level-Months, but a "month" for a miner is 170 hours, the average number of hours per month a miner spends in the mine. A person spending a month at home is there 720 hours, so to compare the home-dweller to the miner, the number of months the home-dweller has lived in the house must be multiplied by the factor 720/170.

To make a long and complicated story short, a person living in a house with a radon concentration of 4 picocuries for twenty years (240 months) receives a total exposure of about 80 Working Level-Months (0.02 x 4 x 240 x 720/170). Of course people "living" in a home do not spend every minute of the day there; a rough estimate is that 70% of the time is spent at home so that in twenty years of residence, the exposure would be 56 Working Level-Months. Miners in uranium mines have been known to receive lifetime exposures of many hundreds of Working Level Months, but the higher exposures found in homes just about overlap the lower exposures among the miners.

A CLOSER LOOK: RADIOACTIVITY AND ISOTOPES

By the end of the nineteenth century the chemical properties of various substances were explained by an atomic theory of matter. Almost one hundred different elementary substances or "elements" had been discovered by that time, out of which all known chemical compounds were composed. The elements occur in the form of atoms, and each atom of any given element was believed to be identical in all ways with every other atom of that element. Each element had its own distinct chemical behavior: which other elements it could combine with, how strong or weak the combination was, and how many atoms of each element was present in the combined unit, called a "molecule." The chemical formula for water, for example, is H_2O, implying that two atoms of the element hydrogen are combined with one atom of the element oxygen to make a single molecule of water. Just as every atom of hydrogen was believed to be identical to every other atom of hydrogen, each molecule of water was believed to be identical to every other molecule of water.

The elements occur in chemically similar groups. For example, the metals lithium, sodium, and potassium belong to one group; all three oxidize readily when exposed to air; and when they combine with chlorine, which they do very readily, they form substances with one atom of the metal for each atom of chlorine. Calcium, strontium, barium, and radium are metals and are members of another group; when they combine with chlorine, each atom of metal combines with two atoms of chlorine. Because strontium and radium are chemically similar to calcium, the bones, as they take up calcium from foods, take up small proportions of strontium and radium as well. Chlorine, a nonmetallic, green, and very corrosive gas, is in a group with the nonmetallic, pale yellow, and very corrosive gas fluorine, the nonmetallic, red, and corrosive liquid bromine, and the nonmetallic, purple, and somewhat less corrosive solid iodine.

Electricity and magnetism had been studied as far back as the fifth century B.C.E. By the nineteenth century it had been concluded that there are two kinds of electricity, called "positive" and "negative," so called because they have the power to neutralize each other. It had been speculated earlier that the two kinds of electricity might be composed, like the atoms of the elements, of individual particles. One of the great twentieth-century discoveries was to confirm this guess: negative electricity consisted of one kind of particle, given the name "electron," and positive electricity consisted of a different kind of particle, named "proton." The negative charge on one electron is just great enough to neutralize the positive charge on one proton. When the two are brought together, the resulting pair has no net electric charge. There is a complication though: protons are not just the mirror image of electrons; they are much heavier. The mass of a proton is about two thousand times the mass of an electron.

Once electrons and protons had been discovered, it was quickly shown that atoms were made up of them. Since under normal conditions, atoms are electrically neutral—they do not move in an electric field—they must be composed of equal numbers of electrons and protons. The protons in an atom are contained in a tiny space called the nucleus; the electrons are spread out in something like orbits (like planets circling the sun) around the much heavier nucleus. The number of protons in the nucleus of an atom of an element is called its "atomic number." The chemical properties of each element are uniquely determined by its atomic number.

The next discovery was that there was a third kind of fundamental particle in the nucleus, electrically neutral, called the neutron, about as heavy as a proton. Electrons are so light compared to either protons or neutrons that the mass of an atom is almost all contained in the nucleus. Since the masses of the proton and the neutron differ so little—less than 1%—and the electrons are so light, the mass of the atom is proportional to the sum of the numbers of protons and neutrons. This number is called the "mass number" of the atom.

The chemical properties of an element are essentially completely determined by the number of protons in the nucleus of an atom of that element. The number of neutrons makes very little difference. With the discovery of radioactivity it became clear that the atoms of any element need not be identical: although the number of protons in any atom of a particular element must be identical—it would not be the same element otherwise—the number of neutrons can vary. Two atoms of the same element may therefore have different masses because they have different numbers of neutrons, but they will still have the same chemical properties. Atoms differing only in the numbers of neutrons in the nucleus, but chemically identical because the number of protons is the same, are called "isotopes."

The neutrons do make a difference, however, not in the chemistry of the atom, but in its stability—determining whether it undergoes radioactive disintegration or not, and how fast. The simplest atom, hydrogen, has a nucleus that consists of one proton, and no neutrons. It is not radioactive. There is a heavy form of hydrogen, called deuterium, with one proton and one neutron in the nucleus. It is also not radioactive. It occurs naturally in normal hydrogen in very small amounts, about 0.02%. Finally, there is an even heavier form of hydrogen called tritium, with two neutrons in the nucleus. It is radioactive, and its half-life, the time it takes for half of any given quantity of tritium to undergo decay, is 12.5 years. Because of the short lifetime of tritium it is very rare in nature, but can be made in the laboratory.

There are a number of different types of radioactive decay: they differ in the type of high-energy radiation emitted and in how fast the decay occurs, as measured by the half-life. The two main types of interest here are alpha decay, the emission of a helium nucleus, which consists of two protons and two neutrons, and beta decay, the emission of an electron. In alpha decay, the atomic number decreases by two (the number of protons emitted) and the mass number by four; in beta decay, the atomic number increases by one and the mass number does not change. Radioactive decay is usually also accompanied by gamma radiation, which because it is electromagnetic radiation rather than the emission of a particle, does not lead to changes in either atomic number or mass number. Figure 3-5 in this chapter gives the sequence of radioactive decays that starts with the isotope of uranium that is most common in nature and ends with a nonradioactive isotope of lead. The kind of radiation emitted by each element in the sequence and the half-life is also given. The various isotopes mentioned in this book are identified by the chemical name of the element followed by the mass number of the particular isotope: uranium-238, iodine-131.

In the scientific literature and in some other sources a different notation is used. Each isotope is identified by the symbol of the chemical element: U for uranium, Rn for radon, Po for polonium, and so on. Preceding this symbol is a superscript giving the mass number: ^{238}U is the symbol for the isotope of uranium with a mass number of 238, which we have symbolized by U-238. In some tables a preceding subscript giving the atomic number is added, so that this isotope of uranium would be written $^{238}_{92}$U. Since all uranium isotopes have the same atomic number of 92, this subscript does not give any information not implied by the symbol U, but not every physicist or chemist knows all the atomic numbers by heart, so it is sometimes helpful to have it.

In this appendix, we have so far described only spontaneous radioactivity. Radioactivity can be made to occur also by bombarding the nucleus of an atom with particles of high energy. In the bomb dropped on Hiroshima the isotope uranium-235 was made to undergo fission by bombardment with a neutron. Fission means that instead of emitting alpha or beta particles, the uranium atom breaks up into smaller atoms of barium and krypton, and at the same time emits gamma radiation and three neutrons. The emitted neutrons cause the fission in turn of other uranium-235 atoms, thus initiating a chain reaction.

4

CHILDHOOD LEUKEMIA NEAR NUCLEAR PLANTS

WINDSCALE: THE NUCLEAR LAUNDRY

In 1983 a television crew was making a documentary film about the health of the employees of a nuclear fuels reprocessing plant in England on the coast of the Irish Sea (fig. 4-1). This plant had previously been the site of a facility for the production of plutonium for nuclear weapons until it was converted to fuels processing after a fire in the reactor in 1957, during which there had been some release of radioactive material to the environment. The crew, filming in a town called Seascale 3 kilometers from the plant, where a number of the employees lived, was shocked to learn from the townspeople that there had been a surprising number of cases of leukemia among their children. Childhood leukemia is a rare disease, but in this small town there had been five cases in the preceding few years, ten times the number of cases that would have been expected from the average rate elsewhere in Great Britain. The focus of the film was changed from the health of the staff of the nuclear facility to the childhood leukemia in Seascale. Shown on television later that year, it aroused national attention and concern, making its points forcefully with shots of rapidly clicking Geiger counters in the neighborhood of the plant, claims that the coastline there is "the most radioactive environment on earth," interviews with the anguished parents of sick or deceased children, reports of

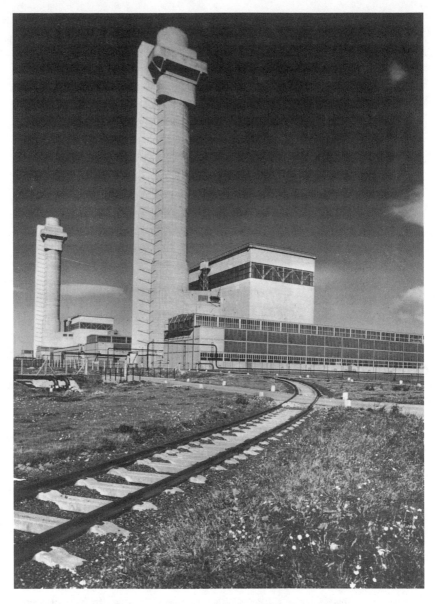

FIGURE 4-1 The first official photograph of the Sellafield plutonium factory in Cumberland, England. Copyright Bettman/Corbis.

cows on neighboring farms born with malformations, and scenes of children playing on the beach with the smokestacks of the plant in the immediate background. It also reported that there had been some 300 other accidents at the plant in which radiation had been released, though the amounts were all of lesser magnitude than in the 1957 fire.

The process for recovering plutonium from spent fuel from power plants does not recover all the plutonium, and some has to be disposed of as waste, along with other radioactive elements. Those responsible for the design of the plant had made the decision, based on both economic considerations and what was then known about the health hazards of radiation, to discharge much of this radioactive waste into the Irish Sea. Analysis of the flow patterns in the sea in that area convinced them that the radioactive wastes would spread out into the sea and pose no risk to people living on the coast nearby. The plant continues to dispose of wastes into the sea to this day, although countries with coasts on the Irish Sea or on adjacent waters have demanded that it stop. A portion of the radioactive waste is discharged into the air also.

Living Near Nuclear Plants

People prefer not to live near nuclear facilities, such as power plants, weapons factories, or waste disposal centers, and if not actually employed in them object to having such facilities built in their neighborhoods. Such concerns have been heightened by reports that rates of childhood leukemia were higher near some of them, even before the discovery of the excess cases in Seascale. The agencies responsible for such facilities have usually claimed that the exposure of the surrounding population to radiation is much too small to cause any illness, being only a small fraction of the natural background radiation. These claims have not always been reassuring to people who know that governments and other interested parties have been known to be less than candid on issues of nuclear safety. They have not even been reassuring to some scientists, who are aware that the claims of harmlessness are not based on direct experiments with low-level radiation but rather on extrapolations from studies in which exposures were much higher. (See discussion of extrapolation in chapters 2 and 3.)

The increases in the leukemia rate noted around some British nuclear plants prior to Seascale had been at most about 15%. Interestingly and confusingly, increases this great had also been noted at sites in Great Britain and in Germany where nuclear plants were planned but not yet built. In Great Britain, on the average about four out of every hundred thousand children get leukemia each year. The number of cases expected in a population the size of Seascale and during the time period 1968 to 1985 was 0.5, or half a case, meaning that on the average in a period twice as long, one case would have been expected. Hence the five observed cases represented a tenfold increase (in percentage terms, 1000%). As this was much larger than any previously observed increase in leukemia around any nuclear facility, it not only aroused great concern but was taken seriously by the authorities and was given a careful investigation.

The Windscale Fire

The nuclear waste processing plant had been built on the site of one of Great Britain's first plants for the production of weapons-grade plutonium. It was known as the Windscale plant at that time, named after a bluff on a river nearby. In 1957 a fire broke out in one of the two piles used for preparing the plutonium, and radioactivity was released to the environment. It was the first publicized major accident in the nuclear industry: one occurring at a Soviet facility at Chelyabinsk in the same year was kept secret by the Soviet authorities. The radioactivity released in the Windscale fire was much greater than in the 1979 Three Mile Island accident in the United States, but a thousand times less than from Chernobyl in 1986. Fortunately, the fire was extinguished by heroic efforts of the staff in a few days, with no deaths and minimal exposure to high-energy radiation.

As the Windscale plant was on the verge of obsolescence anyway, it was decided after the fire to discontinue the production of plutonium there and create a new facility for reprocessing spent fuel. The plant was renamed Sellafield, after a royal ordnance factory that had occupied the site during World War II. It is not surprising that the authorities responsible for the plant wished to change its name, nor is it surprising that the television documentary used the original one (fig. 4-2).

The Secret History Exposed

As noted earlier, the television documentary aroused great concern, and the British government promptly appointed a committee of outside scientists to investigate the leukemia cases. It was soon revealed that the plant authorities and the British government had not been honest in reporting

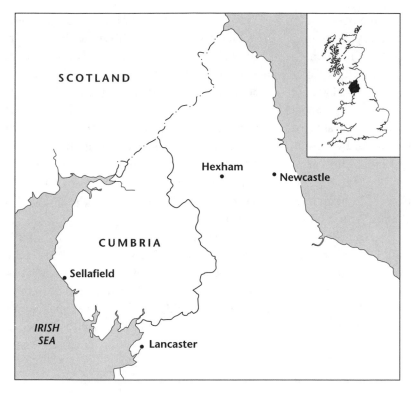

FIGURE 4-2   Map of Cumbna (Cumberland) showing its location in relation to England, Scotland, and the Irish Sea. Reproduced from the article "Stillbirth Rates" by T. J. B. Dummer et al. in the *International Journal of Epidemiology*, v. 27, p. 75 (1998) with the permission of Oxford University Press.

emissions from the plant. The first official report they issued following the Windscale accident did not mention that considerable quantities of radioactive polonium and some plutonium had been released during the fire, in addition to the radioactive iodine and cesium they acknowledged. On another occasion prior to the fire they had reported an accidental discharge of several hundred grams of uranium; during the committee's investigation they admitted that the actual discharge was 20 kilograms.

How Much Harm Was Done?

One of the first conclusions reached by the committee was that in spite of the dumping of waste into the sea and the air, in spite of the under-reporting of emissions, and in spite of the fact that plutonium takes thousands of years to decay, the radioactive material released to the environment did not come anywhere near accounting for the excess leukemia cases. Contrary to the claims made in the documentary the radioactivity in the immediate environment had been increased by only about 25% above the natural background radiation. Put another way, the radiation exposure in Seascale due to discharges from the Sellafield plant would have had to be two hundred times greater to have caused the five cases of leukemia. This calculation was based on the relation between radiation dose and subsequent leukemia found in the Life Span Study in Japan (see chapter 2), assuming that that relation is a linear no-threshold one. (See chapter 3 for a fuller discussion.)

An interesting possibility was suggested by one scientist, Dr. Martin Gardner, who noted that the fathers of the five children with leukemia worked in the Sellafield facility. Could exposure of the fathers to radiation before their children were conceived have caused leukemia in some of those children? A study he initiated showed that the fathers of the leukemia victims had had on the average a greater exposure to radiation, as shown by the doses of X-rays and gamma rays recorded by the film badges they wore at work, than a control group of Seascale fathers of children who had not gotten leukemia, and who were also employed at Sellafield.

Nuclear Energy on Trial

When they learned of this result, two of the parents of affected children sued the British Nuclear Fuels Corporation in 1992. One of the children had died at the age of ten months of leukemia and the other as a young adult had developed a type of cancer called non-Hodgkin's lymphoma believed related to leukemia, and was in remission after treatment.

The case was not tried before a jury; the judge made the final decision. Although both sides called in scientific experts to support their cases, the judge exercised his right to call in experts of his own choosing. Most of the scientists who had studied the Sellafield cluster as well as internationally recognized specialists in relevant fields such as genetics, molecular biology, radiation physics, and epidemiology participated in the trial. The experts on both sides were able to agree on many of the basic facts of the case, more so than one familiar only with the more adversarial U.S. tort system would have expected. The trial therefore provided the occasion for a broad overview of all the scientific evidence then available.

Scientists on both sides at the trial agreed that—even using the most stringent standards for radiation safety, derived from studies of the Japanese bomb survivors and people exposed to medical X-rays (see chapter 2)—the known releases of radioactive material by the Sellafield facility to the environment did not come anywhere near accounting for the leukemia cases. This is notwithstanding the dramatic scenes in the television documentary of scientists wielding clicking Geiger counters on the beaches near the facility.

The judge's ruling was that radiation from the facility was highly unlikely to have caused the cancer of the children, either directly through radioactive emissions, or indirectly through preconceptional exposure of the fathers: the parents lost their case.

This, however, did not end the controversy or the intensive scientific study of why there were so many cases of childhood leukemia in Seascale, and research is still continuing today.

COULD IT HAVE BEEN RADIATION?

Leukemia

What is leukemia, and what is known about its causes?

A child once full of energy, with a hearty appetite, and growing fast, starts to show fatigue more often and loses her appetite. She gets a sore throat, as children often do, but it hangs on longer than any she had before. She becomes pale and begins to bleed easily. Her cuts do not heal as fast, and she develops "petechiae," little hemorrhages under the skin. Her worried parents take her to the doctor, who immediately orders a blood test. What is the doctor looking for?

The leukemias are cancers of the blood-producing system of the body, and as with all cancers, involve rapid proliferation of cells without the normal controls (see discussion of the molecular biology of cancer in chapter 6). Blood consists of a colorless fluid called serum in which both red and white cells are suspended. The red cells (erythrocytes) give blood its color and are the carriers of oxygen to the tissues, and the white cells (leukocytes) fight bacteria and other foreign bodies. There are several types of leukocytes, whose origin, appearance, and function differ. The different types of leukemia are defined by which type of leukocyte undergoes rapid and uncontrolled proliferation. The different types tend to occur at different ages and may best be thought of as different diseases. The abnormal blood cells characteristic of these different types are readily distinguished under the microscope from normal blood cells (fig. 4-3).

Cancer is most often a disease of old age, again reflecting the multiple mutations that must occur before it develops into a clinical case. Leukemia is the most common of childhood cancers: in the United States and Great Britain about four to five children per 100,000 develop it per year. In contrast, the number of adult men who die of lung cancer in the United States in a year is 75 per 100,000, and the number of adult women who die of breast cancer is 27 per 100,000. Until a few decades ago most children who got leukemia died, but current treatments, using either chemotherapy or radiation or both, save over three-quarters of them.

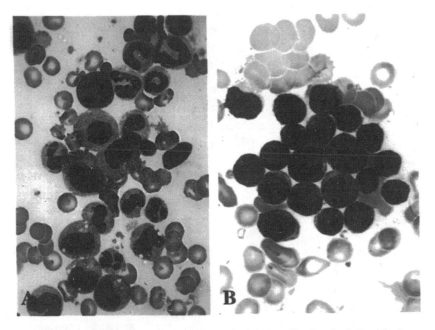

FIGURE 4-3 Comparison of normal and leukemic cells. On the left, cells from healthy bone marrow have been stained to better distinguish them. The presence of a number of different cell types is typical of normal marrow. On the right, cells from the marrow of a patient with acute lymphocytic leukemia; only one type of leukemic blast cell can be seen. Courtesy of the Leukemia and Lymphoma Society.

Causes of Leukemia

Only a small fraction of childhood leukemias are accounted for by inherited genes, unlike some other much rarer childhood cancers of the kidney or the eye.

Exposure to ionizing radiation increases the risk of leukemia for both children and adults. Leukemia in children has occurred as an unintended consequence of X-ray therapy used in the past for certain childhood diseases. It can be shown, from studies of the Japanese bomb survivors and those of children exposed to medical X-rays, that background radiation from natural sources like radon and cosmic rays can account for only a few percent of the cases of childhood leukemia. The relation between leukemia and radiation exposure is more precisely known than for other cancers for two reasons. One is that the time interval between exposure and the appearance of the disease is shorter than for most other cancers— five years or less—and the other is that the relation between leukemia and radiation has been studied more carefully than for other cancers. The long time-interval for most cancers is explained by the fact that six or seven successive mutations must take place for the disease to appear clinically. For leukemia, fewer mutations are needed: one hypothesis is that acute lymphoblastic leukemia (ALL), the most common form of childhood leukemia, requires only two. In Western countries, ALL is most common among children between two and four years old.

Adults exposed to certain chemicals in the workplace, most notably benzene, have a high risk of leukemia. In addition, people treated with chemotherapy (or with radiation) for other cancers have a somewhat elevated risk of developing leukemia years later. Some antibiotics, now used only if there is no alternative in a life-threatening situation, also increase the risk. As most children with leukemia have not been exposed to excessive radiation, or chemical substances like benzene or chemotherapeutic drugs, we cannot as yet say what caused their illness.

The rate of childhood leukemia is greater in Western countries than in the less developed world, and in those countries it is greater among families of higher income and social status, for reasons that are not yet fully understood.

Putting It All Together

The evidence considered in the trial came from many different scientific disciplines—radiobiology, epidemiology, statistics, clinical medicine, genetics, molecular biology; scientific conclusions are more convincing the more the evidence from different fields hangs together to form a coherent picture.

The dose of radiation received by people living near the plant was estimated from data on the known discharges from the plant, measurements of radioactivity in the soil and water in the neighborhood of the plant, combined with some measurements on human tissues taken from inhabitants of Seascale. Both sides in the litigation agreed that the discharges from the plant added only about 25% to the natural radiation present, which of itself is responsible for only a small percentage of cancers. Put another way, the discharges would had to have been 200 times larger to have caused the leukemia cases. Further, the direct measurements on tissues of people living in Seascale showed that their actual exposure was less than estimated from the known radioactive discharges. No excess of other known health effects of radiation, such as miscarriages, birth defects, or other cancers, were observed in Seascale, further evidence that the exposures are not likely to have been high enough to cause a tenfold increase in leukemia.

Most scientists concerned with the issue are now in agreement that the direct radioactive pollution of the surroundings by plant discharges is unlikely to have caused the leukemia cases.

Exposure of the Fathers

Could the exposure of the fathers to radiation at work prior to conception of their children have caused the children's leukemia? To investigate this possibility it was necessary to measure the exposure the men received at work. Some jobs involved heavier exposures than others. Was the chance of the child getting leukemia greater, the greater the exposure of the father before the child was conceived?

The employees at Sellafield wore dosimeters that measured their exposure to X-rays and gamma rays, but not to neutrons, so it was necessary to estimate their neutron doses from what was known about levels of neutron radiation in the plant. In addition, an estimate had to be made for any radioactive elements they might have absorbed—inhaled or otherwise ingested—while working at the plant. Such exposure would not have been recorded by the monitors they wore, which detect only radiation falling on the monitor film. It was possible to make these estimates in a fashion that satisfied both sides in the litigation. The estimated doses from neutrons and from ingested radioactive substances were combined with directly measured doses of gamma and X-rays recorded on the monitors to calculate total doses to male employees. Hence the total radiation exposure to the testes of fathers of children who developed leukemia could be compared with that of all the other male employees who lived in Seascale and had children while working at the plant. The fathers of four out of the five leukemia victims had had total preconceptional exposures during their employment of about 100 millisieverts or more (see chapter 2), while only about one-tenth of the control fathers—men who also worked in the plant and lived in Seascale, but whose children had not gotten leukemia—had had exposures that great. This result initially gave strong support to the hypothesis that exposure of the fathers was responsible for the excess leukemia of the children.

On the Other Hand . . .

Although the exposures in Japan to fathers of children born after the bombing, averaging 400 millisieverts, were much greater than those received by any of the employees at Sellafield, no detectable increase of leukemia among their children was found. Some studies at other nuclear facilities also showed no effect of the radiation received by fathers on their children, but the numbers of people involved and the doses, although comparable to and sometimes greater than at Sellafield, were much less than in Japan, so the results were not as convincing.

Even more strikingly, Seascale was only one of the towns where Sellafield plant employees lived. Many more employees lived in other parts of West Cumbria, their range of exposures was comparable to that of employees living in Seascale, and many children were born to them. There were in fact more than ten times as many children born outside of Seascale than in Seascale to fathers employed at Sellafield, but there was no excess number of childhood leukemia cases except among children born in Seascale itself. Further, for West Cumbria exclusive of Seascale, the average exposure of fathers of children who did get leukemia was no greater than the average exposure of fathers of children who did not.

Long after the trial it was noted that the number of cases of childhood leukemia and non-Hodgkins lymphoma in Seascale continued to be high for about a decade after the initial discovery of the excess. By 1991 there had been a cumulative total of seven cases of leukemia and four of lymphoma, again about ten times the number expected for these diseases combined. However, the fathers of these later cases had not been employed at Sellafield prior to the conception of their children.

It was suggested at the trial that there might be some unique factor present in Seascale but not in the rest of West Cumbria, perhaps an infectious disease episode or a chemical exposure, that interacted with the irradiation received by the fathers to produce the excess cases, but no specific factor that might have acted this way was actually identified.

As a result of the intensive studies stimulated by the discovery of the excess leukemia at Sellafield, a closer look at leukemia rates around other nuclear facilities in Great Britain was taken, and a cluster of leukemia cases was found in a small town, West Thurso, near another facility at Dounreay, on the northern coast of Scotland. There were six cases, about double the number expected from the national rate. Although many of the employees of the Dounreay facility lived in Thurso, most of the fathers of the children who got leukemia were not employed there.

Of Mice and Men

Additional evidence on the health hazards of radiation comes from animal experiments in which the dose is more precisely known, and both the numbers of subjects and the doses are larger than in most human populations studied, so that there are fewer statistical and other kinds of uncertainties. Most studies have shown no greater incidence of leukemia or cancerous tumors in the descendants of irradiated male mice; however, some recent and still controversial ones reported that the descendants of male mice exposed by injecting plutonium into the bloodstream are more susceptible to leukemia and other cancers when exposed to high energy radiation or chemical carcinogens. Also, we can estimate the probability of a hypothetical leukemia-causing mutation in a male mouse's sperm cells from the number of mutations of other kinds produced by a given dose. The evidence so far is that the dose received by the Seascale fathers was much too low to have caused leukemia in their children.

CHANCE AS AN EXPLANATION

No Answer Yet

In spite of the efforts of a number of scientists working on the problem during the past fifteen years, no one explanation of the Seascale cluster has been accepted by scientific consensus. Some still believe it was caused in some way yet to be explained by exposure to high-energy radiation. One speculative idea, unsupported by any direct evidence, is that the radioactive discharges of the plant included one particular radioactive element that is absorbed by the body in some unexpected way, just as radioactive iodine is taken up by the thyroid and radium and radioactive strontium, which have chemical properties similar to calcium, are preferentially absorbed by the bones and teeth. Perhaps when more biological markers of radiation exposure are identified, we may be able to determine whether any particular case of leukemia is caused by radiation or something else. We may have to wait until this happens before we can explain the cluster in Seascale.

There is little doubt that the number of cases there greatly exceeded what would be expected from the average rate in the United Kingdom. The town is just 3 kilometers from a nuclear facility. If the cause was not radiation, what was it? There are some scientists who attribute the excess cases to chance. Chance is of course not a "cause" of disease, but it could be an explanation of the Seascale cluster. How could chance have produced the cluster, and how would we decide when such an explanation is plausible?

Clusters of Disease

A cluster is defined as a group of cases of a disease occurring in a localized area, in a short time period, or among a particular group of people, that greatly exceeds the number expected. Often a disease cluster has revealed a hitherto unsuspected hazard to health. Asbestos was shown to be a health hazard when an unusual number of cases of mesothelioma, a very rare cancer of the lining of the lung cavity, were noted among asbestos workers in a New Jersey city. Similarly, the discovery of a few cases of liver sarcoma among workers in a plastics factory, again an extremely rare cancer, implicated vinyl chloride, the chemical substance from which the harmless polyvinyl chloride is made. Subsequent experiments on laboratory animals showed vinyl chloride to be a powerful carcinogen. Clusters of bladder cancer among workers in the dye industry pinpointed certain other industrial chemicals such as naphthylamine as potent human carcinogens.

On the other hand, the majority of reported clusters of leukemia (to be described in more detail on pp. 127–128) or other cancers remain unexplained, although a lot of time and effort have been spent studying them. One view is that many of them are due to chance alone. How can "chance alone" cause the number of cases to differ so much from the average?

Chance and Disease

What does it mean to talk of diseases occurring at random or by chance? Do not diseases have causes?

To visualize a random process, think of tossing a coin a large number of times, or drawing a series of names from a hat. Each toss of a coin is independent of previous tosses; the chance of heads on each trial is 50%, no matter how many heads have come up in the preceding tosses. Each name drawn from a hat is independent of the preceding names drawn; there is no tendency to draw the names of neighbors any more than the names of people who live far from each other.

Can such processes have anything at all to say about a child getting leukemia? Most child victims of leukemia have not been exposed either to much radiation or to high levels of carcinogenic chemicals, so we must assume there are other causes as well, although we do not know them yet. A child does not get leukemia because his name has been drawn from a hat.

It is our ignorance of most of the causes that makes the idea of chance useful in describing who gets a disease. While national health statistics tell us the number of cases that will occur on the average in a year, we do not know enough about the causes of leukemia to predict which particular children will become ill, or how many cases will occur on any particular street, in any particular community, or in any particular month. In our ignorance, we assume that all children have an equal chance of getting the disease, and that the way the cases will be distributed is something like what we would get if we drew names at random from a hat. Drawing names from a hat is a possible model of what the actual distribution of leukemia—or any other disease whose causes we are ignorant of—may be. Many times the results will, on the average, be about the same as those we actually find. Many times, however, they will not be: there certainly are diseases that are not distributed randomly, for example, contagious diseases like chicken pox, cases of which cluster together in space or time more than they would if they occurred at random. How can we distinguish a random from a nonrandom distribution?

Much of epidemiological research is a search for nonrandom patterns of disease, a search for differences from the average, that provide clues to the causes of disease or test hypotheses about them. We hope that in time we will identify the causes and prevent the disease. Then we will no longer need to assume that the disease is distributed by drawing names from a hat.

Treating disease as a chance event, as impersonal as tossing coins, is objectionable to many people, and especially so when they or members of their families are victims. It is natural to ask, why us? Why should I or my child suffer? It is natural to feel that something has caused the disease: a virus, or some chemical in the environment, some action that the child's doctor should have taken but did not, even, in some cultures, the malice of an envious neighbor giving a child the "evil eye." We would rather believe with Hamlet that "there is a special providence in the fall of a sparrow," than with Solomon that "the race is not to the swift, nor the battle to the strong . . . but time and chance happeneth to them all."

The assumption of randomness is a confession of ignorance. When we make it we are not saying that there are no causes for a disease but rather that whatever the unknown causes are, the chance of any one person being exposed to them is, as far as we in our ignorance can tell, the same as that of any other person.

Chance Is Lumpy

One might guess that if cases of a disease are distributed "at random" the result would be a perfectly uniform distribution. For example, if the rate of the disease were 5,000 cases per hundred thousand people per year (a 5% rate), then there should be just five cases in any group of 100 people. Unfortunately such a simple result is not what occurs "by chance."

While coin tosses and drawing names from a hat are examples of random processes, a more flexible example for our purposes is an "urn" model—a large container or urn filled with an enormous number of small beads—say a billion—most of which are white, but with 500,000 red beads very thoroughly mixed in. The proportion of red beads is therefore five per 10,000. Now we draw 10,000 beads from the urn and count the red beads. We expect five, but we find in practice that often we get four or six, sometimes three or seven, and less often two or eight. In fact, experience shows us, and the mathematical theory of probability confirms, that five red beads in a drawing of 10,000 beads will occur less than 20% of the time.

In the first two colomns of table 4-1 on page 117 we give the results of a treatment of the problem developed in the early nineteenth century by the French mathematician S. D. Poisson, using the theory of probability. We imagine drawing 10,000 beads at a time, returning them to the urn, mixing the beads, drawing a new batch of 10,000, and repeating this process a very large number of times. We list the percent of the drawings that give a specific number of red beads, from zero to fifteen. While outcomes of four or five red beads occur more often than any other single outcome, six occurs almost as often, and outcomes as extreme as one or ten occur 2 or 3% of the time.

The Waiting Line at the Cash Machines

This example of a billion-bead urn may seem remote from any real world problem, but there are real world situations that behave much like it. Consider the waiting line at the automatic teller machines of a particular bank. Suppose the machines average 300 customers an hour during the noon hour, so that, on the average, five arrive every minute. But anyone who has ever waited on lines knows that people do not arrive with such clockwork regularity. Sometimes eight or nine will arrive in a single minute, sometimes a minute will go by with no one joining the line. If the arrival of each individual were random, independent of the time that any other individual arrives, we can use Poisson's treatment to calculate the probability that any particular number of people will join the line in any one-minute interval. When the average rate at which people arrive is five per minute, the results are exactly the same as given by the urn model with five red beads per 10,000 (table 4-1 on page 117). Similarly, if childhood leukemia were distributed at random, with no specific factor that causes it to be higher in some places than in others, and if the overall average rate in a large country were five cases per 100,000 children per year, then the same table gives the probabilities of observing any specific number of cases in any community with 100,000 children, in a particular year.

Getting back to the cash machines, the probability that four people will join the line in a particular one-minute interval (17.55% of the time) happens to be just the same as that for five people (the average) joining the line.

TABLE 4-1 The Poisson Distribution When the Average Outcome Is 5

Possible Outcomes	Probability in % of Each Outcome	Expected Number of Times Each Outcome Occurs in 25 Trials	Observed Number of Times Each Outcome Occurred in the 25 Trials of Figure 4-4
0	0.67	0.2	1
1	3.37	0.8	1
2	8.42	2.1	5
3	14.04	3.5	2
4	17.55	4.4	2
5	17.55	4.4	2
6	14.62	3.7	5
7	10.44	2.6	3
8	6.53	1.6	1
9	3.63	0.9	0
10	1.81	0.5	2
11	0.82	0.2	1
12	0.34	0.1	0
13	0.13	a	0
14	0.05	a	0
15	0.02	a	0

aFewer than 0.1 times in 25 trials, i.e., we would have to perform 250 trials rather than 25 to have a good chance of getting an outcome of 13 or more.

Note: The "possible outcomes" can refer equally well to (1) the number of red beads in a drawing of 10,000 beads, (2) the number of people arriving in the cash machine line in one minute, (3) the number of dots in one square of figure 4-4, (4) the number of leukemia cases in a group of 100,000 children in a particular year, (5) the number of raisins in a slice of raisin cake (see chapter 8). The observed numbers of outcomes in the last column is for the random placement of dots on the squares of figure 4-4. All these situations need have in common is that the events of interest occur at random, and that the average number of events in an interval is five. The Poisson formula can of course be applied to any average value, not just five. It is given in textbooks on probability. In chapter 8 some of the results of that formula are given for an average outcome of ten (raisins per slice of cake).

The probability of ten people arriving in a particular minute is 1.8%, making it a fairly rare event. But there are, after all, 60 minutes in an hour, and 1.8% of 60 is about 1.1, so the unlikely appearance of 10 people in a minute will happen on the average once during every noon hour.

Note that while we have treated the arrivals of customers at the automatic teller machine as "random," each individual would deny that there has been anything random about his arrival time. If we were to ask him why he happened to arrive at 12:17 on Tuesday, March 11, he would tell us some story of having planned to come before going to work in the morning, but his little girl was sick and could not go to school, so he had to arrange for a baby-sitter, and therefore had to come during his lunch hour, but the elevator in his building got stuck for ten minutes, otherwise he would have arrived closer to noon, and so on. Add together 300 different stories and you are close to a random process.

The False Law of Averages

In short, getting exactly the average is less common than getting either more or less than the average. There is a popular belief that there is something called the "law of averages" that ensures that the average is actually what one will observe most of the time. There is no such law. Toss five heads in a row, and the chance of a head on the next toss is still 50%. The fact is that chance is lumpy, not smooth.

This is a feature of chance that people not experienced in its actual workings do not expect. There is an interesting anecdote to illustrate it, about a statistics professor who, wishing to make his students more aware of lumpiness, divided his beginning class into two groups. The members of one group were asked to toss a coin 100 times and record the outcomes. The members of the other group were asked to write down a sequence of 100 tosses of a coin as they imagined it might come out. The students then handed their lists in to the professor, who was able to correctly distinguish the real from the imaginary ones about 95% of the time. His trick was simple: in a sequence of one hundred tosses, there will almost always be one group of five heads or five tails in a row, but people ignorant of the lumpiness of chance and trying to imagine the outcomes of such a sequence will almost never put five heads in a row. In fact they will tend to make heads and tails alternate too regularly, an extremely nonrandom and improbable result, nowhere near the real lumpiness of reality.

Dots and Squares

Because chance is lumpy, even if the cases of a disease really occur at random, they will often seem to cluster. To give some feeling for how this happens, we have placed 125 dots at random (using a computer program) on a diagram divided up into 25 squares (fig. 4-4). The squares may be thought of as "communities," and the dots as "cases of a disease." The average number of dots per square is five, but a glance at the figure shows that some squares have more and some less. Again table 4-1 gives the probabilities of finding any particular number of dots in any square. It

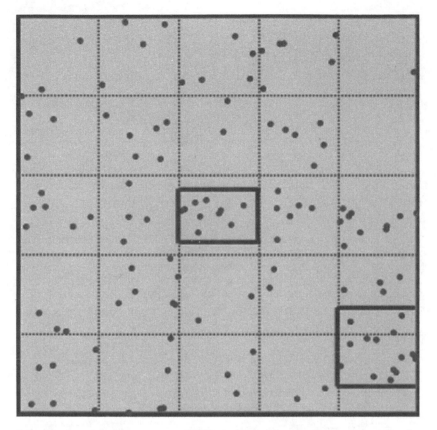

FIGURE 4-4 The dots represent 125 "cases" of a disease, distributed randomly among 25 "towns." The square with a heavy outline has fourteen "cases," a highly improbable event; by shifting boundaries, apparently improbable events can be made to occur. Figure prepared by Professor Andrew Rundle, Columbia University, and used with his permission.

should be remembered that a probability of 100% is equivalent to absolute certainty that the event will occur, and a probability of 0% means the event has no chance of happening. By multiplying the probabilities of getting a certain number of dots in a square by 25 (the number of squares), we obtain the number of squares we expect to find, on the average, with that number of dots (Column 3). We have not calculated the numbers of squares with more than fifteen dots because these numbers are very small.

Note that there are two squares with ten dots, and one with eleven. If these were communities, and the dots were leukemia cases, the three communities would each have double the expected rate. This chance result shows just how lumpy chance can be. In fact, the numbers of squares with any given number of dots in this example do not on the face of it seem to agree well with the Poisson formula, but they should not be expected to. It is only the average of a large number of such experiments that should. For example, on average only one square out of fifty should have ten dots, yet in this experiment three squares out of twenty-five had ten dots or more.

When we combine outcomes into small groups, counting the number of squares with zero to three dots as one group, and the number with four to seven as another group, and so on, and compare this grouping with the predictions of the Poisson formula, the results agree much better (fig. 4-5). Grouping several outcomes together is something like averaging, so the improved agreement is not surprising.

We easily produced a doubling of the "leukemia rate" by chance because the expected number of cases was only five. If the expected number were twenty, both the Poisson formula and experience show that a doubling is less likely to occur by chance alone.

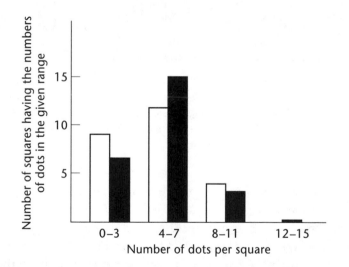

FIGURE 4-5 The comparison of the numbers of "towns" with given numbers of "cases" (white bars) with the numbers predicted from probability theory (black bars). The numbers of squares have been grouped, so that the first white bar shows the number with anything from 0 to 3 cases. The agreement is, in general, good but not perfect, which is what is expected in a single trial. If the "experiment" were repeated thousands of times the agreement would be almost exact.

Signals and Noise

We discuss in chapters 3 and 8 the problem of distinguishing a real increase in the rate of some disease from a random variation. We have compared this to the problem of detecting a signal over a noisy background. In the discussion here, we have shown how randomness is one source of noise.

Nonrandomness and How to Detect It

Let us return to the automatic teller machine line. We have assumed up to now that each person arrives randomly, independent of anyone else, and could arrive at any time during the noon hour. However, people do not really arrive in a random fashion, with an equal probability of arriving at any time. We have already acknowledged this by considering the noon hour only, because the average rate of arrival will be greater than for other hours of the day. Also, there will be a higher average rate of arrival on Fridays and the days before holidays. There could be other reasons for nonrandomness as well. Some of the customers of the bank might live in other neighborhoods and have to come by bus. If we did not know this, we would be surprised to find that at fairly regular intervals twelve or fifteen customers arrive almost simultaneously. There will be real "clusters": the number of one-minute time intervals in which twelve people arrive could not plausibly be accounted for on the assumption of random arrival.

Nonrandomness in Disease

Are there departures from randomness in the distribution of diseases? The answer is that there almost invariably are. There is no medical condition known that everyone has an equal chance of suffering. The rates of most diseases vary markedly with age, particularly for but not limited to cancer. They often depend on other risk factors such as sex, diet, smoking habits, sexual behavior, and ethnicity (see chapter 5). We have mentioned that childhood leukemia rates peak between ages two and three, are slightly greater for boys than girls, and are higher among children of higher social class.

An epidemiological study usually starts with some hypothesis about a possible cause of a disease. First, we identify a group exposed to that presumed cause, and then choose a control group as nearly like the exposed group in all respects known to be relevant to the risk of the disease except that it has not been so exposed (as was done in the study of survivors of the atomic bombing in Japan described in chapter 2). Then we compare their disease rates. If the exposed group has a higher rate than the control group, we may feel encouraged about the hypothesis, but are not yet ready to conclude that it is strongly supported. We know that the numbers of cases in both groups are subject to chance variations, and we have to show that chance alone is not likely to have caused the difference. The test used is a test of "statistical significance." We calculate the probability that the difference could be produced by chance alone. If that probability is less than 5%, chance is considered too unlikely an explanation for the difference, and we believe the evidence supports the hypothesis (see discussion of statistical significance in chapter 8).

When the study starts instead with the observation of a cluster, ruling out chance as responsible is harder. We did not start with a hypothesis and then test it by looking for an excess number of cases, but rather started with an excess number of cases and then looked for a hypothesis to explain it. Before we look for a hypothesis, though, we still want to rule out chance as an explanation. We can certainly calculate an expected rate for the community where the cluster was found, from knowledge of the makeup of the community by age, sex, and so on, and from knowledge of the usual rates of the disease in these categories. But when we proceed to the next step, the test of statistical significance for the difference between the observed and expected rates, we encounter a problem, one we encounter often in daily life without being aware of it. We will use our dots and squares figure to illustrate it.

The Texas Sharpshooter

In figure 4-4 we deliberately selected a square in the lower right hand corner slightly displaced from the original squares, marking it with heavy borders. We selected it because it contains fourteen dots, a number about two and a half times the average, an event with a "probability" of less than one in a thousand. The quotation marks indicate that this is not the correct probability. It is tempting to draw the squares where the dots cluster, but if we are free to draw the squares wherever we want, it is easy to produce events that appear highly improbable. It is like arranging the cards in a deck in preparation for a magic trick. A more extreme example is shown by the small rectangle, also drawn with heavy borders, in the center of the figure. Here we have captured ten dots in one half of the area of the original squares. If we think of the squares as representing one square mile, the number of dots per square mile in this rectangle is twenty, an event with a "probability" of less than one in a million. Again, by drawing the boundaries the way we did we have stacked the deck.

We have spoken of "stacking the deck," but let us switch the metaphor from card tricks to target shooting. Turning a purely chance event into a cluster by moving its boundaries too freely has been termed "The Texas sharpshooter approach." The mythical Texas sharpshooter shoots at the side of a barn, then paints a target around the bullet hole (fig. 4-6).

Kinds of Boundaries

We have been using the word "boundary" in its literal sense, referring to geographical boundaries. There are boundaries in time as well: when the cluster is thought to begin and when it is thought to end. Should we consider only calendar years or calendar decades, or should we take the decade preceding 1983, the year the television crew discovered the high leukemia rate in Seascale, or the decade following 1957, the year of the Windscale fire? Or why use a decade at all? A notorious cluster of childhood leukemia in Niles, Illinois, to be discussed in more detail later in this chapter, was observed between 1957 and 1960. If we had used a decade starting in 1957, the number of cases there would have seemed less striking (though it still would have been unusually high) as after 1960 leukemia reverted to the normal U.S. rate. We can see that there is some elasticity in choosing the time boundaries, just as there was about where to draw the square or how large a square to draw.

Still other boundaries concern the definition of the disease itself. The probability that the Seascale cluster could have occurred by chance is different if we include cases of non-Hodgkin's lymphoma, a cancer related to but not identical to leukemia. There is good medical reason to include the lymphoma because of the close relation between the two diseases, but there have been other reports of clusters in which several unrelated forms of cancer and even other noncancerous diseases have been lumped together (see chapter 7).

When we want to test a hypothesis about the cause of a disease, the hypothesis itself provides reasons to draw the boundaries one way rather than another: to limit the area studied to the vicinity of a known pollut-

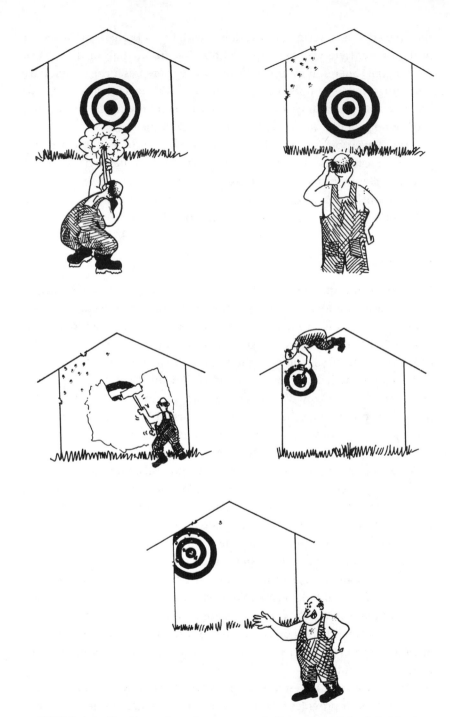

FIGURE 4-6   The Texas sharpshooter at work. Drawn by Michael Goldstein.

ing source, to choose the time period based on the time a hazardous substance was emitted, and to study only diseases plausibly related to the suspected hazard.

Finding Patterns Where There Are None

Sometimes the human tendency to see patterns even in randomness leads us unwittingly to draw boundaries that turn a chance occurrence into a cluster, as we did quite wittingly by moving the boundaries of the square in the diagram to capture fourteen dots in one square. Even one case of leukemia, to its victim and those close to him, is "more than expected from chance alone." If, say, four cases occur in one's own immediate neighborhood, one has a right to be alarmed. The problem comes when we ask the necessary further question, is this likely to have occurred by chance, or not? We can easily calculate how likely it is that four cases of leukemia would occur in one year in a neighborhood with this population, picked at random out of the whole country. All we need to know is the national statistics for leukemia by age, sex, and so on. But we are not picking a neighborhood at random. Instead, we have picked a neighborhood precisely because we noticed that its leukemia rate was high. Having picked it because the rate was high, it is difficult to decide if the high rate could have occurred by chance alone. The bullet hole may be in the bull's eye because we painted the target around it.

How to Distinguish

This is not an argument for ignoring such perceived clusters. There are, after all, real clusters of disease—of mesothelioma, of bladder cancer, of chicken pox—that should not be dismissed as chance occurrences without further investigation. Certainly, the leukemia cluster in Seascale, a town 3 kilometers from a nuclear plant known to have discharged radioactivity into the air and the sea, deserved to be taken seriously. It was not picked at random from all British communities, but because of its proximity to the Sellafield plant. The problem is how to distinguish clusters that might have identifiable causes from those that arise by chance.

One test of whether an apparent cluster is an artifact of chance or not is to look for additional data to confirm its reality. Does it continue as time goes on? As we noted earlier, the excess of leukemia and non-Hodgkin's lymphoma did continue in Seascale for another decade after the initial report. Another is to identify situations like the one being investigated: if we suspect proximity to a nuclear facility is responsible, look for similar excesses around other nuclear facilities. Indeed, small excess rates of leukemia had been observed around some nuclear plants, and during the Seascale investigation, a leukemia cluster was found in West Thurso, near another nuclear facility. However, these effects have not been consistently found near most nuclear facilities, have been observed in the absence of such facilities, and, as we will see, may well have other explanations.

Seascale and Chance

Could the Seascale cluster be simply an example of a chance occurrence magnified out of all proportion by the focus on one small town and one disease out of many?

There are several ways to answer this. The distribution of a number of cancers affecting children among communities in north England was studied to see if the high rate in Seascale was really unmatched in any other community. The conclusion was that the rate of childhood leukemia in Seascale really was highly unusual. It was not only higher than in any other community in north England, but much higher than the rate in the community with the second highest rate. Calculating the probability that this high rate could have occurred by chance does depend on how the rate in Seascale is defined: the answer depends on where we draw the boundaries in time and in diagnosis. But no matter how the choice is made, and putting all the evidence together, chance seems an unlikely explanation.

LEUKEMIA AND CHILDHOOD INFECTIONS

What Then Caused the Leukemia?

The evidence against the view that the irradiation of the fathers caused the leukemia cases in the children is strong. Studies on exposed human populations and on irradiated laboratory animals, together with what is known about leukemia as a disease and what can be inferred from genetics, all cohere in making it implausible.

Yet there is little doubt that the number of cases in Seascale was far greater than we would expect of a town that size, even considering the lumpiness of chance. The town is just 3 kilometers from a nuclear facility that employed the fathers of the victims. If the cases of leukemia were not caused by radiation, what did cause them?

Other Hypotheses

Could childhood leukemia be a contagious disease? If it were, it would not be surprising to find it occurring in clusters, rather than being randomly distributed. Indeed, cats and cows do suffer from virally caused forms of leukemia, spread from one animal to another. Many physicians have observed what they have interpreted as clusters of leukemia among their patients and have suggested that the disease might be contagious. The earliest reported example was in 1905, about the time leukemia itself was recognized as a distinct disease.

Some Notorious Clusters of Leukemia

In the town of Niles, Illinois (population 18,000), in the vicinity of Chicago, in the years 1957 to 1960, there was an extraordinary cluster of childhood leukemia, eight cases, seven of them associated with one particular school, when one or two would have been expected if the usual rate in the United States applied to a community the size of Niles (fig. 4-7). This observation drew national attention. A careful study failed to find any definite reason for the cluster, and in subsequent years the rate of leukemia reverted to its usual value.

Although no cause of the Niles cluster has been clearly identified, it was noted by the scientists studying it that there had been an epidemic among children in Niles of a flulike disease with rheumatic symptoms about the same time as the cases of leukemia occurred. It was not possible in retrospect to determine the precise nature of the disease— whether viral or bacterial—or even to show that the leukemia victims had all suffered from it. Many, but not all, scientists believe that the flulike disease could not have been related to the excess cases of leukemia because the time interval between the two events was, in their view, too short.

Another dramatic cluster was reported in a small Irish village with a population of 415: six cases of leukemia, five of them in children or young people, three of them employed in the same shop. This corresponds to a rate about 200 times the national average for Ireland.

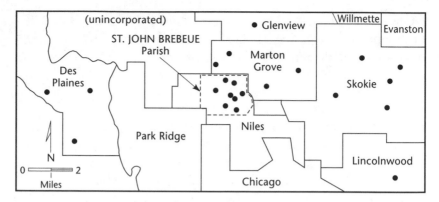

FIGURE 4-7   The leukemia cluster in Niles, Illinois. The map shows the area within the town of Niles corresponding to the Catholic parish of St. John Brebeuf. Most of the leukemia cases were among students or siblings of students attending the school of this parish. Reproduced from the article "Leukemia among Children in a Suburban Community," by C. W. Heath, Jr., and R. T. Hasterlik in the *American Journal of Medicine*, v. 34, pp. 796–812 (1963) with the permission of Excerpta Medica, Inc.

In spite of the dramatic impression these apparent clusters make, it is not a simple matter to show that they are not consequences of chance alone. While such an excess in any one community is very improbable, when we consider how many communities there are in the world, excesses this great occurring *somewhere* are less surprising. The fact is that leukemia cases, by and large, do not often occur in such marked clusters.

A Link with Infections?

It is clear today that leukemia is not itself contagious. On the other hand, there is evidence of a relation between one or more as yet unidentified childhood infections and susceptibility to leukemia. Different scientists have suggested somewhat different hypotheses for such a relation. Some have suggested that childhood leukemia may be a rare response to a common as yet unidentified childhood infection, leukemia being a more likely outcome the older the child is when first infected. This idea could explain some aspects of the distribution of childhood leukemia in different countries, and among different social or ethnic groups within one country. Children growing up in industrialized societies, living in less crowded and more sanitary conditions, are less exposed to infections at very early ages and therefore are more likely to contract them later on. So, for that matter, are children of higher social classes, compared with the children of the poor. Indeed, the childhood leukemia rates are higher in more industrialized societies, and higher in the higher social classes of such societies. Something similar is seen in paralytic poliomyelitis; children in less developed countries living in unsanitary conditions and at high population density get infected with the virus at an early age and do not suffer paralysis, which appears to be associated with infection at a later age. There was an unusual epidemic of multiple sclerosis in the isolated Faroe Islands off Scotland, when British soldiers were stationed there during World War II. It has been suggested that the British soldiers introduced an infectious agent to which they themselves had been exposed at an early age but to which the Faroe Islanders had not. While multiple sclerosis is not a contagious disease, the risk of getting it may be increased by some as yet unidentified infection.

One current view is that the immune system has evolved over time is such a way that it actually needs early infections—by the first year or two of life—to stimulate its proper development. The specific infection, whether bacterial or viral, may not matter; what matters is the challenge. If infectious challenges do not occur in the fetal stage or in infancy, the immune system's normal development is distorted, and the lymphocytes, the white blood cells involved in childhood leukemia, become more susceptible to a carcinogenic mutation. (See chapter 9 for a discussion of early childhood infections and asthma.)

Evidence from Epidemiology

One study of childhood leukemia found that children who were in day-care centers from an early age, and presumably exposed to infections earlier than children who were not in such centers, had a lower risk. Interestingly enough, a similar pattern applies to asthma. It had been known for several decades that the oldest child in a family has a higher risk of leukemia than his younger siblings and that there is a "dose-response" relationship between the risk and birth order: the second child has a slightly lower risk than the first, the third still less, and the fifth child only about half the risk of the oldest. An explanation in terms of the infection hypothesis has been recently offered: firstborn children are likely to get infectious diseases only when they are big enough to play with other children, and then they infect their littler brothers and sisters.

In Japan immediately following World War II the childhood leuke-mia rate was lower than in Western countries, but since the 1970s has risen to Western levels. Researchers suspected a relation between improv-ing sanitary conditions and this increase. As a marker or indicator of sani-tary conditions, they used a blood test for past exposure to a certain type of hepatitis infection but did not assume the hepatitis infection itself was the infection predisposing to leukemia. Rather, the hepatitis infection, transmitted by what is unappetizingly known as "the fecal-oral route," was assumed to correlate with all other infections transmitted this way. Just after World War II, sanitary conditions in Japan were very poor, partly as a result of wartime conditions but also because human waste was com-monly used for fertilizer. At that time, most Japanese women of child-bearing age tested positive for exposure, but decades later the proportion of women of childbearing age who had been exposed was much smaller. A close relation was found between increasing childhood leukemia rates and this evidence of improving sanitation. A similar relation had been found between the age at first infection with this hepatitis virus and the rate of leukemia in children both in white Americans earlier in this cen-tury, and among African-Americans several decades later.

Testing the Hypothesis

Testing the hypotheses of an infectious origin of childhood leukemia is not a simple matter.

If a common but as-yet-unidentified infection could cause some cases of leukemia, one would still not expect to find a large number of children coming down with leukemia all at once, unlike what we see with infec-tious diseases like measles or chicken pox. First, if infections do predispose to leukemia, they do so only in a very small fraction of cases. Second, many childhood infections do not produce clinical symptoms in every affected child: the child has the infection, but neither the child nor the parents notice it. It is said to be "subclinical." We would therefore not be able to identify which children suffered a prior infection. Nor can we do this by blood tests for antibodies to the infection without knowing which spe-cific infectious agent is responsible.

With infectious diseases like chicken pox or measles, there is a short and fairly uniform incubation period of several days or weeks after expo-sure. However, our experience with cancers initiated by radiation suggests that there are likely to be variable time periods between the infection and the onset of leukemia, and between the onset and the actual clinical appearance and diagnosis of the disease. Cases of leukemia might only appear much later, and spread out in time, among a group of children who suffered a predisposing infection at a particular time.

Population Mixing

It occurred to Dr. Leo Kinlen, an epidemiologist at Oxford University who was concerned with the Seascale cluster, that if leukemia is a rare response to a common childhood infection, it ought to be more common under conditions that favor the occurrence of epidemics. In particular, epidemics would be more likely to occur in communities where there has been considerable recent mixing of populations—for example, a mixing of an urban population with a rural one. More generally, if people living in one area are not commonly exposed to some particular infection, the number of susceptible individuals in that group will be high. Among people from an area where the infection is common, there will be a small proportion of them actually suffering from the infection at any one time. When the two groups, one with susceptible individuals and one with infected individuals, are brought into close contact, conditions for an epidemic are created. It is certainly plausible that in the vicinity of nuclear facilities, which are usually built in rural areas to avoid exposing large urban populations to the danger of accidents, and which employ large numbers of people from outside the area, there could have been just such population mixing.

Kinlen examined rates of childhood leukemia in many different areas of Great Britain where marked population mixing had occurred, and found that all of them had significantly increased leukemia rates. They included the evacuation of city children to rural areas to escape bombing in World War II; the stationing of large numbers of young men in military camps around Great Britain in a national service program just after the war, new towns built in rural areas, and communities that underwent large increases in their proportion of commuters. A particularly striking example concerned workers in the North Sea Oil industry, who had been drawn from urban and rural areas all over Scotland. Their working schedule involved three weeks on a major construction project on the North Sea, where they associated with workers from many other areas of Scotland, alternating with one week at home with their families. Those rural towns in Scotland where the highest proportions of such workers lived had higher than normal rates of childhood leukemia; presumably the oil workers living in rural areas brought some infection home with them. One such rural town with a high proportion of oil workers turned out to be Thurso, near the nuclear plant at Dounreay, where as we noted earlier a high rate of leukemia had previously been observed, and which drew particular attention because of its proximity to a nuclear facility.

Other scientists found similar effects. One study in Great Britain showed that communities that had undergone as much as a 50% population influx in the course of a decade had an increased leukemia rate, and others in Greece and Hong Kong found clustering of childhood leukemia cases in areas where population mixing had taken place. Quite strikingly, Kinlen has pointed out that Niles, Illinois, had undergone a period of explosive population growth just before the leukemia cluster was observed.

Back to the Seascale Cluster

It was also noted by Kinlen that the town of Seascale specifically had not only undergone considerable population mixing, but also was isolated geographically and had a population of high social class, many from the scientific and engineering staff at the Sellafield facility. As mentioned earlier, such communities usually have a somewhat elevated rate of childhood leukemia, though nowhere near the excess in Seascale. Although the western part of Cumbria, the county in which Seascale and Sellafield are located, does not have an elevated leukemia rate, one other town only 8 kilometers from Seascale, North Egremont, had a rate almost as high as Seascale. North Egremont is not a residential town for Sellafield employees, but is a center for construction workers in the area, who by and large are a mobile group of people and come from many different areas of the country.

In the studies just described, the concept of population mixing had not been given a quantitative meaning. Communities were classed as either "mixed" or "not mixed" and their leukemia rates then compared, but no category of mixing between "mixed" and "not mixed" was considered.

A more precise quantitative measure was devised in a study by H. Dickinson and L. Parker of childhood leukemia throughout Cumbria: First, they defined any married couple with children as "incomers" if both husband and wife were born outside of Cumbria. Then the fraction of incomers among all married couples with children in each community was taken as a quantitative measure of population mixing in that community. They found that the rate of childhood leukemia in each of the communities in Cumbria (leaving out Seascale for the time being) was closely related to the fraction of incomers, a relationship that could be called one of "dose-response," although being born in London or Glasgow is not, strictly speaking, a dose of anything.

Only then did they apply their approach to Seascale for the time period of the cluster. They included not only the population mixing fraction but all other known risk factors for childhood leukemia, such as social and economic status. Seascale proved to be unusual as far as both the fraction of incomers—70%, a higher fraction than in any other community in Cumbria—and the high social status of its inhabitants. Their model predicted that there should have been about half as many cases as had actually been observed. The "excess" in Seascale would thus be about twice the expected rather than ten times as high, one that could also occur by chance.

This remarkable result led Sir Richard Doll of Oxford University, one of the world's leading epidemiologists, to write an editorial in the same issue of the journal that carried the Dickinson-Parker article stating that Kinlen's hypothesis can be regarded as established: population mixing is a risk factor for childhood leukemia. Doll also suggested that the biological problem of identifying the causative agent (or agents) may prove exceptionally difficult, if the agent is a common one and the leukemia a rare response.

The evidence for a relation between childhood leukemia and common childhood infections is so far primarily epidemiological, based on population studies. Independent confirming evidence might come from microbiological identification of the infective agent, though as noted by Doll, such evidence may be hard to come by.

With all the uncertainties, and with all the work remaining to be done, one must recognize that this evidence of a connection between common infections and leukemia, and that leukemia clusters may be explained by it, is important.

CONCLUSION

No single explanation for the leukemia cases in Seascale has been accepted by everybody concerned. Known radiation exposure, of either the children or the fathers, has not been shown to have been great enough, and most but not all scientists rule out the possibility that in some as yet unexplained way radiation is responsible. It is not considered likely that the cluster is a result of chance alone, without any other factor being involved. The hypothesis that common childhood infections bear some relation to childhood leukemia, as an explanation of clusters both in the vicinity of nuclear plants and in other places where population mixing has occurred, is currently being taken seriously.

The End of Sellafield?

As the final pages of this book were being written, Sellafield was once again in the news. The reprocessing of spent nuclear fuels from power plants around the world was a highly profitable business for British Nuclear Fuels, the company that operated the Sellafield plant, and for Great Britain also: according to the British financial journal *The Economist*, This company has been the United Kingdom's largest single exporter of services, bringing in almost half a billion dollars a year. Recently a number of public relations disasters have clouded its future. It was discovered that documents relating to shipments of reprocessed fuel to both Japan and Germany had been falsified by workers at the plant to conceal unsafe defects in the shipment. Both Japan, sensitized by a recent nuclear accident of its own, and Germany plan to return the material. Independently, some of the operating equipment in the plant was sabotaged, presumably by a disgruntled employee. The governments of Ireland and Denmark, objecting to the continued dumping of radioactive waste in the Irish Sea, have demanded that the reprocessing facility be closed. Meanwhile, changes in the nuclear power industry make reprocessing spent plutonium fuel less profitable.

It has been proposed that the reprocessing plant be closed and Sellafield converted to a nuclear waste management facility, a step that would cost the West Cumbria region about 10,000 jobs. An environmental activist group in the area has said it would welcome the closing, but most people there are not happy with the prospect. The cases of childhood leukemia and lymphoma, still perceived by many to have been caused by radioactivity leaking from the plant, no longer loom so large to them.

5

BREAST CANCER, PART 1: THE RISE OF
ACTIVISM AND THE PESTICIDE HYPOTHESIS

WHAT WE KNOW AND DO NOT KNOW
ABOUT BREAST CANCER

Why Us?

The *New York Post*, a New York City daily, ran a sensational headline on the front page of its April 12, 2000, issue: "Breast Cancer Hot Spots" (fig. 5-1). The news story reported that statistics and maps of breast cancer rates just released by New York State health authorities showed unusually high rates of breast cancer on the Upper East Side of Manhattan, as well as on Long Island and several other areas in New York City and upstate. These high rates were described by the state authorities as "not likely due to chance."

The residents of the Upper East Side, one of the most affluent areas of the city, were understandably alarmed. One woman interviewed was considering whether to move elsewhere, but had not yet decided. A second demanded that the two major party candidates for the U.S. Senate state their positions on the high rate. A third noted that there were no obvious sources of pollution in the neighborhood, no pesticide spraying or toxic waste dumps, that could explain why the breast cancer rate was high.

Many people believe that breast cancer is caused by toxic agents in the environment. Victims of breast cancer we have met at sessions of

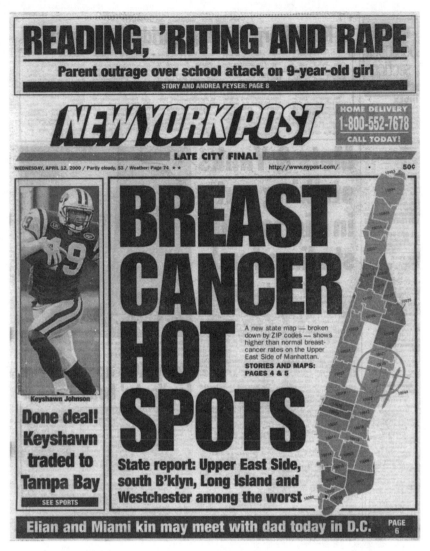

FIGURE 5-1   Front page of the *New York Post*, April 12, 2000. Reproduced with permission of the *New York Post*.

support groups have described vividly the pains and discomfort of chemo-therapy, radiation, and radical surgery; the nagging anxiety about a possible recurrence, the sense of disfigurement, of mutilation; the ignorance and insensitivity of many of the so-far healthy; the strengthening or weakening of bonds to those close to them: husbands, sons, daughters, parents, who either grow in understanding and compassion or fall short. But there is one common thread that runs through their stories: each of them feels there must be a reason why she, at this particular point in her life, should have gotten this terrible disease. Why me?

Lucia D., in her late thirties, remembers that as a child of eight or nine growing up in Panama she and other children used to run after the truck that periodically sprayed DDT in their neighborhood and dance around in the spray. She is convinced that this childhood exposure is the reason she has breast cancer at such an early age.

Martha W., sixty-seven, does not understand why, having been a vegetarian most of her life, she should have gotten breast cancer at all, unless it is because she lives near a U.S. government nuclear research laboratory from which leaks of radioactive material had been reported.

Miriam L., fifty-nine, recently diagnosed with the disease, knows of eight women in her own immediate circle of acquaintances, women of about her own age, who have had breast cancer. Her elderly mother knew of only one case of breast cancer among her own friends. She is sure that chemicals in the environment are causing this increase in the disease.

Susannah G., in her seventies, had a double mastectomy ten years earlier and appears free of the disease. She has lived for the last forty years in a small community on Cape Cod surrounded by the bogs in which cranberries had been grown at the time she moved there. She believes that pesticide residues from spraying the cranberry bogs have leached into the underground water table and reached the wells in her community, not only causing her breast cancer but also increasing the rate of breast cancer throughout the Cape.

Karen B., forty-four and a Long Island resident, now undergoing radiation and chemotherapy, wonders whether the electric power line cutting across the rear corner of the lot on which her house stands was responsible for her early cancer. She says she can detect a kind of hum from the wires when she stands near the line.

These women express common perceptions about cancer in general and breast cancer in particular: there is more of the disease than there used to be, there are neighborhoods where there is more of it than elsewhere, and breast cancer and many other cancers must be caused by something in the environment. Perhaps it is pesticides, perhaps preservatives added to the unnatural and highly processed foods we eat today, or electromagnetic fields, or radiation from nuclear plant emissions or weapons tests.

An activist movement has grown out of such concerns, that by demanding answers to the question "Why us?" has changed the playing field on which struggles are fought out both for scientific funding and for control over the direction scientific research should take.

Some scientists also believe that a portion of breast cancer is caused by environmental pollutants, including pesticides. What is the evidence for this view? Do studies to test it confirm it? Given what has been found

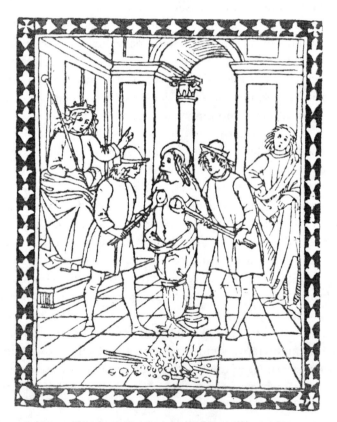

FIGURE 5-2   Florentine woodcut of the Martyrdom of Saint Agatha, an early Christian martyr, tortured by having her breasts cut off. They were miraculously restored to her subsequently. Copyright Bettman/Corbis.

so far, what should be done next to prevent women from dying of breast cancer?

Causes of Breast Cancer

Smoking causes 90% of lung cancer. High liver cancer rates in certain third-world countries, one hundred or more times greater than those in the developed West, are known to result from exposure to aflatoxin, a substance produced by molds that grow on grain stored in humid environments. A dramatic increase of a rather rare type of vaginal cancer occurred in young women whose mothers had been given the drug diethyl stilbestrol, a synthetic hormone, during pregnancy to avoid threatened miscarriages. These forms of cancer for which causes are known that account for the majority of cases are atypical.

On the other hand, breast cancer is like most other cancers: only a small proportion of cases can be accounted for by known exposures. The only environmental cause we are sure of is high-energy radiation, as shown by studies of survivors of the nuclear bombing of Japan and of tubercular women who underwent repeated X-ray examinations of the chest. Women today are not exposed to enough high-energy radiation to account for any appreciable number of cases.

Clues to Causes

An important observation about breast cancer was made at the beginning of the eighteenth century. In 1713 the Italian physician Bernardino Ramazzini, in his book *De Morbis Artificum*, or *Diseases of Workers*, described the various diseases that workers in different industries and occupations suffered from, essentially inventing the field of occupational medicine. In a chapter on the diseases of wet-nurses he mentions that nuns are more subject to cancer of the breast than other women, which he attributes to their celibacy. He writes that nuns he treated for cancer of the breast had regular menstrual periods, apparently because some other physician had speculated that suppression of the menses might cause breast cancer (fig. 5-3).

What Ramazzini observed in the early eighteenth century is true today: nuns still have a higher risk of breast cancer than women in general. So for that matter do single women and married women who have not borne children, so it is not celibacy as such that is responsible.

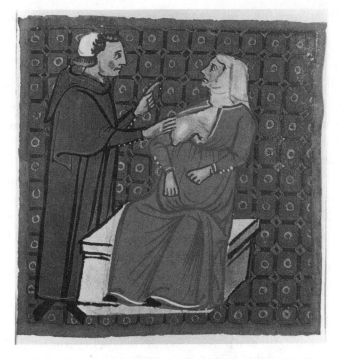

FIGURE 5-3 Nun having her breast examined by the surgeon Teodorico Borgognoni, thirteenth century. Courtesy of the New York Academy of Medicine.

Why should having children protect a woman against breast cancer? As we will see, it has been explained in terms of the reduced exposure of a woman to her own sex hormones during pregnancy and the effect of the first pregnancy on the development of the breast cells, but the precise mechanism is controversial. We cannot say that not having had children "causes" breast cancer because we are not sure of how the two are related; instead the term "risk factor" was coined for such a relationship.

Risk Factors

People can be divided up into groups in an unlimited number of ways: by age, by occupation, by ethnicity, by diet, by social class, by education, by life and medical history, by where they live and what they are exposed to in their neighborhoods. The risk of getting any disease will vary from one such group to another, although often we do not know why. We use the term "risk factor" for any group property—age, occupation, childbearing, or whatever—that is statistically associated with an extra risk of some particular disease.

A risk factor may or may not be a cause of the disease. The term implies only that someone who has this risk factor has been found to have a greater chance of getting the disease than a person who does not. For example, poverty is a risk factor for tuberculosis: on the average, poor people are more likely than middle-class or rich people to suffer from it. Poverty is not the "cause" of the disease: it is a risk factor presumably because poor people live under more crowded living conditions with more exposure to other victims and have poorer nutrition so that they are more vulnerable.

Children from families on Medicaid have three times the risk of having high lead levels in their bodies than other children, and federal law mandates that they should undergo blood tests to ascertain if they have been exposed to lead and need treatment. We conclude that being on Medicaid is a risk factor for lead exposure, though clearly it is not the cause. Families on Medicaid are more likely to live in old housing with old lead paint flaking off the walls.

Risk factors may provide clues to causes, but even when their relation to the causes is not clear, knowing risk factors may help prevent disease. Smoking a pack a day of cigarettes was identified as a risk factor for lung cancer long before the evidence that smoking causes it became overwhelming. Giving up cigarettes was saving lives before that evidence was available. Whenever risk factors are avoidable, prudence requires that we do what we can to avoid them. We need not always wait for causation to be proved.

Who Gets Breast Cancer and Who Does Not?

A number of risk factors for breast cancer have been reported in the scientific literature. Age and sex are among the most important, as they are for most cancers. Men do get breast cancer, but only at less than one-hundredth the rate of women. Rates in women are low before menopause, and then increase: the rate at ages fifty to fifty-four is almost ten times the rate at ages thirty to thirty-four. The rate after menopause continues to increase with age, but much less dramatically than before menopause, and much less dramatically than with most other kinds of cancer.

Women with first-degree relatives—mothers or sisters—who have had the disease have about twice the risk of other women. Some of this risk may come from a shared environment and a shared lifestyle; some is surely genetic. Jewish women of European origin (Ashkenazi Jews) have a slightly increased rate of breast cancer, so being Jewish is a small risk factor. It has been suggested that this small risk occurs because a higher percentage of Jewish women than women in general have a particular genetic predisposition to the disease, but this is still under investigation. Among those women, Jewish or not, who share this genetic predisposition, as many as 50% will get breast cancer. The predisposition is associated with mutations on one of two different genes and can be detected by blood tests. Having such a mutation is therefore a large risk factor. Because it is rare in the population in general, it is responsible for only a few percent of cases of the disease.

Most of the other risk factors for breast cancer so far reported have to do with the reproductive life of women. Not having had a baby early in life is one of the most well established. Nursing one's babies has been reported to be protective, but there has been some controversy about it. A number of factors are related to the menstrual cycle: early age at menarche (the beginning of menstruation) is a risk factor, as is late age at menopause. The greater the total number of menstrual periods in a woman's life, the higher her risk, which implies a higher risk the shorter the time interval between periods and the more regular the cycle. Often when menarche is delayed, especially if it is delayed as a result of poor nutrition, the cycle is irregular, and becomes regular only after some time. Women who exercise or do hard physical work—for example, ballet dancers and joggers—have more irregular cycles, and, in the case of dancers starting ballet in childhood, undergo menarche as much as three or four years later than other girls. It appears that exercise in general is protective, and how much and why is currently under study. The older a woman is when she has her menopause, the higher her subsequent risk of breast cancer. Women who undergo artificial menopause by surgical removal of the ovaries have a lower risk.

Avoidable and Unavoidable Risks

These reproductive risk factors, unlike cigarette smoking, are, practically speaking, unavoidable. Either women cannot choose them—such as the age at menopause—or they are too much part of our modern lifestyle to surrender. Women today marry later than they used to, delay childbearing, and nurse their babies less. Should they sacrifice careers or other personal goals to reduce breast cancer risk? Poor nutrition in childhood is believed to be one cause of a delayed menarche, but we do not starve little girls to decrease their risk of breast cancer later on. Taking up ballet at an early age should not be forced on children; there is no surer way to make them hate it for life.

Are there other risk factors, not necessarily related to the reproductive factors, which might be avoidable?

International Differences in Rates

The United States has one of the world's highest rates of breast cancer, so living there is a large risk factor (fig. 5-4). Less developed countries in Africa and Asia have relatively low ones. Although Japan is a highly industrialized country, up to a few decades ago the rate there was about one-sixth the U.S. rate; it has been rising rapidly recently, but is still about one-third

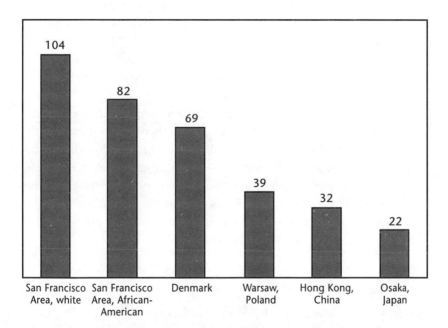

FIGURE 5-4   International breast cancer incidence (new cases per 100,000 women per year) by geographical area. The rate in San Francisco, United States, was almost five times the rate in Osaka, Japan, for the period 1980–1990. Data from *Cancer Incidence in Five Continents, Volume VI*, by D. M. Parkin et al., International Agency for Research on Cancer, Lyon, France, 1992.

to one-half. Why are there these differences? Are Japanese and other Asians and Africans genetically less susceptible to breast cancer than Caucasians? A relatively simple observation rules it out as a major factor: Japanese women who moved to the United States as young adults suffer a slightly increased rate compared to women of their age in Japan, and their ethnically Japanese daughters and granddaughters born and raised in the United States suffer breast cancer at almost the Caucasian rate. If the difference in rates had a genetic origin, the low rates in Japanese women would not disappear in one or two generations any more than those genetic traits that make them look "Japanese." The breast cancer rate among women in Africa is also very low, but African-American women suffer from breast cancer at a rate only a little lower than Caucasian women in the United States rather than at the rate of women in Africa. This relatively high rate among African-Americans is not accounted for by the fact that most people to whom the term "African-American" is applied have a mixed African-Caucasian set of genes.

We have mentioned that there are rare genetic defects that predispose a very high proportion of the women who have them to breast cancer, but they account for only a few percent of cases in the United States. In addition there appear to be some more common genetic sensitivities to specific exposures that increase the breast cancer risk only slightly. These will be described in more detail later.

It follows that if genetic heritage is not very important in explaining differences in cancer risk, environmental or lifestyle factors must play the major role. Many of the U.S.-Japanese differences can be accounted for by differences in the reproductive risk factors described earlier: age at menarche and menopause, age at birth of first child, and so on. A few scientists believe all of the U.S.-Japanese differences can, but there is no consensus on this. Are there other factors? If we could identify them we might hope to reduce breast cancer rates drastically. What might they be?

Other Risk Factors

One of the first guesses about U.S.-Japanese differences was that diet might explain them. The traditional diet in Japan was very different from the U.S. diet: more fish, less meat, rice instead of wheat and corn, less fat, more fiber, and so on, but it has been getting more like the U.S. diet in recent years. We said earlier that poor nutrition in childhood delays menarche, but aside from this, could diet play a role in breast cancer?

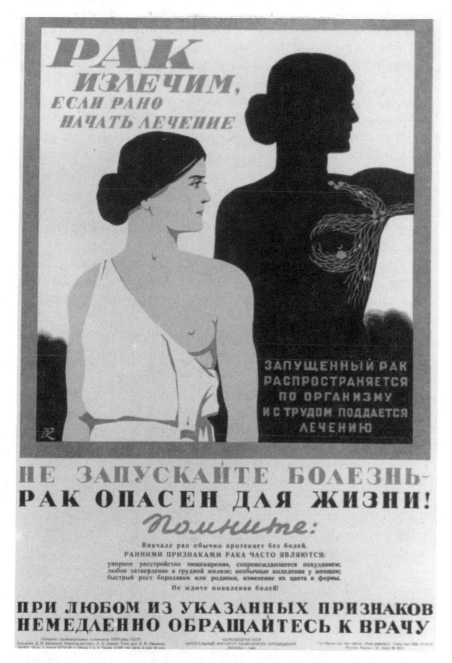

FIGURE 5-5 This Soviet-era poster carries the message that cancer is treatable if detected early. From the National Library for the History of Medicine, National Institutes of Health, Bethesda, MD.

Striking evidence that it does not comes from a study of Seventh-Day Adventists in the United States, who as a group eat almost no meat. Their colon cancer rate is 50% of that of the U.S. population as a whole, but their breast cancer rate is 90%. Other studies have also found that a high-meat or a high-fat diet during adult life does not appear to have a great influence on the risk of breast cancer. It has been suggested but not yet confirmed that reducing body fat to an extremely low level might reduce the risk. Research has shifted to the effects of diet of the mother during pregnancy, diet in early childhood, and on the precise effect of these on the age at menarche. What happens in childhood deserves special attention: it is noteworthy that women in Hiroshima and Nagasaki who were five years old or younger at the time of the bombing had a lifetime risk nine times that of women not exposed at that age.

One additional risk factor is body weight. Japanese women, especially postmenopausal women, weigh much less, on the average, than their American counterparts, and at least some of the U.S.-Japanese differences are attributed to this.

Alcohol consumption is believed to increase the risk slightly. Smoking does not appear to confer much risk, except that some studies suggest that there is a subgroup of women with a specific type of genetic sensitivity; among this subgroup exposure to somebody else's tobacco smoke does increase risk.

Women of different social classes live different lifestyles and therefore differ with respect to the known risk factors: women of higher income and education have fewer children and have them later, have better nutrition and therefore earlier menarche, and so on. This would suggest that they would have more breast cancer and in fact they do. Whether the excess rate among higher social class women can be completely explained by the known reproductive factors is not clear, but that there is an excess among them is not surprising.

THE ESTROGEN EXPOSURE HYPOTHESIS

Risk and Estrogens

What clues to the causes of breast cancer do the risk factors we have so far discovered give us?

The most important ones so far identified are those related to the reproductive life of women. An explanation for their importance has been offered that is consistent with many biological observations: all of these reproductive risk factors are related to the total lifetime exposure of a woman to her own estrogens and other sex hormones. Estrogens are a group of female sex hormones that stimulate cell proliferation in the breast and uterus. A hormone is a chemical produced by one organ of the body that affects the function of other, sometimes distant, organs. Sex hormones are produced in women mostly by the ovaries and to some extent in fatty tissue, and in men by the testicles. Most of the sex hormones are members of a class of chemical compounds called steroids, which are composed of carbon, hydrogen, and oxygen. They are small compared to proteins, and more soluble in fat than in water.

The peak production of estrogens during adult life takes place during a particular phase of the menstrual cycle, the follicular phase, in the first half of the cycle, after the actual menstrual period. The more years that lie between menarche and menopause, and the more regular and frequent a woman's periods are, the greater her cumulative exposure to estrogens. Events that decrease the number of menstrual cycles between menarche and menopause, such as pregnancy and nursing a baby, are believed to reduce the risk of breast cancer. Alcohol consumption, a minor risk factor, does increase estrogen levels temporarily. After menopause, the ovaries gradually cease producing estrogens, but they continue to be produced in fat tissue, and this may explain why body weight after menopause is a risk factor.

The effect of women's exposure to their own estrogens appears to be more important at younger ages. The delay of menarche by one year has a stronger protective effect than menopause occurring one year early, and birth of a first child at an early age is more protective than later births. Cells of the body start out alike, and only mature into the cells characteristic of different organs—breast, liver, lung, muscles—later. Immature cells are more vulnerable to mutations, and the first pregnancy matures the breast cells.

Many women take supplemental estrogens after menopause to alleviate some of its more unpleasant symptoms. These supplemental estrogens are synthetic substances, not the natural kind produced in the human body. This hormone replacement therapy (HRT) has been reported to produce only a slightly increased risk of breast cancer, which must be balanced against the fact that HRT protects against osteoporosis, a crippling porosity of the bones that affects elderly women more than elderly men, and possibly against Alzheimer's disease as well.

Biological Evidence

There is considerable biological evidence that exposure to one's own estrogens increases breast cancer risk. We have already mentioned that early removal of the ovaries reduces risk (first shown in 1895), and also that while the rate of the disease increases with age after menopause (when estrogen production decreases), it does so less dramatically than with other cancers. Breast cancer patients have been found consistently to have higher estrogen levels in their blood than do women of the same age and with otherwise the same risk factors but who have not gotten breast cancer. The amounts of estrogen excreted in urine during particular phases of the menstrual cycle are lower in young women in Asia, where breast cancer rates are low, than in America. Cultures of breast cancer cells in test tubes grow faster when exposed to estrogen. Male transsexuals taking estrogens to increase breast size have a higher rate of breast cancer than men in general.

Feeding estrogens to rats increases the incidence of mammary tumors as well as the size of the tumors formed. If rats are given a carcinogenic chemical known to produce mammary tumors and then fed estrogens, the time to development of the tumor is shortened.

So the evidence for a relation between a woman's lifetime exposure to her own estrogens and breast cancer risk is strong, but knowing this does not suggest a simple way to reduce the rate of the disease. The body's production of estrogen responds to certain life events like childbirth and nursing, and even exercise, but is otherwise not under a woman's control. Is the occurrence of breast cancer like a natural disaster, something we can do nothing to prevent?

Estrogens and Evolution

Why should a woman's exposure to her own estrogens kill her? The idea is offensive, reminiscent of a past era, when menstruation was called "the curse," and an even more distant era, when the use of anesthetics for women in childbirth was opposed by clergymen who quoted the biblical judgement on Eve, "in sorrow shalt thou bring forth children." Some scientists have argued that there is an evolutionary basis for this paradox. The British cancer researcher M. Greaves put it this way:

> The stark reality is that females of our species are burdened
> with a five-million-year-old genetic programme that anatomi-
> cally and physiologically primes them for regular pregnancy

and lactation. But then our rapid social development as a species has produced a schism between our socialized reproductive behaviour and our evolutionary heritage—nature and nurture in conflict.

Put bluntly, one important component of evolutionary survival fitness is reproductive success. Greaves points out that an aboriginal woman typically has six children compared to the Western modern woman's one or two, and nurses them for years instead of a month or two. As a consequence the aboriginal woman has about 150 menstrual cycles in a lifetime, compared to her modern sister's 450. Evolution has selectively designed the female body for the first pattern, and in advanced societies today women have chosen a different pattern. Even if this idea is correct, it need not mean that breast cancer is inevitable, but we defer discussion of this until we have explored the extent to which environmental agents account for the disease.

Silent Spring *and the Rise of Environmental Activism*

In 1962 the biologist Rachel Carson published her book *Silent Spring*, a turning point in awareness of threats to the environment from the chemical products of an industrial society. She described damage to wildlife from indiscriminate use of pesticides, particularly DDT, and envisaged an eventual springtime in which there would be no birds singing because none would be left alive. In spite of violent attacks on her book by representatives of the chemical industry, who regarded her claims as exaggerated and a threat to progress, her warnings prevailed, and in the 1970s DDT was banned in the United States and other Western countries. DDT is still used in less developed nations because it protects the population from malaria and other serious insect-borne diseases, although there is current controversy on whether it should be banned even for this use.

The harm to wildlife noted by Carson was not only the death of exposed animals and birds but damage to their ability to reproduce their kind. For example, birds in areas where DDT had been sprayed failed to lay eggs, or if they did, the shells of the eggs were so thin they did not survive for the young birds to be hatched. Carson was very concerned about dangers to human health as well: she gave examples of death or permanent harm suffered by individuals accidentally exposed to large amounts of pesticides, and speculated about the possible cancer-causing potentials of widely used chemicals. She noted that among the ways the chemicals might cause cancer was through their ability to damage the liver. The liver regulates the concentrations of sex hormones in the bloodstream, eliminating excessive concentrations if they should happen to build up. She suggested that if the liver is unable to do this job, excessive hormone concentrations could cause certain cancers of the reproductive system. She mentions cancer of the uterus, but not breast cancer, as a demonstrated outcome of exposing animals to high concentrations of sex hormones.

Her perspective is finely illustrated by this quotation from her book:

> [T]here is an ecology of the world within our bodies. In this unseen world minute causes produce mighty effects; the effect, moreover, is often seemingly unrelated to the cause, appearing in a part of the body remote from the area where the original injury was sustained. "A change at one point, in one molecule even, may reverberate throughout the entire system to initiate changes in seemingly unrelated organs and tissues," says a recent summary of the present status of medical research. [Although this was quoted by Carson in her book published in 1962, it is still true today.] When one is concerned with the mysterious and wonderful functioning of the human body, cause and effect are seldom simple and easily demonstrated relationships. They may be widely separated in space and time. To discover the agent of disease and death depends on a patient piecing together of many seemingly distinct and unrelated facts developed through a vast amount of research in widely separated fields.

Rachel Carson died in 1964 of breast cancer.

Certain environmental pollutants, including DDT, were later reported to produce some of the same effects in wildlife that estrogens do, in spite of the fact that many of them do not have chemical structures resembling estrogens. For example, male fish in rivers contaminated by sewage or certain industrial discharges were "feminized"; their sexual development as males was deficient, as though they had been exposed to female hormones. Alligators in a heavily polluted lake were reported to have undersized penises, though which of the many pollutants present might have been responsible is unknown. Some of these effects have been duplicated in laboratory animals exposed to pesticides. Of more direct concern to humans are reports of declining sperm counts in men in industrialized countries, but these reports have been hotly contested.

The terms "xenoestrogens" (*xeno* being a Greek prefix meaning "foreign," as in "xenophobia") and "estrogen mimickers" were coined to describe substances in the environment that are not estrogens but act like them, although some scientists prefer the less specific term "hormonally active agents." Some scientists, aware that there is a relation between total estrogen exposure and breast cancer, speculated that exposure to pesticides and to other hormonally active agents might account for high rates of breast cancer.

Hormonally Active Chemicals in the Environment

Included among the substances found in the environment that demonstrate some hormonal activity are pesticides, plasticizers, and some additives in commercial household products. Many of the commonly used pesticides are soluble in fats rather than water, and tend to collect in fat tissues of the body. They remain there for long periods of time, years rather than days, but can be released rapidly when stored body fat is being used up rapidly, which happens under conditions of starvation, but also during lactation. Babies may therefore be exposed to them in breast milk. (See "Chemicals in the Environment" [p. 166] for more details on chemicals in the environment.)

The Search for Avoidable Causes:
The Role of Breast Cancer Activists

The National Breast Cancer Coalition, an umbrella organization, has over 500 affiliated organizations and a total membership of 60,000. It has stated as its goals in breast cancer research "to promote research into the causes, optimal treatments, and cure for breast cancer through increased funding; recruitment and training of scientists, and improved coordination and distribution of research funds." Its other goals include improving access to screening, diagnosis, treatment, and care, and expressing the concerns of both victims of the disease and potential victims to federal and state legislative bodies and regulatory agencies. As a result of its efforts and those of other activists, funding for research on breast cancer has increased from less than $90 million in 1991 to $660 million in 1999.

The activists, as well as others, had been aware of a reported rise in breast cancer over the last fifty years, which suggested the possibility that exposure to chemicals not previously in the environment might be responsible. They were also aware of reports of geographical differences in breast cancer incidence (number of new cases each year) and of breast cancer death rates not just internationally but also within the United States itself. Certain areas stood out, in particular the highly urbanized areas of the northeastern United States. Long Island, New York, had reported incidence rates 15% higher than the New York State average, which in turn was higher than the national average. It is interesting to note that in 1957, Long Island residents had instituted a lawsuit to stop indiscriminate spraying of DDT against gypsy moth infestation. The suit was unsuccessful, although it went all the way to the Supreme Court. Other areas of high incidence were Cape Cod, Massachusetts, with a reported 20% excess over the rest of the state, and the San Francisco Bay area. Concerned women living in these areas were worried that some environmental factors were responsible and that studies carried out there could identify them. Being aware of the hypothesis about xenoestrogens, they suspected pesticides in particular, though they did not rule out other possibilities (fig. 5-6).

Cape Cod and Long Island

When the Massachusetts cancer registry issued a report in 1993 showing that breast cancer on Cape Cod had been unusually high during the period 1982–1990 (the registry began collecting data in 1982), the Massachusetts Breast Cancer Coalition successfully demanded that the state legislature provide money to find out why. The coalition was aware that considerable spraying of insecticides had taken place on Cape Cod. There had been spraying of the bogs where cranberries grew, spraying of golf courses to control weeds, spraying of trees to control gypsy moths. Further, there was a U.S. Air Force base on the Cape that had carelessly discharged fuel wastes, unused explosives, and other chemical wastes, some of which were known carcinogens, in such a way that they seeped into the groundwater. Cape Cod has a sandy soil through which water travels easily. The water table, from which drinking water is drawn, is shallow, and contaminants, including pesticides and other chemicals, as well as the outflow from septic tanks (which includes estrogens from human waste), drain into it. Tests of some of the Cape community drinking water supplies showed contamination from these sources (fig. 5-7).

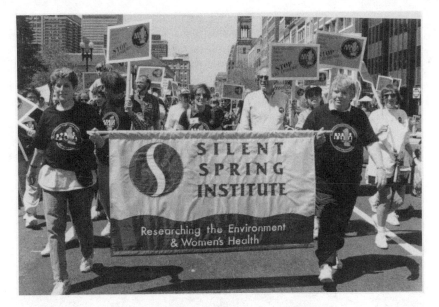

FIGURE 5-6   Activist demonstration. Courtesy of the Silent Spring Institute, Newton, MA.

The Silent Spring Institute, a research institute committed to studying possible links between environmental hazards and women's health,
particularly breast cancer, was funded by the State of Massachusetts to
study breast cancer on the Cape. A number of scientists at universities in
the Boston area are collaborating in the study. The goal is to find out if
the breast cancer rate on Cape Cod is related to exposure to environmental
agents, particularly hormonally active agents and mammary carcinogens
among the pesticides, detergents and other household products, and toxic
wastes from the Air Force base and other sources that people on the Cape
have been exposed to, as well as electromagnetic fields from power lines
and house wiring.

The story on Long Island was similar. A state-financed study there
had reported excess breast cancer in the vicinities of a number of industrial toxic waste dumps. The study was based on only a small number of
cases and had been criticized for various weaknesses, but it aroused attention and concern. When New York State figures on breast cancer rates
showed that Long Island had one of the highest rates in the state, breast
cancer organizations began a successful campaign to persuade Congress
to appropriate funds for a study on Long Island (fig. 5-8).

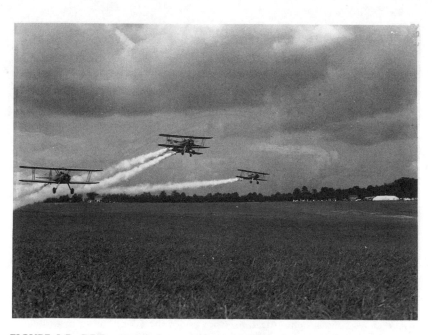

FIGURE 5-7   DDT spraying from airplanes in 1945. Copyright Bettman/Corbis.

The study mandated by the U.S. Congress gave the authority to the National Institutes of Health to invite scientific institutions to submit competing proposals on how they would carry out such a study. The National Institutes of Health then had them evaluated by a committee of scientists specializing in the field. A large grant was awarded to Columbia University, together with a consortium of scientists from other universities and medical institutions in the New York City area, to evaluate the role of pesticides and other suspected agents in relation to breast cancer on Long Island.

ARE THE RATES REALLY HIGH?

Before we describe how these studies are being done, we have an important question to answer. How do we tell that there really is more breast cancer, or for that matter more of any disease, in one place, or at one time, or in one group of people, than in another? This question comes up

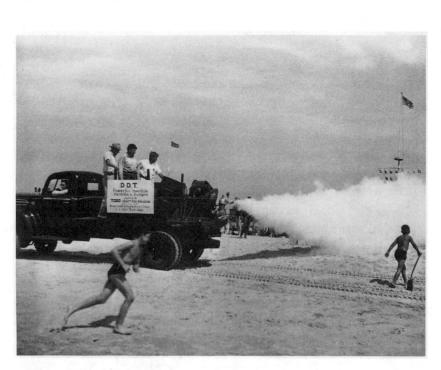

FIGURE 5-8   This shows the first public use, in July 1945, of an "Insecticidal Fog Applicator," at Jones Beach on Long Island, New York. A stretch of four miles was blanketed with DDT oil fog as Sunday bathers ducked out of the way. Copyright Bettman/Corbis.

whenever an unusual "cluster" of disease is noted, such as leukemia near a nuclear plant (see chapter 4) or around sites where chemical wastes have been dumped (see chapter 8).

The statements "Women on Cape Cod have more breast cancer than women in the rest of Massachusetts" and "Women today have more breast cancer than fifty years ago" are simple-sounding statements, but showing that they are a cause for concern is not so simple and takes a lot more work than just counting breast cancer cases. We want to know if the rates are high for a particular reason: to test the possibility that exposure to something in the environment, perhaps pesticides or other chemicals, has caused them to be high. "More" in this sense therefore means more than can be accounted by things we already know about—those risk factors we have already discovered. How can such risk factors account for higher rates of breast cancer in some areas than in others? The following quotation may help: it is from *An Introduction to Logic and Scientific Method*, by

Morris R. Cohen and Ernest Nagel, the textbook in a course one of us took at the City College of New York many years ago:

> There is always a danger from an unwitting selection of material in comparing different groups. A recruiting sergeant will convince most people with the following argument. The death rate in the United States Navy [Cohen and Nagel apparently assumed that the U.S. Navy used "recruiting sergeants"] during the Spanish-American War [of 1898] was 9 per 1,000, while the death rate in New York City for the same period was 16 per 1,000; it is therefore safer to be a sailor in the navy during a war than a civilian in New York City. But an examination of the evidence for this conclusion soon shows that the two death rates have not the significance which they appear to have. For the New York City death rate includes the mortality of infants, old people, people in hospitals and asylums; and it is well known that the death rate for the very old and the very young, as well as for the sick, is relatively high. On the other hand, the navy is composed of men between the ages of 18 and 35, each of whom had been judged fit in a rigorous physical examination. It follows that the two death rates do not warrant the conclusion that the navy is a safer place than New York City. Adequate evidence for such a conclusion would require the comparison of two groups which are homogeneous with respect to age, sex, and health. (p. 319)

Age and Disease

Obviously, the numbers of new cases of breast cancer in Massachusetts will be greater than the number on Cape Cod because there are more women in Massachusetts than on Cape Cod. We need to know the *proportion* of women in both areas who get breast cancer, rather than the numbers of cases. Breast cancer "incidence" is defined as the number of new cases diagnosed per 100,000 women per year.

When we want to know whether breast cancer rates in two areas are similar, or whether one area has a suspiciously higher rate, we need to know first if they are similar in their proportions of people of various ages, and if they are not, to correct for the difference.

The breast cancer incidence rate in U.S. women between the ages of seventy and seventy-five is double the rate in women between fifty and fifty-five, and twenty times the rate between thirty and thirty-five. This implies that if the proportion of older women on Cape Cod or on Long Island is greater than in the areas to which they are being compared, Cape Cod and Long Island will have a higher rate of breast cancer, but not because of pesticide exposure. Indeed, there is reason to expect women on the Cape to be older: lately a lot of people have chosen Cape Cod as a good place to retire.

When the rates of some disease in two groups of people are being compared, correcting for the possibility that they may not have the same age distribution and therefore different rates of the disease is called "age-adjusting."

Age Adjustment: Why and How

To show how age differences between two different communities might confuse the question of whether there is more disease in one rather than the other, we will give a simple example, using some made-up numbers, and two hypothetical areas, Cape A and the state in which it is located, State B. First, consider just women in the age group fifty to seventy, and imagine it subdivided into the two age groups fifty to sixty and sixty to seventy (table 5-1). The approximate U.S. incidence rates for breast cancer in these two age groups are 200 and 400, respectively (per 100,000 women per year). Let us assume that these rates apply to State B, and further, that there really is nothing unique to Cape A causing increased breast cancer there, so that the same rates apply equally to each age group in both Cape A and State B. Let us further assume that the women of Cape A are somewhat older than in State B, so that of any 100,000 women in State B between fifty and seventy, 60% of them are in the younger age group between fifty and sixty, while in Cape A with its older average age only 40% are. We can now easily calculate that the breast cancer incidence rates for women fifty to seventy in the two areas are 280 and 320, so that, yes, there is more breast cancer in Cape A, 14% more, but it is because women on Cape A are older, and older women everywhere have more breast cancer.

Doing the Arithmetic

To "age-adjust" the data to make a proper comparison of breast cancer rates in the two towns, we can calculate what the Cape A incidence would be if its age distribution were the same as that of State B. The calculation

TABLE 5-1   How Age Differences Affect Breast Cancer Incidence
(a Hypothetical Example)

Age Subgroup	Number of Women in Subgroup	Incidence in Age Subgroup, per 100,000 Women per Year	Number of Cases in Each Subgroup, per Year	Incidence in Area Among Women Aged 50–70 (Cases Per 100,000 per year)
State B[a]				
50–60	60,000	200	120	
60–70	40,000	400	160	
				280
Cape A[a]				
50–60	40,000	200	80	
60–70	60,000	400	240	
				320

[a]100,000 women aged 50–70 in both State B and Cape A.

is simply the reverse of what we did in the table. For anyone interested in the details, the next paragraph gives them.

We multiply the incidences for the two age groups in Cape A by factors representing their relative differences from the age distribution in State B. We multiply the incidence of 80 in the fifty-to-sixty group by 60/40 (the proportion of women in that age group in State B, divided by the proportion of women in that age group in Cape A) to get an adjusted incidence of 120. Then we multiply the incidence of 240 in the sixty-to-seventy group by 40/60 (again, the proportion of women in that age group in State B, divided by the proportion of women in that age group in Cape A) to get an adjusted incidence of 160. Then we add the two to get a total incidence for the fifty-to-seventy-year age group in Cape A of 280, the same as in State B, as it should be. This gives us what the incidence in Cape A would be if its age distribution were the same as that in State B.

In the United States it is common practice to use the U.S. population as the reference, so both Cape Cod and Massachusetts rates would be age-adjusted accordingly.

Sex and Disease

We have taken for granted in discussing breast cancer that we are talking about women. Male breast cancer is a very rare disease, with an incidence rate less than one one-hundredth that of women.

Certain diseases are unique to members of one sex: only women get cancer of the uterus, only men cancer of the prostate. Most cancers, however, regardless of the organ involved, are not distributed equally by sex any more than they are distributed equally by age, although we do not always know why. For example, men in the United States suffer stomach cancer at twice the rate, and bladder cancer at four times the rate, that women do.

More Risk Factors to Worry About

The age-adjusted breast cancer incidence rate among women on Cape Cod in recent years has been 20% higher than in all of Massachusetts, and the rate on Long Island 15% higher than in all of New York State. So there is more breast cancer in these areas than in the rest of the state they are being compared with. Can we yet conclude that there must be some environmental agents—pesticides, other chemical toxins, electromagnetic fields, or something else—responsible for the excess? We have already shown why age differences alone might account for different breast cancer rates in different places, which is why we adjust the crude rates for age. Could there be other reasons, not connected with pesticides, the careless waste disposal practices of the U.S. Air Force base on the Cape, or toxic waste sites on Long Island, for the higher rates? The answer is yes: differences in the risk factors we described earlier.

When Ramazzini in the eighteenth century observed that nuns have more breast cancer than expected, there were no pesticides in the environment. Though nuns in the twentieth century still have more breast cancer than women in general, we know better than to blame it on pesticides. It can be explained by the fact that they have not borne children. Before we assume that there must be some environmental explanation of the greater rates on Cape Cod or Long Island, we must first show that there is more than we can account for by those risk factors that we have already discovered: childbearing, menstruation history, and so on. If women now living on Cape Cod happen to differ from women in the rest of Massachusetts in respect to these, they can have different breast cancer rates, just as if there were age differences.

Some of these risk factors involve personal choice, like when to have a baby or whether to drink a martini; others do not, like when to have one's first period or having a sister with breast cancer. Women differ with respect to them, and some of the differences are related to social class, education, ethnicity, diet, and so on. We must expect, therefore, when we compare breast cancer rates in two different communities, that the rates may differ because the social makeups of the two communities differ.

To take a specific example: African-American women have an age-adjusted incidence rate for breast cancer about three-quarters that of the Caucasian-American rate. If there are fewer African-American women living on Cape Cod than in the rest of Massachusetts, the breast cancer rate will be somewhat higher than in the rest of Massachusetts for that reason alone, again without having to take pesticides into account.

How We Adjust

Adjustment for age and sex is relatively simple to do. The U.S. Census data provides detailed information about the age and sex distribution not only in the whole United States but in all of its subdivisions, like states, counties, and towns. Adjustment for all the other risk factors is fraught with problems. The goal of such adjustment is to compute an "expected" rate, with which the actual rate is to be compared. This "expected" rate is the rate we would observe if the study population were exactly the same with respect to all the known risk factors as the population it is being compared to. Except for age and sex adjustment, there are no prescribed procedures for the adjustment, and different scientists often disagree about whether any one risk factor is important to include or not. Also they may disagree about how to describe a risk factor. Is "early age at menarche" under twelve, or under thirteen? In studies of hormone replacement therapy, women are often divided up into three categories: nonusers, short-term users, and long-term users. How long is long-term? Different scientists draw the line in different places. Things are made more difficult by the fact that many of the studies involve small numbers of women and are therefore subject to large statistical uncertainties. Inevitably, different scientists come up with different expected rates. In turn, it follows that there will be some range of uncertainty for the expected rate—a 95% confidence interval, for example (see chapter 8)—within which the true value is likely, but not certain, to lie. This range is itself not easy to calculate for risk factor correction, and it is not often given.

In a preliminary and unpublished study by Harvard scientists, the excess breast cancer rate on Cape Cod for women over 50 was found after adjustment for risk factors to be 20% higher than in the rest of Massachusetts (outside of metropolitan Boston), but the 95% confidence interval calculated ranged from 4% to 40%. In other words, the excess rate on Cape Cod could be as low as 4%, an almost negligible difference, or as high as 40%, a considerable one. Which is it? At this point we do not know and might be justified in feeling that the 20% excess is maybe at the margin of what we can possibly establish with confidence. Scientists at Harvard are doing a more careful analysis, but have not yet published their results.

So we see that correcting for known risk factors other than age (and sex, when relevant) is difficult and uncertain.

Can We Trust the Data?

Another problem is the reliability of data. While government agencies, including cancer registries, collect statistics on diseases, including ages of the victims, they do not collect statistics on when women first menstruated or when their menopause began. This kind of information must be obtained either by asking the subjects of the study or their families, or by consulting medical records. It is a time-consuming job, and is subject to various errors, including those that arise from faulty memories. A woman who learns she has breast cancer will want to know why, and think about every possible event in her life that may have exposed her to risks. A woman who does not have the disease may not think as hard about everything she has ever done. This selectivity of memory could make the breast cancer victims seem to have been exposed to more environmental hazards than the control group, when in fact they need not have been.

In a study of whether oral contraceptives increase breast cancer risk, both cases and controls were asked whether they had or had not used the pill. The study found that oral contraceptives increased the risk in younger women by about 25%. The longer the time since the women had been off the pill, the lower their risk became, becoming negligible by the time five years had elapsed since they stopped. In a critical examination of this study, Dr. S. Shapiro of Boston University calculated that if only two percent more of the control women than of the women with breast cancer had forgotten that they had ever used the pill, a large part of the apparent excess risk would disappear.

Dr. Shapiro also noted another kind of error that could make the risk appear larger than it really is. Ever since oral contraceptives were introduced, both doctors and lay people have expressed concern that they might cause cancers, particularly of the breast or uterus. As a result, women on the pill have often been urged to monitor their breasts closely, and they were therefore somewhat more likely to be under closer medical surveillance. Once mammography was introduced, they were more likely to undergo mammographies than other women. Since mammograms detect breast tumors more readily, women who have them done will appear to have a higher incidence rate of breast cancer. It would not take more than a few percent of extra cancers discovered by mammography among contraceptive users compared with nonusers, together with a few percent more women who did not get cancer forgetting that they ever used the pill, to account fully for the slightly higher apparent rate of breast cancer among contraceptive users. Dr. Shapiro did not claim that the small increased risk with contraceptive use is not real, but only warned that small increased apparent risks can result from small differences between the ways women with and without breast cancer remember past behavior or seek medical care.

Scientists, aware of the possibility of such sources of error in epidemiological studies, tend to be skeptical of studies that report small increases in rates of disease, say, up to 25 or 50%, even when the difference is "statistically significant." This is one unfortunate limitation of epidemiological studies. When a disease is a common one, affecting hundreds of thousands of people, an increase in its rate of 25% would be of enormous public health importance. If we were really sure that some preventive measures we could take would reduce its rate this much we would surely take them, even if they were very costly. But typical studies are based on small groups of people and subject to such uncertainties that we are not often sure enough to act. The same considerations came up in the problem of electromagnetic fields and childhood leukemia (chapter 7), where the relative risk of leukemia among children exposed to high residential magnetic fields was about 50%.

Is There a Breast Cancer Epidemic?

Breast cancer has been reported to be more common than it was fifty or a hundred years ago, and some observers have spoken about a breast cancer "epidemic." Is breast cancer increasing throughout the developed world and specifically in the United States? If so, how can we account for it? Could pollution of the environment be responsible?

We are now comparing different time periods rather than different geographical areas. Do changes over time in known risk factors account for the increase or, if they do not, should we conclude that some environmental factors might be causing it? Indeed, over the last 100 years patterns of reproductive choices have changed: average age at birth of a first child has been increasing, as has the proportion of childless women. In addition, age at menarche has been decreasing: it was sixteen in the middle of the nineteenth century in the United States and is thirteen today. Women exercise less than they did fifty years ago, in spite of the impression one might get from the number we see jogging today: one might say electric washers and dryers, as well as disposable diapers, are risk factors for breast cancer.

But other things besides known risk factors may change over time. The way physicians diagnose disease has also changed, as well as the practices involved in assigning and recording causes of death on death certificates, our only source of information about breast cancer in the past. The term "breast cancer" has undergone a continuous process of refinement into a number of subtypes, distinguished by where in the breast the cancer is found, the type of cells involved, and the genetic makeup of those cells. New methods of detection, such as mammography, are discovering cases that in the past might have been missed. Also, we keep better records today: physicians in most states must report new cases of cancer to cancer registries, together with other information about the patient. We have to be aware of these changes when we compare the reported incidence and death rates from breast cancer in the United States in the last several decades.

The reasons for the rise in breast cancer incidence over this time period are not fully understood, but many scientists believe that at least part of the increase is not accounted for by changes in known risk factors, or in medical practice. The search for as yet undiscovered causes therefore continues.

More Breast Cancer in San Francisco?

Women of higher social class and with more education were among the first to request mammography, and not coincidentally a rise in reported incidence took place among them first. The San Francisco Bay area was found in the 1980s to have a significantly higher incidence compared to the U.S. average. A large portion of that excess turned out to be the result of early detection by mammography and mostly disappeared by 1995. The remaining excess can be accounted for almost completely by the known reproductive risk factors: women in San Francisco, being of higher social class, have their children later and so on. The breast cancer "hot spot" on the East Side of Manhattan can most likely be accounted for by the higher social class of its residents.

Does Mammography Increase Breast Cancer Rates?

A physician discovering a breast cancer must report it to the local cancer registry, together with the stage of the cancer: is it in an early, more treatable, stage or a later stage? The proportion of early-stage cancers among the reported breast cancer cases in San Francisco after mammography was introduced was larger than the proportion of early-stage cancers found before, showing that mammography was detecting cases earlier. Further evidence is that after an early increase following the introduction of mammography, the incidence rate decreased to about what it was previous to that introduction, but the proportion of late-stage cancers reported among cases of breast cancer at first diagnosis has remained lower, as has the death rate.

It is common for the rate of incidence of a disease to rise when a new, more sensitive method of screening a large population is introduced, but not because in any real sense there is more of the disease. An even more dramatic rise in prostate cancer among men followed the introduction of a specific blood test for this condition. Previously such cancers could be detected only when they were large enough to be felt by the physician during a rectal examination. The new test for prostate cancer is not an unmixed blessing: it detects life-threatening cancers but also responds to the presence of cancerous cells in the prostate glands of many older men who would never have developed a clinical case of prostate cancer in their lifetime. These men may be now subject to considerable anxiety and the possibility of strenuous and debilitating treatment. Autopsies done on men over the age of seventy who have died of other causes have shown that more than half of them have cancerous cells in their prostate glands. It is not known whether they would have developed a clinical case of prostate cancer if they had lived longer.

How Much Do the Risk Factors Explain?

We have described the considerable attention given to high breast cancer rates in three areas in the United States: Long Island, Cape Cod, and the San Francisco area.

The excess breast cancer incidence in San Francisco turned out to be accounted for by the known risk factors, together with the effect of mammography on incidence. This is not to say that the rate in San Francisco is "normal" and nothing can be done about it. We still do not know what causes breast cancer in each individual case, either in San Francisco or anywhere else. All we can say is that if exposures to any environmental agent whatever are causing it to be high in the United States, the women of San Francisco appear to be exposed to the same extent as all the other women of comparable social class in the United States.

If the social class of people living on both Long Island and Cape Cod is higher than the U.S. average, then it is to be expected that at least some of the excess would be explained in the same way as in San Francisco. The scientists doing the Long Island study are investigating how much of the excess rate there can be accounted for by the known risk factors, but have not yet reported their results. Adjustment of the breast cancer rate for them on Cape Cod is not yet completed. We have mentioned the preliminary results from the Harvard School of Public Health, which suggest that there is indeed an excess of about 20% among women over 50, with a 95% confidence interval from 4% to 42%. This result did not include the effect of mammographic screening.

To conclude this discussion, when we find more cancer in one place than another and want to know why, we must first see if known risk factors can account for the difference. But we must be aware that correcting for them is a difficult process, and the results are subject to considerable uncertainty. Will the 15–20% excesses in breast cancer rates on Long Island and Cape Cod turn out to be explained by such factors? Even if not, are they so large, given the range of uncertainty in correcting for them, that they should be taken seriously as clues to as yet undiscovered environmental causes? These are questions on which scientists might well disagree.

SUMMARY

The known risk factors for breast cancer, many of them related to the reproductive life of women, are for the most part not under their control. These risk factors have suggested the idea that the greater a woman's exposure to her own estrogens, the greater her risk of breast cancer. In turn, certain chemical pollutants in the environment, such as pesticides, seem to act like weak estrogens, raising the question whether exposure to them is a factor in breast cancer. It may also provide a clue to why certain areas of the United States have above-average breast cancer rates. Studies have been started, in response to the demands of activists, on Long Island and Cape Cod, where breast cancer rates are high and where it is believed that residents have had considerable exposure to pesticides.

In the next chapter we will summarize the evidence from epidemiological studies on possible relations between pesticides and breast cancer, and describe other studies now in progress, among whose goals are to find what factors not yet known might be involved in breast cancer, and what can be done to avoid them.

A CLOSER LOOK: CHEMICALS IN THE ENVIRONMENT

In the modern world we are exposed to chemical substances—hundreds of thousands of them—that were newly created in this or the previous century. The substances found to show hormonal activity, and that are therefore under suspicion as possible factors in breast cancer, can be classified by their chemical names—organochlorines or alkyl phenols, for example—or by what they are used for—pesticides, plasticizers, or detergents. Pesticides are of particular concern because they are present not only in the fruit and vegetables we eat but in the meat of exposed animals that are part of our diet.

Only a small fraction of the 15,000 organochlorines in common use are pesticides, and not all pesticides are organochlorines. For that matter, some industrial products that show hormonal activity are neither organochlorines nor pesticides. They include components of common household detergents, and chemicals added to plastics to improve their mechanical properties ("plasticizers"). Plasticizers do escape from plastics over time and can be found in food or water stored in plastic containers. Last and not least, there are real estrogens in the environment, either natural estrogens or those from pharmaceuticals such as the birth control pill and compounds given as postmenopausal hormone therapy, that are excreted in urine and may eventually find their way into drinking water.

Organochlorines

Organochlorines are compounds composed of the elements carbon (which is what chemists mean by the term "organic"), chlorine, and, usually, hydrogen. There may or may not be other elements such as oxygen in the compound. They have all sorts of uses in industry, commerce, and homes; as raw materials for industrial syntheses and as solvents for dry-cleaning and for removal of oil-based paints. The common plastic polyvinyl chloride is an organochlorine, as is the pesticide DDT and the mixture of substances known as PCB, once used as a pesticide and fungicide, and as a flame-retardant in children's clothing. Many organochlorines are carcinogenic in animals, causing tumors of the liver and other organs, but not of the mammary glands. DDT, in particular, produces liver tumors.

The class of substances known as dioxins, almost always a mixture of many chemically similar substances, occur as contaminants in other industrial organochlorines and as a product of their combustion. There is evidence that dioxins are carcinogenic, but they also have antiestrogenic activity and have been shown to reduce the risk of mammary tumors in rodents. Two common dioxins bear the acronyms TCDD and PCDD, one letter D in each term standing for "dioxin."

Many of these substances as prepared for commercial use are not single compounds but mixtures of a number of different compounds that are chemically similar but not identical. Estrogenic activity, and hormonal activity in general, is highly specific to particular molecules: a slight change in chemical structure may make a big difference. PCB is a mixture of over two hundred different chlorinated biphenyls; some show estrogenic activity, some are antiestrogens, and some are inactive. We cannot assume that molecules that are chemically similar act like each other in living organisms and, in particular, have the same influence on the development of breast cancer. One molecule may act as a promoter, and a very similar one may inhibit promotion of cancer.

One important property of organochlorines is that they dissolve more readily in fats or oils than in water. This means that when they are absorbed in the body, they are preferentially stored in fat tissues, from which they are slowly released to the blood. Hence, there is a balance between their concentrations in fat tissues and in the blood. Since chemical analysis can detect them at very low concentrations, the total amount in the body can usually be estimated from tests on blood. The fact that they dissolve in fat also provides a mechanism by which humans are exposed to them through the diet: cows grazing on contaminated grass concentrate organochlorines in their fatty tissue and in the fat of milk, and we eat beef and drink milk.

Polyaromatic Hydrocarbons

Polyaromatic hydrocarbons, referred to by the abbreviation PAH, are a class of substances that have chemical structures that resemble some of the sex hormones. In spite of this resemblance, it is not yet clear whether they are hormone mimickers. One in particular, benz-alpha-pyrene, is a mammary carcinogen in laboratory animals but is not hormonally active; it is carcinogenic by some other mechanism. PAHs in general are known to be direct carcinogens, causing types of cancer unrelated to estrogen activity. They are present in coal and other fossil fuels and are emitted to the air in the form of small particles when such fuels are burnt in the internal combustion engines of cars and trucks, particularly from diesel engines. They occur also in cigarette smoke, and traces of them are found in foods.

Substances from Detergents and Plastics

Certain detergents or breakdown products of detergents, known as alkyl phenols, are also hormonally active. They differ chemically from organochlorines or PAHs, being compounds of carbon, oxygen, and hydrogen, and are more soluble in water rather than in fat. Because they are used for washing dishes and laundry, traces of them remain after rinsing, and they show up in the groundwater and sometimes in the water supply.

Ironically, additional xenoestrogens were discovered in the course of developing tests for estrogenic activity. Plastic tubes used in the laboratory were found to release small quantities of plasticizers that had considerable estrogenic strength. Plasticizers are added to plastics during manufacture because they improve the mechanical properties of the final product. They are also compounds of carbon, oxygen, and hydrogen, and most of them are derivatives of a substance called phthalic acid.

From Plants and Vegetables

There are substances having weak estrogenic activity that occur naturally in plants and vegetables. These are called "phytoestrogens," *phyto* being a Greek root meaning "plant." They are common in the fruits and vegetables we eat and are believed to be protective against certain cancers, including breast and colon cancer.

The Future of the Xenoestrogen Hypothesis

The epidemiological studies carried out so far on the xenoestrogen hypothesis have tested only a few substances known to be hormonally active, specifically DDT and PCBs. A much larger number of substances present in the environment have been shown to have such activity in laboratory tests, a number so large as to be daunting.

The National Research Council committee, which wrote a report on hormonally active substances and breast cancer we quote from in the next chapter, recommended the use and further development of laboratory tests of hormonal activity.

Tests on laboratory animals are time-consuming and therefore expensive to do. Alternate tests on living cell cultures in vitro (in glass vessels) have been devised. In one such test, for example, a substance is classed as a xenoestrogen if it promotes cell proliferation in cell lines taken from breast cancers.

Such tests can be done not only on suspected individual chemicals but also on the complex mixtures of substances that we find in the environment, mixtures in which many of the ingredients are not yet identified and which may act differently (synergistically) when they are together from what one would expect knowing how they act alone.

Given the extraordinary number of hormonally active chemicals in the environment that laboratory tests have discovered and the high cost of doing epidemiological studies, it is urgent that some criteria of selection be set up, some way to pick plausible candidates to look at. Certainly, one such criterion, perhaps the first to use, should be how much estrogenic activity a substance shows in the laboratory.

While there is no single generally accepted screening system to estimate estrogenic activity, the combined result of several tests could serve to provide a rough-and-ready separation of the tested substances into two classes: those worth investigating further, and those that for the time being should be disregarded.

To summarize briefly, hormonal activity has been demonstrated in a number of compounds that are not hormones and are found in the environment. Among them are plasticizers, pesticides, and some additives in commercial household products. Some of them persist in the body and can be detected long after exposure, others are metabolized and excreted quickly. They have not for the most part been shown to be mammary carcinogens in animals. The few that have been studied in humans have not been shown to play an important role in breast cancer.

6

BREAST CANCER, PART 2:
TESTING THE PESTICIDE HYPOTHESIS

A NEW APPROACH

We do not yet know how much of the excess rates of breast cancer on Long Island or on Cape Cod will ultimately be explained by the known risk factors. We do know that pesticides have been sprayed in both these areas, and toxic chemicals carelessly disposed in them. Has breast cancer been increased by such exposures? The studies in progress on Long Island and Cape Cod are not the only ones that have tried to answer this question: a number of completed studies, carried out in other locations, have also done so, and we will describe them in this chapter.

These studies rely to a considerable extent on recent discoveries in molecular biology. This rapidly advancing field has already contributed enormously to our understanding of cancer as well as other diseases, and it will contribute even more in the future. We have learned from it how to identify certain individuals who have genetic sensitivities to particular environmental agents. It may in some cases provide means to determine which environmental hazards have caused a particular case of cancer, from the genetic makeup of the cancer cells. With knowledge of that genetic makeup, physicians who treat cancer are helped to choose the most effective therapy in any given case of the disease, without having to go through a process of trial and error. Future research into the causes, prevention, and treatment of cancer and other diseases, whether in the clinic, the research laboratory, or in the epidemiological field study, will rely more and more on the perspectives and techniques of molecular biology.

We will review briefly some of the basic concepts of this field before we describe the studies, completed or in progress, of environmental agents and breast cancer.

MOLECULAR BIOLOGY OF CANCER

Who Is Susceptible?

In general, even when dramatic increases in the rate of some disease have been clearly linked to an environmental agent, only a fraction of the people exposed ever suffer the disease. Most people who survived the bombing of Hiroshima and Nagasaki have not suffered health effects from their radiation exposure. Cigarette smoking causes 90% of lung cancer today, but only 10% of heavy smokers will die of lung cancer. It is reasonable to conclude that people differ in sensitivity, most probably reflecting genetic differences. Both environmental and genetic factors must interact to produce the disease.

There are certain genes that confer a very high risk of breast cancer, but only 5–10% of breast cancer is believed to be due to them. In addition, genetic sensitivities to environmental agents that play a less dramatic role have been identified, and more may be discovered. These and other aspects of the molecular biology of cancer are increasingly important factors in breast cancer research. What determines genetic sensitivity, and what is a gene?

What Is a Gene?

The inheritance of organisms—tomato plants, mice, or people—depends upon DNA molecules in the cell nucleus (DNA is an abbreviation of the chemical name of the molecules), each such molecule containing "instructions" for making all of the proteins that the organism needs to function. The portion of the DNA molecule that carries the instructions for making a particular protein is called a gene. Estimates of the number of genes in human DNA have varied; currently, with the decipherment of the human genome completed, it has been found that there are 30–35,000 genes.

One of the essential properties of the DNA molecule is that it can be copied: with the aid of enzymes in the cell another DNA molecule carrying exactly the same instructions can be made, using the original DNA molecule as a template, somewhat as a photographic negative can be used to make a positive transparency, which, in turn, can be used to produce a new negative. This takes place during cell division, permitting each of the two daughter cells to have DNA molecules identical to the DNA molecules of the original cell.

Another time the DNA is copied is when a protein is made according to the DNA instructions. First, a chemical signal, a specific molecule, must attach itself to the DNA molecule next to the gene itself, to permit the copying of the instructions from the DNA for making the protein. The copying process involves producing a new molecule, similar to DNA, called RNA, put together with the help of enzymes from smaller molecules available in the cell. Only a short section of the DNA need be copied to make the protein, so the RNA is a much smaller molecule than DNA. This RNA molecule then wanders to a site in the cell where proteins are synthesized according to the instructions copied, with the help of other enzymes. When the whole process ending in the production of the desired protein molecule has taken place, the gene is said to have been "expressed."

Mutations: How Cancer Gets Started

Occasionally a DNA molecule in one particular cell is damaged. Such damage may occur as a result of exposure to toxic chemicals or to ionizing radiation, but also can occur spontaneously, because all molecules are in constant motion at ordinary temperatures, and sometimes the motion is energetic enough to break them down. The DNA is most vulnerable during cell division, when it is being duplicated to provide DNA for each of two daughter cells. Sometimes damage can be repaired by the cell, and at other times it is so severe the cell dies, but sometimes neither extreme occurs: the cell survives damaged, and when it divides it passes on its damaged DNA to the two daughter cells produced. When this happens, the cell is said to have undergone a mutation.

Among the many proteins that the genes of normal human cells carry instructions for are proteins that tell the cell when to divide, or that regulate the process of cell division, or that repair damaged DNA, or that determine when the cell dies. As a result of mutations in the corresponding genes, the cell may fail to produce some of the needed proteins, or it may produce the "wrong" protein, one chemically altered from the normal protein the undamaged gene codes for. There are also mutations that cause the cell to make too much of a normal protein. In any case the way the cell functions is altered. Such cells and their descendants may thus gain a reproductive or a survival advantage over ordinary cells; this is the first step—called initiation—in the process of carcinogenesis. The reproductive advantage benefits the mutated cell line, but harms the organism.

The "Multistep" Process of Carcinogenesis: Fingerprinting the Disease

One mutation is never enough, however, to produce "cancer". Carcinogenesis is said to be a "multistep" process: it usually requires six or seven different mutations, each conferring an additional small reproductive advantage to the cell line or removing natural limits on how long the cells live, before the cells grow sufficiently out of control to produce a clinical case of the disease.

Current techniques of molecular biology permit us to detect the presence of many of the genes in the DNA of any organism, and to distinguish between the normal form of the gene and a mutated one. This means that to some extent we can now distinguish which mutations have occurred in a particular case of cancer, and our ability to do so will increase as time goes on, which has important practical considerations for both the study and the treatment of the disease. When a physician diagnoses a case of breast cancer, the diagnosis is always more specific than "breast cancer": the most common diagnosis currently in the United States is "neoplasm of the ductal epithelium," which accounts for about 90% of cases. As we noted earlier, the development of a clinical case of cancer usually requires six or seven mutations. There are more than one set of possible mutations that can give rise to a case of "neoplasm of the ductal epithelium," which means that with the aid of molecular biology we can distinguish different patterns of mutated genes in different cases of what we have previously considered a single disease.

The mutational pattern observed in the cells of any one tumor may reflect both particular exposures to environmental agents or individual sensitivities to them. Genetic fingerprints of exposures to environmental agents causing a few cancers are known, such as exposure to aflatoxin, a naturally occurring liver carcinogen; to vinyl chloride, an industrially produced liver carcinogen; and to ultraviolet light, an initiator of various skin cancers. Being able to "read" the history of environmental exposures in each case of cancer would provide epidemiology with a precise and powerful tool. By analogy to the term "molecular biology" this new approach can be called "molecular epidemiology." As an example, in some but not all breast cancers a particular gene called the p53 gene is defective. This gene is called a tumor suppressor gene; when it functions properly it codes for a protein that prevents damaged DNA from being duplicated.

Another of the practical consequences is that the particular pattern of mutations in a case of the disease may determine how the disease will respond to treatment. One genetic difference among breast cancer tumors is the number of "estrogen receptors" in the cells. Estrogen receptors are protein molecules that bind to hormone molecules that enter the cell. The resulting complex of receptor and hormone activates a gene carrying instructions for making a protein that induces cell proliferation in the breast tissue. The cells of breast tumors do differ in how many receptor molecules they have, so the individual cells are classed as "receptor positive" or "receptor negative." Those tumors in which more than 10% of the cells are receptor positive are classed as "receptor positive" tumors. It is the receptor positive tumors that respond well to the drug tamoxifen (fig. 6-1).

Nature and Nurture in Cancer Risk

The overwhelming majority of human genes are identical in all individuals on the planet. We would not be members of the same species if they were not. A small minority of genes do differ from one person to another, which is why some of us are men and others women, why we do not all look alike, and why we do not have the same sensitivities to foods, allergens, or environmental agents. The different forms of a gene that occur naturally in human populations are called "polymorphisms." The less common and usually disadvantageous genes are often called "variants." It follows that genes predisposing to cancer not only come into existence by mutation during the life of the individual, but also may be inherited from his or her parents. The DNA of any individual is a combination of portions of the DNA of mother and father: each cell has two copies of each gene, one from each parent. Most of the time both genes are identical, and code for the same protein, but sometimes the two genes differ. One or the other may predominate, and the individual's body will function much as though both genes were the same as the dominant one. Sometimes, however, both exert an influence.

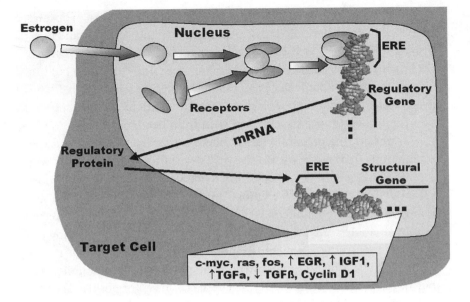

FIGURE 6-1 An estrogen molecule entering the nucleus cannot bind to DNA and lead to the expression of a protein unless it binds to two estrogen receptor molecules first. The bound complex then can attach to the DNA. Figure prepared by Professor Andrew Rundle, Columbia University, and used with his permission.

This matters tremendously if either or both genes involve sensitivities that predispose to cancer. There is a particular gene that makes an enzyme that repairs damaged DNA, known as the AT gene. It is not common to have a defective version of this gene, and it is very uncommon for an individual to have both genes defective. The unfortunate rare individuals that do suffer a condition called ataxia-telangiectasia, characterized by muscular dysfunction and immunodeficiency. Its victims have an unusually high risk of cancer. The individuals who have one defective gene and one normal one are at a somewhat higher risk of cancer than people who do not have this gene defect and are thought to be more sensitive to radiation.

Two genes (designated BRCA1 and BRCA2) have been discovered with rare polymorphisms that strongly predispose to breast cancer: of the women who have either variant gene, half will develop breast cancer by the age of 70. There are two known variants of BRCA1 and one variant of BRCA2 that are predisposing. The variants occur in only one woman in a thousand in general, but among Jewish women of European (Ashkenazic) ancestry 25 in a thousand do. Because of their rarity the variant genes are believed to be responsible for only a few percent of cases.

Other Genetic Susceptibilities

There are other genetically based sensitivities that increase a person's cancer risk only slightly, but because they are much more common may have a significant effect on cancer incidence rates. Enzymes are proteins that speed up certain chemical reactions. In particular there are "detoxifying" enzymes that speed up ("catalyze") the chemical alteration of foreign toxic substances, to make them easier for the body to excrete. Other enzymes govern the synthesis and metabolism of estrogens. Some individuals may have detoxifying enzymes that do not function as well, or that metabolize estrogens to products that promote considerable growth of breast tissue. Individuals with such genetic traits would be at greater risk of cancer. For example, smoking is not a risk factor for breast cancer in most women. It has been reported that a small subgroup of women have a variant gene, perhaps involving a faulty detoxifying enzyme, that increases the risk of breast cancer if they smoke. Women with this defective gene who are heavy smokers have been reported to have a much higher risk of breast cancer than do heavily smoking women without it. (Of course, heavy smokers without this defective gene still have a greatly increased risk of lung cancer.)

There is one particular set of genes that are believed to play a role in many other cancers as well as breast cancer. These genes, known as cytochrome P450 genes, code for the production of a number of detoxifying enzymes. Unfortunately, sometimes this "detoxification" converts a noncarcinogenic substance into a carcinogen. There are a number of variant forms of the P450 genes that are fairly common in human populations, which may account for an individual sensitivity to environmental toxins. The frequency of occurrence of the variant genes, normally a few percent of the population, does sometimes differ between different ethnic groups.

Some less common genetic variations are protective rather than predisposing: while nursing a baby has been reported to be protective against breast cancer, recent research suggests that it may be so only among women who have a particular less common form of a certain gene.

Estrogens and Promotion of Cancer

Not all the events in the progression of cancer are mutations. There are certain substances that do not cause mutations directly, but create the conditions under which mutations are more likely. Cells are more vulnerable to mutation when during the course of cell division, the DNA molecules are being duplicated to provide DNA for the two daughter cells being formed. There are occasions when rapid proliferation of cells takes place in one organ or another. Sometimes this is part of the normal function of the body, as when hormones speed up development of breast tissue in puberty or pregnancy. Sometimes it is what happens in response to a toxic chemical or a virus infection that destroys cells, either of the skin or of a vital organ. The body compensates for the damage by turning on the mechanisms that induce cell division in the damaged area, but unfortunately in doing so increases the risk of mutation, and hence of cancer. Both hepatitis and heavy alcohol consumption damage liver cells and are risk factors for liver cancer.

Substances that are not mutagens but increase the opportunity for cancerous mutations in this manner are called "promoters." Their action can be demonstrated in the laboratory on animals that are either genetically susceptible to cancer or else have been previously exposed to cancer-causing mutagens: when exposed to promoters they develop more tumors, or develop them faster. Estrogens act as promoters in cancer, rather than as direct carcinogens.

The first mutational event that starts a cell line on the path that leads ultimately to cancer is called "initiation." Cancers in humans usually require decades after initiation, decades needed for the additional mutations that convert a slight reproductive advantage into an overwhelming one. Provided initiation has already occurred to create a precancerous state of affairs, promotion can convert it very rapidly into a clinical case of the disease.

Estrogen Receptors and Breast Cancer

That estrogens, which enable a woman's reproductive system to function, should also play a role in causing cancer, is part of the tragedy of cancer itself. Cancer is a disease in which the capacity of organisms to adapt to change through evolution is turned against the organism and, unchecked, destroys it. Estrogens stimulate maturation and proliferation of breast cells and of the cells that line the uterus; that is their job, but during proliferation cells are more vulnerable to mutations. As cells mature they differentiate to become, for example, muscle cells, liver cells, or breast cells. Breast cells in childhood and to some extent in adulthood before the birth of a first child are immature and are more susceptible to DNA damage than differentiated cells. An example of the sensitivity of immature cells is the greatly increased risk of breast cancer, many years later, to young girls exposed to ionizing radiation.

Estrogens, like most sex hormones, are smaller molecules than proteins, and unlike proteins are more soluble in fat than water. Before menopause they are formed mostly in the ovaries, and afterward mostly in fat tissue, and have to travel through the blood system to reach the breasts. Once they enter a breast cell they must bind to a protein molecule called a receptor to start the process leading to the expression of a target gene, for example, the production of a protein signal for breast cell proliferation. The effectiveness of the drug tamoxifen in preventing recurrences of breast cancer after surgery or other treatment, and its use as a breast cancer preventive for women at high risk, is related to its ability to bind to the estrogen receptors in breast cancer cells. It is believed that the tamoxifen, by binding to the receptor, blocks the binding of the body's own estrogens. Although all normal breast cells have estrogen receptors, only about 60% of breast cancer tumors are receptor-positive, and those are the cancers that the drug works for. This percentage is an average over all ages of breast cancer victims; older victims have a higher proportion of receptor-positive tumors. Fortunately, there are simple laboratory tests to determine whether a tumor is receptor-positive. Whether the cells of a particular breast tumor are or are not receptor-positive is determined by the particular mutational sequence causing the tumor.

Molecular Biology and Pesticides

We can now suggest what impact molecular biology might have on research on cancer generally and breast cancer specifically, and more specifically, on testing the xenoestrogen hypothesis.

First of all, we should be able to classify breast cancer more and more according to the particular patterns of mutations and variant genes associated with each case, which will make it possible to distinguish the roles of different kinds of exposures, different risk factors, and different genetic sensitivities. Some mutations have already been shown to result from particular exposures, and no doubt more will be discovered as time goes on.

Molecular biology has a role in cancer therapy through its ability to distinguish the particular mutational pattern in individual cases of cancer. How well a cancer responds to any one kind of treatment depends on this particular pattern. One example is the use of tamoxifen to prevent recurrence of cancer after receptor-positive breast tumors have been surgically removed. The possibility of selecting the optimal treatment in advance without having to go through a trial-and-error process with a potentially fatal disease is a great blessing when there are available treatments to choose from.

STUDIES ON HUMAN BEINGS

Pesticides: Who Has Been Exposed?

Now we turn to tests of the hypothesis that exposures to pesticides or other chemicals that may be hormonally active are responsible for a certain proportion of breast cancers. To do such tests requires that we compare the exposures to these chemicals of women who have gotten breast cancer with the exposures of women who have not.

Exposures to potentially toxic chemicals are usually much greater in workplaces, and convincing evidence of harm easier to come by. We have mentioned some examples in other chapters: asbestos as a cause of cancer of the lining of the lung cavity, aromatic amines in bladder cancer, vinyl chloride in liver sarcoma, benzene causing leukemia in shoe-manufacturing workers, melanoma and leukemia among radiologists exposed to X-rays.

Women have only recently entered the workforce in large numbers and are still underrepresented in blue-collar jobs in chemical industries. Studies have not yet consistently shown any breast cancer risk associated with a particular kind of work. In particular, studies so far of women employed in agricultural occupations in which pesticides were used, or who worked in plants where pesticides or polychlorinated biphenyls (PCBs) were manufactured, have not shown any elevated breast cancer risk. However, the numbers of women in such occupations has so far been too small to detect anything but extremely large effects, and no large effects have yet been found. Studies of women exposed to pesticides because they either live in farming areas or work on farms are now in progress, and results on them should be available soon. One such study will be described in a later section of this chapter.

The Estrogen Connection: Pharmaceutical Estrogens

In the preceding chapter we discussed the hypothesis that a woman's exposure to her own estrogens throughout life increases her risk of breast cancer, and the more speculative hypothesis that pesticides and other chemicals in the environment may increase that risk further because they produce some of the same effects in the body as the natural estrogens. It is worth asking if synthetic estrogens women take as medication, although they are not identical to those produced in the body, increase breast cancer risk.

Two types of synthetic estrogens taken by large numbers of women have been carefully studied for possible cancer risks: birth control pills and hormone-replacement estrogens used to control some of the unpleasant effects of menopause. Since these synthetic estrogens have similar activity to the natural estrogens produced by the body, their effects on breast cancer rates are of particular interest.

A number of studies have reported an increased risk of about 20–30% in women who have used the birth control pill for at least ten years, compared to nonusers of the same age. We discussed in the previous chapter the view of one scientist that even this small effect may not be real, but could be an artifact of biases in the studies—differences between the way breast cancer victims and healthy controls remember their use of medication, and differences in how often they get breast examinations.

When hormone-replacement therapy was first used with postmenopausal women, estrogen alone was used. There was an abrupt increase in the rate of endometrial cancer (the endometrium is the lining of the uterus), which was eventually attributed to this use of estrogen. The therapy was changed to include progestin, a steroidal hormone that counteracts some, but not all, of the effects of estrogen, and the endometrial cancer rate dropped to its previous level. Studies of women taking hormone replacement therapy for ten or more years showed an increased risk of breast cancer of about 30%, which did not change much when progestin was added to the medication (many women who use the medication do so for only one or two years). It is possible that some of this increase is a result of more intensive medical surveillance of women taking the medication, just as with women using oral contraceptives. An increase of 30% in breast cancer among postmenopausal women, whose breast cancer rate is already high, would be a serious matter. Some positive benefits of hormonal replacement therapy that were not originally anticipated have been reported: a reduction in osteoporosis, and a possible decrease in the risk of Alzheimer's disease.

Dioxins, Pesticides, and Industrial Accidents

A major accident occurred in Seveso, Italy, in 1976, involving a dioxin compound known as TCDD (fig. 6-2). A study of the heavily exposed population published in 1993 did not find any significant increase in breast cancer, or for that matter in any other cancers, but the time elapsed since the accident has not been long enough to rule out a definite effect of exposure on cancer rates. It is interesting that dioxin actually shows anti-estrogenic activity in laboratory tests, and perhaps no increase of breast cancer should be expected. There is some weak evidence, not statistically significant, that dioxin exposure actually reduces the risk.

An accidental contamination of cattle feed with polybrominated biphenyls (PBB) took place in Michigan in 1973. Thousands of people were exposed through eating contaminated meat and dairy products. A study in 1991 of over three thousand exposed individuals showed that no elevation of cancer rates, including breast cancer, had yet occurred. Polybrominated biphenyls are chemically similar to PCBs, except that they contain bromine rather than chlorine. They have not been studied for hormonal activity.

Pesticides and the Rest of Us

People not employed in the pesticide industry, or not exposed unwittingly as a result of industrial disasters, are not exposed to large quantities of pesticides or other chemical agents, but there are, after all, many more such people. Even if the risk from low exposure is small, so many are exposed that a large total number of cases of breast cancer could result. Women are exposed through their use of garden products like weed killers and plant insecticides, by various other household products like roach or rodent poisons, or by aerial spraying for mosquitoes or agricultural pests.

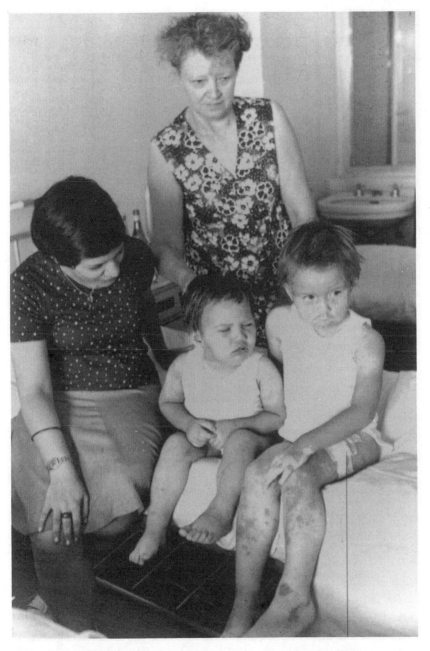

FIGURE 6-2 Children exposed to dioxins and other chemicals as a result of an industrial accident in Seveso, Italy, in 1976. These chemicals typically produce skin rashes in exposed individuals, clearly visible on the legs of the children. Copyright Bettman/Corbis.

To find out whether they have been harmed by such exposures, we need to compare exposed groups with control groups of lesser or preferably no exposure. Because the exposures of the general population to pesticides are usually relatively low, only a small number of cases could result, unless the exposed group is extremely large. As breast cancer will occur anyway in an unexposed population—no one has ever seriously suggested that all breast cancer is a result of chemicals in the environment—we face the usual problem of detecting a small excess number of cases in the exposed group. To study very large groups is very, very expensive.

Epidemiologists have developed the "case-control" study to get around this difficulty. Instead of asking if there is more breast cancer in a group of exposed women than in a group of unexposed women, they ask if there has been more exposure in a group of breast cancer victims than in a similar group of women without breast cancer. It is far easier and cheaper to start by identifying 200 women with the disease and a few hundred without it for comparison, than it is to identify 200,000 women who have been exposed to DDT and compare the number of breast cancer cases among them with the number among 200,000 less exposed women. (We say "less exposed" rather than "unexposed" deliberately. Chemical analysis for DDT is very sensitive, and has shown that it is ubiquitous in the environment, though usually at very low concentrations.)

Exposure to Pesticides and Risk

In a case-control study, one starts by selecting cases of the disease from some specific population, for example, all cases diagnosed in a certain community or by a certain hospital. Then one compares their exposures to the exposures of a "control" group of people without the disease, but from the same population, that is, from the same community or using the same hospital but not having gotten the particular disease. This makes it more likely that both cases and controls are similar. The ideal is that the two groups should be similar with respect to the known risk factors for the disease, a requirement that is easier to state than to satisfy. If we find that women with breast cancer have been more exposed to DDT than the control group of women without breast cancer, we can then say that there is an "association" between exposure to DDT and the disease.

In a number of case-control studies, exposure to DDT or to PCBs has been measured either in the blood or in the fat tissue of cases and controls. DDT exposure is usually estimated from the concentration in the blood of DDE, a chemical formed by metabolic breakdown of DDT in the body. Fortunately, blood levels of DDE usually give a good estimate of total body DDE.

The results of such studies have not been very consistent. Some showed higher exposure to DDT or the other organochlorines tested for among the breast cancer victims than the controls, and some did not. Questions have been raised about these studies. In many of them known risk factors, such as lactation or body weight, were not fully corrected for. In most of them, the number of cases is so small that chance cannot be ruled out as a factor (see discussion of statistical power in chapter 8).

It is also possible that a high DDT level might be a result of treatment for, rather than a cause of, the disease. Sometimes the blood analysis was done after treatment for the cancer had begun, and radical treatments might have drastic effects on metabolism. The conflicting results of these studies, and the flaws critics have noted, do not mean they have been useless. They have at least pointed to ways of improving the design of later studies.

Getting a Better Handle on Past Exposures

Case-control studies are sometimes done by "piggy-backing" them on to studies started for other, more general, purposes. A study may begin not with cases of a particular disease but rather with a young and healthy group of people, whose health and whose lifestyle factors (childbearing, exercise, diet, etc.) will be monitored at intervals over a long time period. As time passes, individuals in the group get various diseases: forms of cancer, heart and vascular conditions, diabetes, and so on. It is possible to look at factors that play a role in the onset of the diseases long before the individuals get sick, because the members of the group have been under surveillance before these conditions appeared. Blood samples, for example, may be taken at frequent intervals and frozen for long periods, so that tests not yet invented or not yet recognized as important to do at the start of the study can be done later. In particular, women in the group who develop breast cancer can have past exposures to organochlorines determined from the frozen blood samples, to compare with women in the group who did not develop breast cancer. This type of case-control study is said to be "nested" in the broader study.

The first such study on the possible relation between organochloride exposure and breast cancer was carried out by Dr. Mary Wolff and associates on a group of some 15,000 participants in a women's health study of diet, hormones, and breast cancer. These women were to have mammograms at regular intervals as part of the study, and blood samples were taken when they had their first mammograms. Fifty-eight women in the group were diagnosed with breast cancer within six months after they entered the study. The stored blood samples of these cancer victims, and of women in the same study who had not gotten breast cancer in this time interval, were analyzed for DDE and PCB. The controls had been chosen to match the cases in age and some other factors, and further corrections were made for differences in other risk factors, such as family history of breast cancer, age at birth of first child, and lactation history. There was a statistically significant correlation between DDE blood levels and breast cancer, but not for PCB.

In a number of such studies, blood samples frozen years before the diagnosis of breast cancer are available. Examples include a study of nurses carried out by Harvard University scientists, going on for almost a quarter of a century, and a study of members of a large health maintenance organization, the Kaiser-Permanente group in California. The Harvard nurses study began in 1976 with 120,000 married registered nurses from eleven states, who filled out questionnaires every two years thereafter, reporting their health status and other relevant factors. A large subgroup of them gave blood samples in 1989 or 1990 that were frozen at the time. By 1992, 240 of the women who had given blood samples had developed breast cancer. Their blood levels of DDE (a metabolite of DDT) and PCB taken years before the onset of disease were compared to levels in a control group selected from nurses in the group who had not developed breast cancer, but were otherwise comparable, by the known risk factors, to the nurses who did. The results were negative: there was no excess of DDE or PCB in the blood of the cases compared with the controls.

In the study of members of the Kaiser-Permanente Group in California, 150 cases of breast cancer were selected, 50 of whom were Caucasian, 50 African-American, and 50 of Asian ancestry. In the group as a whole, there was no relation between breast cancer risk and levels of DDE or PCB in blood samples taken prior to diagnosis. The Caucasian and African-American cases showed greater DDE levels and the Asian group showed lower DDE levels than control groups, but the authors of the paper regarded these differences as not of significance. The point is controversial; other scientists believe the excess exposure among the Caucasian and African-American women who got breast cancer should be taken seriously.

Harmful, Yes, but Do They Cause Breast Cancer?

A committee of the National Research Council evaluated whether hormonally active agents in the environment are causing breast cancer and other diseases of the reproductive system and summarized the evidence on breast cancer from a number of epidemiological studies in a preliminary report published in 1999.

> These studies [of breast cancer] have included large numbers of women and employed internal dose measurements of exposure. In these studies, DDE and PCB's were measured in blood or adipose [fatty] tissue collected from the subjects at varying time intervals before the diagnosis of breast cancer, thus accounting for varying exposure windows and latency periods. . . . These studies do not support an association between DDE and PCB's and cancer in humans.

The committee did recommend additional case-control studies, including a greater use of biological markers of exposure, to finally settle the question.

While the committee concluded that the evidence for a link between breast cancer and those hormonally active agents that have been studied is weak, it stated strongly that such agents in the environment are not harmless. There is evidence, from studies on human populations accidentally exposed to them, on wildlife, and on laboratory animals, that prenatal exposures cause developmental defects, particularly of the reproductive system but also of the nervous system, low birth weight, and IQ and memory deficits.

What Next in Breast Cancer Research?

Studies of women with breast cancer have not offered much support for the hypothesis that xenoestrogens in the environment are responsible for a significant proportion of breast cancer cases. However, some scientists feel that the question is not yet closed. They point out that only a limited number of hormonally active substances, out of the many hundreds known to be in the environment, have been tested. Unfortunately, when one considers the cost and time required for those studies that have been done, doing hundreds more is clearly impossible. Some way is needed to choose a limited number of them as plausible candidates for a link with breast cancer, perhaps by testing which have the greatest estrogenic activity or promote cancer in laboratory animals. As an alternative, tests are being developed to determine the total hormonal activity of the complex mixtures of substances that occur in the environment, without attempting, at least at first, to distinguish which components of the mixture are responsible for any activity found.

Other scientists who study breast cancer believe that the evidence for hormonally active agents or other environmental factors is weak and that the focus of research should be on lifestyle factors related to reproduction, and on the molecular biology of the body's own sex hormones and how they act in the body to increase the risk of the disease.

STUDIES IN PROGRESS

Introduction

The studies of breast cancer on Long Island, mandated by Congress and administered by the National Institutes of Health, and on Cape Cod, funded by the State of Massachusetts, have not yet been completed. Both studies have features in common with the other epidemiological studies we have described earlier; they are case-control studies in which the exposures to suspected agents of women diagnosed with breast cancer are compared to the exposures of comparable women who have not been diagnosed with breast cancer. Although as of this writing their results have not yet been published, it is of some interest to describe how they are being carried out. One reason is that as studies undertaken in response to the demands of activists, and to answer questions the activists felt had not adequately been addressed by other studies, they have drawn much public attention. Another is that they will try to bridge gaps left by earlier studies: one will attempt a surveillance of a broad range of environmental exposures of individual women, and the other will make extensive use of tools provided by molecular biology to link exposure to the disease.

We will also describe another study in progress with a similar goal: to find out if there is a relation between pesticide exposure and breast cancer. This study is being done in an area where it is known that pesticide exposure has been high, and the measures of exposure to them are more extensive than on Long Island or Cape Cod. The area was selected not in response to the demands of activists or mandated by a legislative body, but rather chosen by scientists because they could make accurate assessments of individual exposures to high levels of pesticides and may therefore have a better chance of detecting health effects, if there are any.

Description of the Silent Spring Study

The Silent Spring Institute study, in its initial phase, conducted an investigation of some of the possible sources of contamination on Cape Cod, including wastes from the Air Force base near Falmouth, microwave radiation from a major Air Force radar station, and proximity to a nuclear power plant in Plymouth, very near the Cape, and found no statistically significant excess of breast cancer associated with them. During this initial phase the study identified over 90 substances that might be related to breast cancer, and to which women on the Cape may have been significantly exposed.

At the next stage, now in progress as of this writing, different routes of exposure to these substances through the air, through the food chain, and through drinking water will be examined, to estimate the exposures of both breast cancer cases and controls. Because it is not feasible to do an epidemiological study on so many substances at one time, some selection will most likely be made to narrow down the field of possibilities. The substances to be studied will be those of demonstrated cancer-causing potential in tests on animals and on cell lines, and present in the human environment in large enough concentrations to pose a likely risk. There must also be ways to estimate each individual woman's exposure. Only then will it be possible to compare breast cancer cases and controls, and determine whether the cases have been significantly more exposed than the controls.

The Silent Spring Institute study began by administering a detailed questionnaire to each of the cases and the controls, about her health, personal history, and use of various household products, including pesticides (for example, those used to control termites, ticks and fleas on pets, and mosquito repellants), detergents, sprays to control mildew, bleaches, and personal care products.

To supplement the information to be obtained from the questionnaire, the institute will use a geographic information system (GIS) to provide information about exposures that the women in the study would not necessarily know about: whether they or their homes have been exposed by spraying of pesticides in the vicinity, whether wastewater has contaminated the drinking water, whether there are sources of toxic pollution such as waste dumps in the neighborhood, and how much air pollution there is from nearby traffic. For example, certain types of pesticide were used on cranberry bogs, other types to eliminate gypsy moths, and still others on golf courses. The times and places sprayed and the kind and amount used are to some extent available from recorded information. How much of any of these might have reached a particular home can be estimated from the amount sprayed, the manner of spraying, and the wind direction at the time (fig. 6-3). Further, it is possible, from the known stability of the pesticides, to estimate how much of them are expected to be still present in the home and how much has disappeared over time. The geographic information system stores all such information and permits one to estimate a contamination history for each residence on Cape Cod (figs. 6-4, 6-5, 6-6). Each woman's exposure history can be obtained from knowledge of when and where she resided.

To see how well information on exposure from both the questionnaires and the geographical information system agree, the Silent Spring Institute study plans to select 145 homes from the 2,500 cases and controls and directly measure concentrations of the ninety different substances they have selected, in the air of their homes and in household dust. Urine samples will be collected from these 145 women and tested for the substances being investigated, or for their metabolic breakdown products. The exposures of women in the remaining homes are to be estimated from the questionnaires and the geographic information system data alone; the tests on the 145 homes will show how much confidence can be placed on these estimates.

The intensive surveillance of a large spectrum of environmental pollutants, an innovative feature of this study, is only beginning. The hope is that it will identify hazards, develop new research tools, and provide a basis for further health studies.

The Long Island Breast Cancer Study

The Long Island Breast Cancer Study has many features in common with the Cape Cod study, and many differences. Like the Cape Cod study, it is a case-control study in which all women in the study area who had been

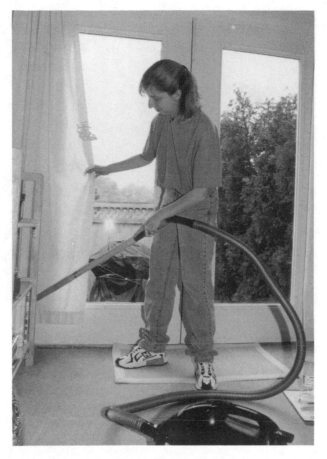

FIGURE 6-3 Laboratory technician collecting dust samples in a home on Cape Cod for the Silent Spring study. Courtesy of Tanya C. Swann, photographer, Woods Hole, MA.

diagnosed with breast cancer within a specified time period were compared to a control group selected to be as similar as possible in known risk factors to the group of cases, but that did not get breast cancer in that same time period. Exposure to a number of hormonally active substances, as well as other substances believed to have carcinogenic potential, are being studied in relation to the risk of breast cancer. Information about the extent of exposure was obtained by questioning the subjects in the study, from monitoring dust, air, and water in homes, and using a geographic information system.

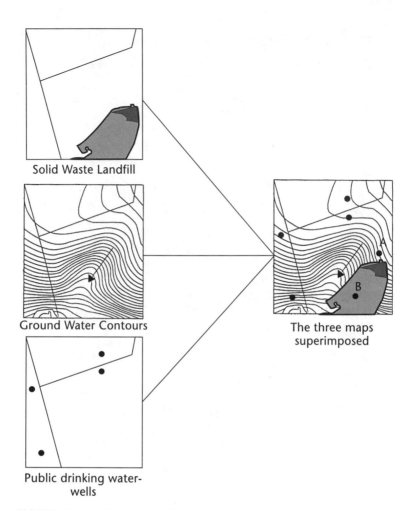

Solid Waste Landfill

Ground Water Contours

Public drinking water-
wells

The three maps
superimposed

FIGURE 6-4 A Geographic Information System (GIS) is a computerized
method of analyzing and displaying information about the environment. Here
three separate maps are combined. The top map shows an area of
contamination from a solid waste landfill, the second the flow of ground water
in the area of the landfill, and the third the location of homes. All three are
combined in a final map shown to the right. Also shown are two homes,
marked A and B. Home A is much closer to the center of the source of the
contamination, but the flow of underground water is such that the more
distant home B receives more highly contaminated drinking water. Courtesy of
the Silent Spring Institute, Newton, MA.

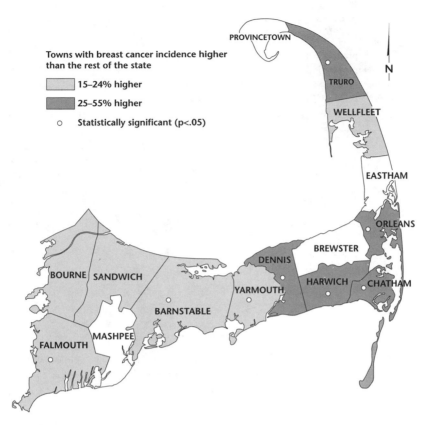

FIGURE 6-5   Breast cancer incidence in towns on Cape Cod, 1982–1994. The shading distinguishes towns with rates less than 15% higher, towns with rates 15–24% higher, and town with more than 25% higher than in the state of Massachusetts as a whole. Courtesy of the Silent Spring Institute, Newton, MA.

There are also important differences. The Long Island study is doing more comprehensive medical and biological tests. In particular, blood and urine were collected from a sample of the subjects, and tested not only for the presence of the suspected chemicals but also for genetic traits related to the development of cancer. The breast cancer cases on Long Island were divided into subgroups according to their specific genetic sensitivities (as determined from the blood and urine samples), to study their responses to specific environmental exposures. Clues to roles for genetic sensitivities were sought in the family and medical histories, nutritional habits, and ethnicity of the subjects.

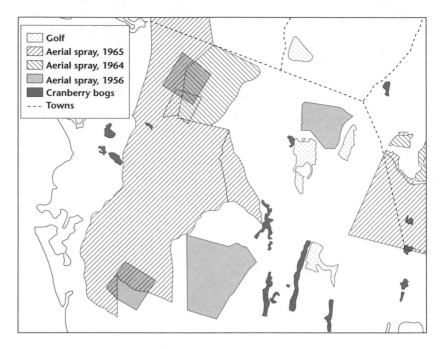

FIGURE 6-6 A GIS map of the area of Falmouth, on Cape Cod, showing areas sprayed with pesticides, the location of golf courses and cranberry bogs, and township boundaries. Courtesy of the Silent Spring Institute, Newton, MA.

The number of suspected environmental hazards to be studied is less than in the Cape Cod study, but they will be studied more intensively. They include two pesticides, DDT and chlordane; PCBs; and polyaromatic hydrocarbons (PAHs).

A relation between electromagnetic fields and any form of cancer has not yet been convincingly established, but the Long Island study is examining this factor also. It is interesting that one speculative hypothesis on how electromagnetic fields might possibly interact with the human body is through an effect on the hormonal system. This is discussed in more detail in chapter 7.

Data for this study have all been collected and are now being analyzed, and the results should be published soon. It is a comprehensive study that, whatever its outcome, should add to our understanding of breast cancer and the environment.

Farmers, Pesticides, and Cancer

Scientists at the National Cancer Institute have begun a study of farmers and their families in the states of Iowa and North Carolina. These states were chosen because they are important agricultural states that require users of pesticides to apply for licenses and undergo some training in their use. Only farmers who applied for such licenses and their spouses and children, together with a number of commercial pesticide applicators, are being studied. At the time of applying for a license, the farmers in the study will be asked about which of some fifty different pesticides they may have used or plan to use, together with information about the crops they grow, and whether they use protective clothing when spraying, as well as other health-related and medical information, for example, about family history, diet, smoking, and alcohol use.

Farm life is a healthy life; farmers live longer, smoke less, get more exercise, and suffer less heart disease and less lung and colon cancer. However, they do suffer more work-related injuries, have more leukemia, prostate and skin cancer, and more respiratory disease and more dermatitis. They are exposed, in addition to pesticides specifically and agricultural chemicals generally, to sunlight, biological agents including animal viruses, dust, fuel exhaust, and animal wastes.

The Agricultural Health Study is not limited to breast cancer though it includes 31,000 farmer's wives as well as 59,000 farmers and 6,000 commercial pesticide applicators: it will cover various cancers that might be related to the exposures just mentioned or to the farmer's lifestyle, and some noncancerous conditions like kidney problems, neurological disease, and various reproductive outcomes.

The exposures will be determined, first of all, from questionnaires filled out by the study subjects about pesticide use, which pesticides, how they were handled, and what protective measures were taken. A group of 200 farm families will have their homes monitored for pesticides and other agents of interest, to see how well exposure estimated from the questionnaires agrees with direct measurement. In addition, a database on pesticide handlers developed by the Environmental Protection Agency, providing information about exposures to workers who manufacture, process, mix, or apply pesticides under various conditions of handling, will supplement information from the questionnaires and from the home monitoring.

In this "nested" case-control study the health of the subjects will be monitored as time goes on, and when a large enough number of cases of any one disease has occurred, a suitable control group from subjects who have not gotten that particular disease will be selected, and the exposures of the two groups compared. In addition, blood DNA tests for genetic susceptibilities will be performed. The exposures of all subjects in the study will be evaluated at regular intervals, again through questionnaires and home monitoring.

It can be seen that the aim of the Agricultural Health Study is similar to that of the Long Island and Cape Cod breast cancer studies. There are important differences: the levels of exposure should be greater than on Long Island or Cape Cod, and the assessment of exposure, because of the regulations the users are required to obey, more reliable. It is hoped that this study, expected to continue many years, will be able to detect effects of such exposures on breast cancer, among other conditions.

SUMMARY

So far, epidemiological studies have not provided much evidence that breast cancer risk is increased by exposure to pesticides, organochlorines, polyaromatic hydrocarbons, or any hormonally active agents other than natural and possibly synthetic estrogens. Although polyaromatic hydrocarbons are mammary carcinogens in rodents, they do not act by mimicking hormones, but less directly, by influencing hormone metabolism.

The search for avoidable causes of breast cancer continues: new studies testing new hypotheses are reported all the time in the scientific literature. U.S. government funding for breast cancer research has increased sixfold over the past decade. At the same time our understanding of the molecular biology of cancer is improving rapidly. We are increasingly able to study the genetic variations, both inherited and acquired, that affect cancer risk. Among those genetic variations are some that reflect exposures to environmental chemicals, and identifying them will supplement what we learn by direct chemical determination of toxic substances in body tissues or in blood.

We have described the achievements of the breast cancer activists. They have created a sense of urgency about a form of cancer that except for lung cancer kills more women than any other, and fought for and achieved a great increase in funding for breast cancer research and treatment, and the initiation of studies on Long Island, Cape Cod, and else-where. They have made many scientists aware of the need to explain their research to those whose health and well being depends on that research. In turn, many of the activists have learned much about science, including its limitations. The two groups, scientists and activists, share a common goal, and the more they listen to each other, the quicker that goal will be reached. Was the communication as good as it should have been when the demands were made for the Long Island and Cape Cod studies?

In funding the studies, legislative bodies accepted certain assumptions held by activists in these areas on how and where to look for links be-tween pesticide and other exposures and breast cancer, and mandated that the studies be done in these areas. Once the studies were mandated, pro-posals submitted were evaluated by peer review boards, in the Long Island study a National Institutes of Health board, and in the Cape Cod study a board selected by the Massachusetts Department of Public Health (which is also funding some studies elsewhere in the state). These boards made their awards on the basis of the scientific merits of the proposals, subject to the conditions of the mandate. These conditions, however, may not have produced the best strategies for research on breast cancer, or even on the relation between hormonally active agents and breast cancer. On both Long Island and Cape Cod the excesses may yet be explained by the known risk factors for breast cancer. This is not meant to imply that some of the cases of breast cancer in these areas could not have been caused by exposure to hormonally active agents, nor that the studies are incapable of showing that there is an increased risk from such exposure, if there is one. It does, however, lead one to ask whether these were the best areas in which to do the research. Many scientists believe that better locations to test the pesticide hypothesis are agricultural areas where spraying is common and exposures can be more reliably assessed, as in the Agricul-tural Health Study we described.

In any event, possible roles of environmental agents in breast cancer are still being studied. So are factors such as diet that influence known risk factors such as age at menarche and frequency of the menstrual cycle. So are the mechanisms by which estrogens act in the body, how they produce both their desirable and harmful effects, and the ways they may be influenced by environmental exposures.

It may, after all, turn out that breast cancer has little to do with hor-monally active chemicals in the environment, but is primarily a result of lifestyle factors, not all of which have been identified, that influence each woman's exposure to her own estrogens. If so, the conflict between what 5 million years of evolution has destined women for and what women today want may be blamed. But there is no need for human beings to be slaves of strict biological determinism. We defy it in so many ways, by warming ourselves with fire, by wearing clothes, by immunizing ourselves against infectious diseases, by cooking our food, by living long past child-bearing age, that there is no reason not to defy it in this.

7

POWER LINES, MAGNETIC FIELDS, AND CANCER

SOUNDING THE ALARM

We are old enough to have had iceboxes in our kitchens when we were children. Every few days an iceman came through our neighborhoods, in Jerusalem leading a donkey cart and in the Bronx in a truck, each full of blocks of ice. Housewives would put a sign in the window or call out to him to let him know how big a piece to leave. We were very proud of our first home refrigerators; not everyone in the neighborhood had one. Refrigerators were easier to use: we did not have to worry about missing the iceman, the food stayed fresh longer, and ice cream could be kept in the freezer compartment.

We cannot imagine modern life without electric power, and not just for the convenience of keeping ice cream. When a study published in 1979 suggested that magnetic fields from the electric wiring in homes and from outside power lines might cause leukemia in children, it was taken seriously, and not only by scientists. Public awareness and concern grew rapidly as these results were publicized in the media, and today they are one of the more controversial suspected environmental hazards. On the one hand, claims have been made that they are responsible for clusters of various cancers, birth defects, and neurological disorders, which are covered up by power companies and government agencies. On the other hand, there have been contemptuous dismissals of such claims with the counterclaim that they could not possibly hurt anyone and that irresponsible journalists are creating a panic. Some examples of extreme positions give the flavor of the controversy.

Magnetic Fields Are Dangerous

A series of articles written by the journalist Paul Brodeur for the *New Yorker* magazine, followed by two books, *Currents of Death* and *The Great Power-Line Cover-up*, describe health problems in a number of neighborhoods and schools in which there was reason to believe high magnetic fields were present. He reports that on one small street of four houses in a Connecticut town, directly across from a power substation, there was a cluster of diseases that he strongly implied were caused by fields emanating from the substation:

1. two malignant brain tumors,
2. a malignant eye tumor,
3. a nonmalignant brain tumor,
4. a nonmalignant ovarian tumor,
5. a nonmalignant tumor on the tibia (bone of the lower leg),
6. two cases of brain seizures,
7. one case of painful ganglion cysts of the wrist,
8. a miscarriage,
9. a surgical removal of the parotid (salivary) gland,
10. a growth on the hand requiring surgical removal,
11. both a serious kidney disease and a dissolving of the fatty tissues under the cheeks in one young woman, each being extremely rare conditions,
12. a suspicious looking cyst in the breast of another woman,
13. a high rate of birth defects,
14. two children with spinal and ligamental developmental disorders,
15. a number of people with recurrent and excruciating headaches.

Brodeur also attributed large numbers of cases of cancer in two schools in California, in one school among the children, in the other in the teaching and administrative staff, to high magnetic fields from power lines or power substations near the schools.

"Electrical Sensitivity," Cellular Phones,
Brain Tumors, Depression

A search of the Internet gave over a thousand "hits" on "electromagnetic fields and cancer." Some of the sites were of commercial organizations offering advisory and remedial services for homeowners, including a small device, costing $19.95, to be worn or carried that was claimed to protect the wearer from magnetic fields. The web site of an organization based in England that offered advisory service to concerned citizens stated that digital cellular phones may cause brain tumors, Alzheimer's and Parkinson's diseases, and eye damage, and describes a condition, "electrical sensitivity" or ES, with symptoms of dizziness, headaches, buzzing, and nausea, as well as the aggravation of allergies. It mentioned the study that reported a relation between residential fields and childhood leukemia, and the claim of a physician that such fields are responsible for depressive illness, headaches, and suicide. A manufacturer of a device to measure magnetic fields stated that they can cause brain, breast, and lymphatic cancers, cancers of the blood-producing and nervous system, birth defects and miscarriages, learning disabilities, depression, and Alzheimer's disease. Still another manufacturer of a similar device stresses the impact of such fields on the resale value of homes, a reasonable concern since the *Wall Street Journal* reported on September 3, 1993, that homes near power lines often sold for 30% less than equivalent homes elsewhere. A sharp decline in the prices of stocks in the cellular phone industry occurred when a man filed a lawsuit claiming that his wife's fatal brain cancer was caused by her heavy use of cellular phones, followed by newspaper reports of two cases of brain cancer in officers of a cellular phone company.

Articles in popular magazines also showed a range of opinions and the extent of public concern. The magazine of the Sierra Club, an environmental organization, recommended that families survey the magnetic fields in their homes. The *Ladies Home Journal* reported that residents of a township in New Jersey attributed a large number of cancers and birth defects, including Down's syndrome, to local satellite antennas that transmit microwave radiation.

Power Line Fields Are Harmless

In contrast, the American Physical Society, the leading organization of American physicists, issued a statement from which the following quotation is taken:

The scientific literature and the reports of reviews by other panels show no consistent, significant link between cancer and power line fields. . . . No plausible biophysical mechanisms for the systematic initiation or promotion of cancer by these power line fields have been identified. Furthermore, the preponderance of the . . . research findings have failed to substantiate those studies which have reported specific adverse health effects from exposure to such fields.

In what follows we will describe how scientists have studied the health effects of electric and magnetic fields, and explain why it has been so hard for them to reach agreement.

Where Do Fields Come From?

Electric and magnetic fields are described in more detail in "What Are Electric and Magnetic Fields?" (p. 230). For the present, we will note that whenever alternating electric currents flow in wires, both alternating electric and magnetic fields are produced in the vicinity of the wires. Since alternating electric currents operate our appliances, run in wires through our houses and in high-tension (high-voltage) transmission lines through our neighborhoods, we are exposed to alternating magnetic and electric fields all the time, though at some times to stronger fields than others. Sleeping under an electric blanket, sitting close to a video monitor, drying our hair with a hair dryer, all expose us. Does the exposure cause cancer? Are our children in danger?

How Fields Might Harm Us

What do the fields actually do to our bodies? First, the fields from power lines or house currents are not ionizing radiation. Some forms of ionizing radiation, such as X-rays and gamma rays, are electromagnetic waves with extremely high frequencies, a billion megahertz and more, and carry their energies in concentrated bundles (photons) of energy high enough to physically disrupt molecules, including DNA molecules, and cause chemical changes in them. The electric and magnetic fields associated with house current, which alternate at 60 cycles per second or 60 hertz (50 hertz in Europe), do not have the energy to cause chemical change directly, so if they cause harm, they must do it some other way. Microwave ovens, although their power is supplied by 60-hertz house current, use that power to produce electric fields at frequencies much higher than the residential frequency of 60 hertz but far lower than the lowest frequencies of ionizing radiation. Therefore microwaves, like 60Hz house current, do not have photon energies high enough to disrupt molecules directly, but they do so in a different way; the total energy they supply to the water molecules in food is enough to raise the temperature of the food and cook it. Microwave ovens are therefore shielded to protect the users from burns. Incidentally, cell phones use radio frequencies, which are also too low to disrupt molecules. High temperature alone may disrupt molecules, but the fields from 60-hertz house current do not raise the temperature of human flesh by any significant amount. How then might such fields act? And why has the focus mainly been on magnetic fields and not electric fields?

Body fluids contain salts, which make human—and animal—bodies good conductors of electricity. When good conductors, such as metal wires or living bodies, are exposed to an electric field, the field causes currents to flow in the surfaces of the conducting body, but it does not penetrate inside. It is not likely that electric currents in the skin can harm our internal organs or our blood. In addition, the walls of buildings have some conducting power and therefore partially shield people inside from electric fields from power lines outside the house. Magnetic fields, on the other hand, do penetrate good conductors, and therefore cause weak electric currents to flow inside our bodies, not only in our skins. This is one way—but not the only possible way—magnetic fields could harm us, if indeed they harm us. The study of health effects has therefore focused on them.

STUDIES ON HUMAN BEINGS

Magnetic Fields and Leukemia

The study that began the tidal wave of research, concern, and controversy was done in Denver, Colorado, in the late 1970's by N. Wertheimer and F. Leeper. It was a "case-control " study (see chapter 6) that compared the exposures to magnetic fields of children living in that city who had died of leukemia between 1950 and 1973 (specifically acute lymphoblastic leukemia, [ALL], the most common form affecting children) to the exposures of a similar group of children from the same area who had not had leukemia. The authors reported that children who died of leukemia had on the average been exposed to higher magnetic fields than children without the disease, and that exposure to the highest magnetic fields found in Denver homes roughly doubled a child's risk of leukemia.

How was this epidemiological study done? What are its limitations? Have subsequent studies confirmed its conclusions?

Pitfalls and Problems

There are a number of things that are known to affect a child's risk of leukemia (the technical term is "risk factors for leukemia": See chapter 5 for a more detailed discussion). Children aged two and three are much more likely to get leukemia than older or younger children so that it is important to compare the cases of leukemia with control children of the same age. Boys are slightly more susceptible than girls, so sex matters also. Matching the controls by age and sex may be done by choosing as a control a child of the same sex as the case child and born in the same hospital during the same week, but who did not later get leukemia. Another procedure is to telephone homes at random in the area of each case, and ask the families if they have a child of the same age and sex as the case child, and if they would be willing to participate in the study. In practice, it has been found to take fifty to seventy-five phone calls to find one suitable control child. The telephone search method has a drawback. If some of the families of the children who got leukemia did not have telephones, and the control group was chosen by telephone contact, then the controls are more likely to have telephones at home and will presumably have a higher average income than the cases they have been supposedly matched to. Why should this matter? Children whose parents have more education and higher incomes generally have a higher rate of leukemia, for reasons not fully understood (see chapter 4). High social class is one "risk factor" for childhood leukemia.

Firstborn children are at somewhat higher risk than later-born, and so are children born to older mothers. Exposures of the mother to X-rays during pregnancy also increase risk to the child. In any event, the rate of childhood leukemia varies from group to group, from place to place, and from time to time, and not all the reasons are known.

It is often difficult to take all of the known risk factors into account in choosing the control group, but some can be corrected for later. Sometimes differences between cases and control groups are discovered after the data has been collected. For example, the homes found in this study to have higher magnetic fields turned out also to be older homes on the average, located in older sections of the city, with higher traffic and population densities. This suggests that if there were an excess rate of childhood leukemia in such homes it might have something to do with the age of the home or the area, or pollution from the traffic, rather than exposure to magnetic fields. This possibility had to be looked into before it could be ruled out.

Another problem in choosing a control group is that families who have a child with leukemia are usually willing to participate in such a study, because they have an emotional stake in helping fight the disease, but families requested to participate as control subjects are often less willing. The factors that influence a family's choice not to participate might include its educational level, income, ethnicity, being in the country illegally, a criminal record, and others, some of which might have a bearing on the risk of leukemia. This is very difficult to evaluate unless the noncooperating families are willing to be interviewed about their reasons for not participating, but the factors that make them noncooperating often make them uncooperative.

In the Wertheimer-Leeper study, 300 controls were selected, to be compared with 300 children who developed leukemia.

Estimating Exposure to Magnetic Fields

The next step was to determine the exposures of both cases and controls to magnetic fields. As we have noted, magnetic fields penetrate the body but electric fields do not. The investigators wanted to compare the total exposure of the case children to magnetic fields (prior to the diagnosis of their disease) to the total exposure of the controls. But like the victims of the atomic bombs in Hiroshima and Nagasaki, the cases and controls did not wear badges or monitors that recorded these exposures. An estimate could have been obtained by a "spot check": going into their present residences and measuring magnetic fields in the rooms where the child spent appreciable time. This is not the same as measuring all the child's lifetime exposure before she got sick: exposure during her mother's pregnancy might be important, the child might have been exposed to fields from various appliances such as electric blankets or television sets in the past, or the wiring in the home might have been changed, all things that would be missed in a spot check. However, even this one-time field measurement would have been expensive to do. As we will see, some later studies did just that, in spite of the expense.

Wire Codes: Estimating Exposure from Power Lines

Wertheimer and Leeper made some preliminary observations that convinced them that the magnetic field in the home of each of the cases and controls came mostly from power lines in the neighborhood, and could be predicted from several characteristics of the lines such as the voltage and the distance from the home. They developed a system for representing these characteristics by a "wire code," and then classified the homes of subjects as "very high," "high," "low," and "very low" in accord with this code (fig. 7-1, 7-2, 7-3).

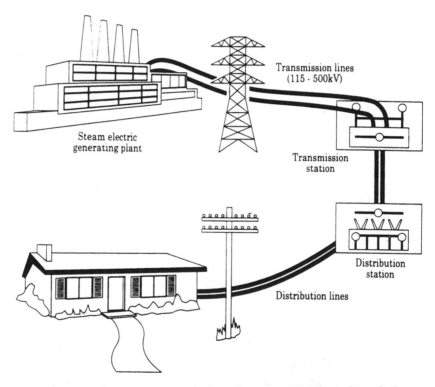

FIGURE 7-1   Utility power network, from the generating plant, through the high voltage transmission system, to the local and residential level. Reproduced from the book *Electric and Magnetic Fields: Invisible Risks?* by Leonard A. Sagan, published by Gordon and Breach, Amsterdam, 1996, with the permission of Gordon and Breach, of the Overseas Publishers Association, NV, and of the Electric Power Research Institute.

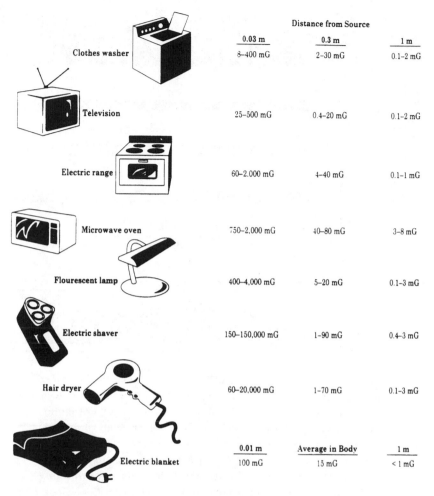

	Distance from Source		
	0.03 m	**0.3 m**	**1 m**
Clothes washer	8–400 mG	2–30 mG	0.1–2 mG
Television	25–500 mG	0.4–20 mG	0.1–2 mG
Electric range	60–2,000 mG	4–40 mG	0.1–1 mG
Microwave oven	750–2,000 mG	40–80 mG	3–8 mG
Flourescent lamp	400–4,000 mG	5–20 mG	0.1–3 mG
Electric shaver	150–150,000 mG	1–90 mG	0.4–3 mG
Hair dryer	60–20,000 mG	1–70 mG	0.1–3 mG
	0.01 m	**Average in Body**	**1 m**
Electric blanket	100 mG	15 mG	< 1 mG

Source: EPRI

FIGURE 7-2 Magnetic field levels near household appliances. Note how rapidly the fields decrease as the distance from the appliance increases. The fields in the figure are given in milligauss (thousandths of a gauss). One milligauss equals 0.1 microtesla. 0.03 meters, or 3 centimeters, is a little over an inch; 0.3 meters is about a foot. Reproduced from the book *Electric and Magnetic Fields: Invisible Risks?* by Leonard A. Sagan, published by Gordon and Breach, Amsterdam, 1996, with the permission of Gordon and Breach, of the Overseas Publishers Association, NV, and of the Electric Power Research Institute.

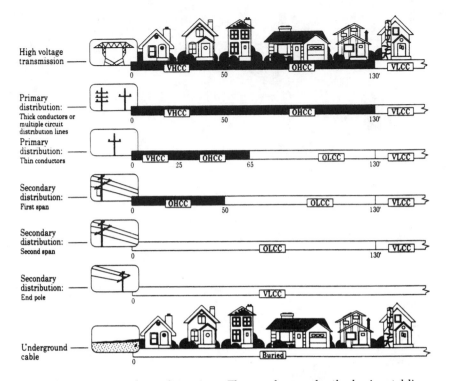

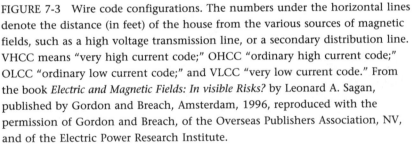

FIGURE 7-3 Wire code configurations. The numbers under the horizontal lines denote the distance (in feet) of the house from the various sources of magnetic fields, such as a high voltage transmission line, or a secondary distribution line. VHCC means "very high current code;" OHCC "ordinary high current code;" OLCC "ordinary low current code;" and VLCC "very low current code." From the book *Electric and Magnetic Fields: In visible Risks?* by Leonard A. Sagan, published by Gordon and Breach, Amsterdam, 1996, reproduced with the permission of Gordon and Breach, of the Overseas Publishers Association, NV, and of the Electric Power Research Institute.

The wire code is a substitute measure for the quantity we would ideally like to know—the child's total exposure to magnetic fields—and is called a "surrogate variable." Use of a surrogate variable is often necessary in health studies on human populations, which are expensive and time-consuming anyway, but such variables sometimes represent the desired quantity poorly, and thus usually makes the health risk seem smaller than it really is or, less often, exaggerate it.

The investigators then compared exposures estimated by wire codes in the case and control groups and found that children living in homes with the "very high" rating of wire code had about twice the risk of developing leukemia than other children. They concluded therefore that exposure of children to high magnetic fields is associated with an increased risk of getting leukemia.

More Studies on Magnetic Fields and Health

Subsequent to the Wertheimer-Leeper study, many epidemiological studies have been or are being carried out in the United States, Canada, Europe, and Japan. There have been studies of the relation of childhood leukemia and some other cancers to the use of certain electrical appliances, and occupational studies of leukemia and brain cancer in workers exposed to high fields in the workplace, and studies in homes of other cancers and of other diseases.

Most studies of home appliances have given ambiguous results. A recent extensive one by researchers from the National Cancer Institute examined childhood leukemia in relation to the use, either by the child, or by the mother when pregnant, of a wide range of appliances including television sets, video games, electric home heating systems, air conditioning, kitchen appliances, sewing machines, hair dryers, and a number of small appliances. Increases in leukemia rates (typically 20–50%) were observed with exposures of the pregnant mothers to electric blankets, heating pads, and humidifiers, and of the children to electric blankets, hair dryers, sound systems with headsets, and video games. However, the authors noted that the excess leukemia rates did not relate particularly to the duration or intensity of exposure to these appliances and concluded that the relationship of excess leukemia to appliance use was probably fortuitous. A number of other scientists commenting on their work disagree with this conclusion.

Electric blankets manufactured prior to the concern about possible carcinogenic effects of magnetic fields exposed their users to magnetic fields of as high as 10 microtesla, about one hundred times stronger than the usual residential fields from wiring and transmission lines (see "What Are Electric and Magnetic Fields?" [p. 230] for an explanation of "microtesla"). As a result of the concern about leukemia, the design of electric blankets has been changed so that the fields are much weaker, but the study covered a time period preceding this change (fig. 7-4).

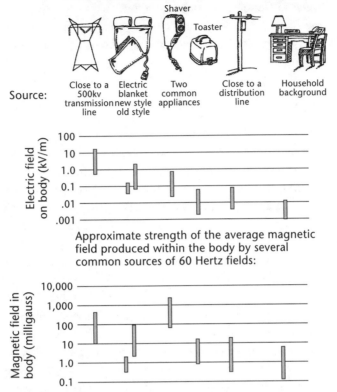

Approximate strength of the average electric field at the surface of the body produced by several common sources of 60 Hertz fields:

Source:

| Close to a 500kv transmission line | Electric blanket new style old style | Two common appliances | Close to a distribution line | Household background |

FIGURE 7-4 Approximate strength of average electric and magnetic fields at the surface of the body, in the vicinity of several common sources of fields. Note that the magnetic field strengths are given in milligauss (one milligauss equals 0.1 microtesla). Note also that electric and magnetic fields are measured in different units. The scale used for the field strengths is logarithmic, meaning that each horizontal line corresponds to a field ten times greater than the line below it. The range of magnetic fields from an electric shaver, for example, is from 100 milligauss (10 microtesla) to about 2000 milligauss (200 microtesla), and from an old-style electric blanket from about 3 milligauss (0.3 microtesla) to about 100 milligauss (10 microtesla). Note, however, that exposures to electric blankets are of much longer duration than to electric shavers. From the pamphlet "More on 'What are 60 Hz fields?' "copyright by Department of Engineering and Public Policy, Carnegie Mellon University, and reproduced with permission of Professor Granger Morgan, Carnegie Mellon University.

Studies of workers exposed to high magnetic fields in the workplace have not found consistent results; some reports of excess brain and breast cancers have not been confirmed by others. The exposures have been to somewhat higher fields than in residential settings, and the failure to find consistent reproducible results means the case for an occupational risk of cancer for adults is weaker than in the childhood leukemia studies.

We will focus our discussion from here on on studies of the relation of childhood leukemia to average magnetic fields in homes, as there have been more of them, and the results have been more consistent.

How Good Are the "Wire Codes"?

One of the uncertainties of the Wertheimer-Leeper Denver study was the extent to which the "wire codes" really represent the magnetic fields in the homes.

In later studies Werthheimer and Leeper refined their wire code classification to take into better account the kind of transmission line (high-voltage, medium-voltage), the thickness of the wires and how close they were to each other, whether the current was two-phase or three-phase, whether the lines were overhead or underground, and very important, the distance from the home to the power lines. Other scientists used similar but not identical wire codes, but more recently direct measurements of magnetic fields have been made in or near the home and compared with those estimated from the wire codes to test how accurately the wire codes represent the fields.

A Paradox—Is It Really the Magnetic Field?

Even accurate knowledge of the magnetic field in a home at one point in time may not be reliable. It would have been desirable to know the total exposure of the case and control children from birth, or even earlier, up to the age at which the children became ill, but this could no longer be done in most studies. Still, it was worth comparing the field measured in the homes at one point in time with the classification of the home according to the wire code. It would show, first, how good the wire code is as a surrogate for the fields from nearby power lines. It would also show whether the preliminary observation of Wertheimer and Leeper, that the main contribution to home magnetic fields is from outside lines rather than from wiring and appliances in the home, is correct.

As this kind of data accumulated, and it came from more than one study, a problem emerged: the measured fields in the homes did not agree well with the fields estimated from the wire codes, except for the wire code category "very high." In other words, the three lower categories of wire code did not correlate very well with the directly measured home magnetic fields.

It also turned out on closer examination of the results of the studies that the wire code did not particularly correlate with an excess of leukemia cases except for the "very high" wire code. While this result still suggests an association of magnetic fields with childhood leukemia, it essentially reduces the four or more categories of wire codes to two: "very high" and "not very high."

Have We Been Measuring the Wrong Thing?

It is also possible that the wire codes or spot measurement of the average home fields after the child has become ill miss some property of the magnetic fields that is more significantly related to the increased risk of childhood leukemia.

Part of the problem is that we do not yet know why or how magnetic fields might affect biological processes in living organisms. We mentioned earlier that 60-hertz alternating magnetic fields do cause 60-hertz electric currents to flow inside the body, but whether this could influence biological processes that lead to leukemia is not known. Most molecules in the body do not have marked magnetic properties, but there are some that do, notably iron compounds like hemoglobin and a kind of molecule often formed as a result of radiation exposure, called a "free radical." Again, how the biological action of such magnetic molecules in living organisms would be affected by weak 60-hertz magnetic fields is so far unknown.

Because we do not know how and where a magnetic field might plausibly act, we do not know what property of the magnetic field should be studied. It may be that the wiring codes and direct field measurements do not represent that property well. Most direct measurements made so far were "spot" measurements, taken in only one or two places, and only for a short time. They certainly need not represent a long-term average exposure. Even if they did, though, it is possible that what matters is short-term exposures to very high fields, such as occur with sudden large changes in the strength of electric currents—surges or "transients"—when appliances are turned on or off. Such momentary high fields would not show up in a measurement of the long-term average field. Even without surges, it might be that only fields higher than a certain minimum level do any harm, again something that might be missed by a long-term average. So we are left with some uncertainty as to what we should really be measuring (fig. 7-5).

Dose and Response

Much can be learned from studies that divide the subjects up according to the two qualitative categories of "exposed" and "not exposed," and then divide up the outcomes into two categories: "sick" and "not sick." If the "exposed" are also more often the "sick," and the "not exposed" more often the "not sick," we can feel we have some basis for believing exposure might be harmful. Often "sick" or "not sick" are the best we can do for the health outcome; a child either has or does not have leukemia, and

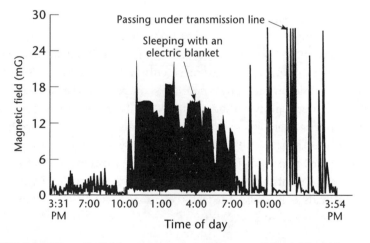

FIGURE 7-5 Magnetic field exposure of an eight-year old girl. The girl wore a field monitor for about 24 hours starting at 3 P.M. During the night she used an electric blanket, and on her way to school walked near electric transmission lines. Reproduced from the book *Electric and Magnetic Fields: Invisible Risks?* by Leonard A. Sagan, published by Gordon and Breach, Amsterdam, 1996, with the permission of Gordon and Breach, of the Overseas Publishers Association, NV, and of the Electric Power Research Institute.

an adult either has or does not have lung cancer. But if we can character-ize exposure in more quantitative terms, so that instead of just two cate-gories of exposure we have four, or ten, or fifty, and then show that the proportion of "sick" subjects is greater the higher the level of exposure, we can have more confidence that the association between exposure and illness is not a statistical accident. This is certainly the case with cigarette smoking and lung cancer, where not only do smokers have a much greater risk but the proportion of smokers who get lung cancer has been shown to be greater the greater the number of cigarettes smoked (see fig. 2–7 in chapter 2). A clear finding of a "dose-response" relationship is one of a number of criteria used to decide whether the association found between sickness and exposure is likely to be a cause-and-effect one. So far the relationship between magnetic fields and cancer has not been shown to be a dose-response one. All that has been found up to now, and in many but not all studies, is that there is more childhood leukemia in homes classified as having "very high" fields. Homes having only "high" fields have shown the same leukemia rate as homes having lower fields.

A Committee Reports

The National Research Council of the National Academy of Sciences, a nongovernmental scientific advisory body, had issued a report in 1997, *Possible Health Effects of Exposure to Residential Electric and Magnetic Fields,* prepared by a committee of leading scientists in the fields of epidemiol-ogy, biology, and physics. The committee compared and evaluated all the studies then done, and concluded that while definitive proof has not yet been given that there is an association between the wire codes of homes and childhood cancer, the studies considered as a whole do suggest that such an association is likely. The report noted, however, that if an asso-ciation were definitively established, it need not mean that exposure to magnetic fields is the cause; the wire codes may correlate fortuitously with an unknown real cause.

A Definitive Study?

In the same year but too late for inclusion in the National Research Council report, Dr. Martha Linet and coworkers at the National Cancer Institute published the results of a large and careful study: over 600 cases and over 600 controls from nine different states of the United States. The authors interpreted the results as showing that magnetic fields had no relation to childhood leukemia.

In the same issue of the scientific journal in which it appeared, another scientist, expressing his own opinion rather than that of the journal itself, commented as follows:

> [T]he weight of the better epidemiologic studies, including that by Linet et al., now supports the conclusion [that there is no convincing evidence that high-voltage power lines are a health hazard or a cause of cancer]. It is sad that hundreds of millions of dollars have gone into studies that never had much promise of finding a way to prevent the tragedy of cancer in children. The many inconclusive and inconsistent studies have generated worry and fear and have given peace of mind to no one. The 18 years of research have produced considerable paranoia, but little insight and no prevention. It is time to stop wasting our research resources. We should redirect them to research that will be able to discover the true biologic causes of the leukemic clones that threaten the lives of children.

As we shall see, this view has been strongly contested.

In the Linet study, great care was taken to consider all other risk factors known or suggested as having a relation to childhood leukemia. Cases and controls were compared to assess any possible influence on the rate of leukemia of such risk factors as the mother's age at the birth of the child, the number of children in the family, the birth order of the child, the type of residence, the degree of urbanization of the neighborhood, or the kind of home ownership.

Direct measurements of magnetic fields were made in the homes. Fields were measured for twenty-four hours in the bedroom of the child close to the child's bed. Spot checks of fields were also made in other rooms of the house, and an appropriate average exposure calculated that took into account the time spent by the child in the different rooms. Unless measurements could be made in the houses in which the case child(the leukemia victim) had lived 70% of the time period prior to the diagnosis of leukemia, the child was not included in the study. It was required that the control child matched to the case child also meet this condition for the same time period.

The magnetic field measurements were made within two years of the diagnosis of the disease, unlike in earlier studies when they were made sometimes as much as a decade or more after diagnosis. This shorter time period meant that the measurements were more likely to represent the child's exposure before he or she became ill.

The authors' conclusions were as follows:

> The risk of childhood [acute lymphoblastic] leukemia was not linked to summary time-weighted average residential magnetic-field levels. . . . The risk . . . was not increased among children whose main residences were in the highest wire-code category. . . . Furthermore, the risk was not significantly associated with either residential magnetic-field levels or the wire codes of the homes mothers resided in when pregnant with the subjects.

More than 80% of the homes were found to have average magnetic fields less than 0.2 microtesla (see "What Are Electric and Magnetic Fields?" [p. 230]), so the homes were divided into two groups, those with less than 0.2 microtesla, and those with more. No statistically significant difference in leukemia risk between the two groups was found by the authors. As we will see, the particular test they used for statistical significance has been criticized. However, using their test they did find a statistically significant excess risk in one narrow range of exposure: in homes in which the magnetic fields were between 0.4 and 0.5 microtesla (fields higher than this are considered to be "very high" for residences). They noted that the number of cases was small and also noted that there was no significant excess risk in the even smaller number of homes with fields higher than 0.5 microtesla, the highest fields observed in the study, and no trace of a dose-response relationship. They therefore concluded that this excess of leukemia in homes with fields between 0.4 and 0.5 microtesla was a statistical fluke, in spite of the fact that it met their test of statistical significance.

The most serious criticism of this study is a technical one, concerning whether the test for statistical significance used by the authors was the right one to use. A number of scientists have argued that the test should have been done differently, and if it is done the way the critics recommend, the excess leukemia risk for homes above 0.2 microtesla would have been statistically significant, not just the risk in homes with fields between 0.4 and 0.5 microtesla. Obviously, if the critics are right, the study supports rather than contradicts the conclusions of earlier studies. Even disregarding this technical point, critics pointed out that the statistically significant excess of leukemia in the children exposed to fields between

0.4 and 0.5 microtesla, an effect unlikely to have occurred by chance alone, was quite in line with preceding studies.

The disagreement between the authors of this study and their critics is therefore not so much about the data as about what the data mean. Linet and her coauthors, as scientists should, published their data and described in full detail how the data were gathered and analyzed, leaving other scientists free not only to disagree but also to use the same results to support a different conclusion.

Less Risk in the United Kingdom

A British study published in 1999, the largest completed so far, compared the exposure to magnetic fields, measured directly in the homes and in schools, of over 2,000 childhood cancer cases with an equal number of control children. The study's conclusion was as follows: "This study provides no evidence that exposure to magnetic fields associated with the electricity supply in the United Kingdom increases the risks for childhood leukemia, cancers of the central nervous system, or any other childhood cancer." An editorial comment in the issue of the journal bearing this article points out that in the United States and Canada, exposures to higher magnetic fields in the home is more common than in the United Kingdom: 10–15% of homes in these North American countries have fields exceeding 0.2 microtesla, while only 2–3% of United Kingdom homes do, a consequence of the differing electric voltages used in homes in these countries. In other words, because of the small number of homes with fields above 0.2 microtesla, this study lacked the power to detect a moderately increased leukemia rate, if such an increase had occurred (see discussion of power in chapter 8). It follows that the study, while reassuring to residents of the United Kingdom, does not really contradict studies showing higher leukemia rates in homes in the highest magnetic field category.

Have These Studies Solved the Problem?

Considering that there is some evidence in the Linet study of a relation between leukemia and very high fields in the homes, it is not likely that if the National Research Council Committee had added that study to the dozen other studies they reviewed, it would have changed their conclusions by much. The same can be said about the large British study, in which there were too few cases exposed to high fields to apply definitively to U.S. conditions. A number of other studies have also been published recently, with the same sort of mixed results described in the National Research Council report.

A 1999 review of the problem by the National Institute of Environmental Health Sciences (NIEHS) came to essentially the same conclusion as the earlier National Research Council report, classifying low-frequency electromagnetic fields as a "possible human carcinogen," rather than a "probable human carcinogen," which in turn is a lower risk category than a "known human carcinogen." The scientific evidence that exposure to such fields might pose a leukemia hazard was described as "weak," and "insufficient to warrant aggressive regulatory concern," though less intensive measures to reduce exposure were suggested.

It is to be hoped that when those studies now in progress are completed, a clearer picture will emerge. Among them are some that consider exposures not only to average fields over time, but also to transient much higher fields, lasting less than a second or so, that occur when large appliances are turned off or on. In addition, a large Japanese study is underway, in which exposures have been very high.

The increase in leukemia found in those studies that reported an increase at all was on average about 50%, smaller than the doubling of the risk (a 100% increase) reported in the original Denver study. Childhood leukemia is a rare disease, affecting about 4 to 6 children per 100,000 per year. While only a small proportion of homes in the world have high magnetic fields, the number of exposed children is very large, and even a small increase in the rate of the disease could add up to a lot of children made to suffer. On the other hand it has not been conclusively demonstrated that magnetic fields are the cause of this 50% increase. There are many reasons for being cautious about such a conclusion.

ASSOCIATION VERSUS CAUSATION

The National Research Council summarized the results of the epidemiological studies by saying that it is likely that an "association" exists between local power transmission wiring and childhood leukemia. We have put the term "association" in quotes because it needs more explanation. If it does not mean that magnetic fields cause childhood leukemia, what does it mean?

Association between two quantities can be either positive or negative. If when one increases the other does also, it is a positive association. If when one increases the other decreases, it is a negative one. An example of a positive association is that between people's education and their income, of a negative association, coffee drinking after dinner and subsequent hours of sleep. If when one quantity increases the other shows no tendency to either increase or decrease, they are said to be not associated. An example of two quantities not associated is the Dow-Jones index and the daily rainfall in Karachi. Certainly, if one quantity is the cause of the other, they will be associated. But the opposite need not be true; two quantities may be associated for many reasons other than a cause-and-effect one. The history of medicine is rich with examples of associations once believed to represent cause-and-effect relationships, which later turned out to be accidental. It is worth citing one example.

When London was suffering repeated epidemics of cholera in the mid-nineteenth century, the germ theory of disease was still a speculative idea, believed by only a few physicians. At that time most of them thought that contagious diseases were transmitted through the air by "miasmas," heavy clouds of foul and disease-causing poisons given off by the bodies of the sick or the dead. A leading London physician, Dr. William Farr, reasoned from this miasma theory that the low-lying districts of London, to which the miasmas would sink, should have higher rates of cholera than the districts of higher elevation. He found the marked (negative) association between the elevation above sea level of London districts and their death rates from cholera that he predicted, and thought, with good reason, that he had proved a cause-and-effect relation.

Dr. John Snow, another eminent London physician and an early believer in the germ theory, found a different explanation for Dr. Farr's association: cholera is spread by a water supply contaminated by the excretions of its victims, the excretions presumably containing a living organism that caused the disease. The drinking water of London was taken from the Thames River, polluted by the sewage of the city, and therefore was more polluted as the river flows down past the city. The lower the elevation of districts of London, the further downstream they were, and the more polluted their drinking water tended to be.

Professors of statistics or epidemiology often make the distinction between "association" and a cause-and-effect relation in their classrooms by the example of a strong negative association, discovered by a clever statistician: in the United States in the early twentieth century, the death rate from typhoid fever declined in close proportion to the increase in the number of telephone poles. Telephone poles, however, do not prevent typhoid fever. Both changes are consequences of the rising standards of living and sanitation and the introduction of new technology at that time.

In Europe, both the birth rate and the number of storks nesting on rooftops have declined together. It is left as an exercise for the reader to figure out why.

In brief, an "association" does not prove causation. Epidemiology works by guessing at a possible cause of a disease and examining human populations to see if the guessed cause is associated with an increased rate of the disease. Sometimes the association is strong, as it is with cigarette smoking and lung cancer, and the guess is supported by other evidence also. The association between magnetic fields, or with wire codes as their surrogates, and leukemia is weak. What other kinds of evidence could we use to establish or refute a causal relationship?

How We Recognize Causes

To define precisely what we mean by "cause" would get us into too philosophical a discussion. Instead, we will simply report how scientists concerned with health and disease use the word. In brief, while an association found in epidemiological studies can suggest a cause, other kinds of evidence are required to confirm it. Are the epidemiological findings consistent with what doctors have learned about the disease in the course of treating its victims? Is there a dose-response relationship? Is there supporting evidence from laboratory experiments on living cells, living tissues, or on animals? Is the hypothesis about the cause consistent with what we know from molecular biology? Specifically, if the illness is cancer, does it fit in with what is known about carcinogenesis? Does the hypothesis violate the laws of physics and chemistry?

It is only when there is coherence among all the relevant scientific disciplines, not just evidence from one of them, that scientists are willing to use the word "cause."

As an example, how do we know that ionizing radiation "causes" cancer (see chapters 2 and 3)? First of all, the many studies of cancer in human beings exposed to ionizing radiation, either from nuclear bombs or from medical X-rays, give fairly consistent results, and there is a dose-response relationship between the risk and the amount of exposure. Second, studies on laboratory animals and cell cultures show cancer risks in accord with what has been found from studies of human exposures. Third, our current understanding of molecular biology is consistent with the idea that ionizing radiation could cause cancer: at least some of the damage to the DNA molecules in the chromosomes produced by ionizing radiation is directly observable in the microscope. Fourth, the damage produced is consistent with what physics tells us about the disruption of chemical bonds by ionizing radiation. Everything hangs together; the different sciences increasingly shed light on different aspects of the question, and what they tell us is coherent.

Is there such a coherent picture on the health effects of magnetic fields?

Testing Coherence: Magnetic Fields in the Laboratory

What has been found in experiments exposing animals, cells, and living tissues to magnetic fields?

Such experiments have certain advantages compared to studies of human beings, among them that the strength and duration of the exposures can be chosen by the experimenter, and the animals may be given large exposures if necessary to produce detectable effects. Another advantage is that large numbers of animals can be used, many more than the numbers of people in typical episodes of radiation exposure, especially important when the disease under investigation is a rare one, like leukemia or brain cancer. Still another advantage is that animal populations used in laboratories are much more homogeneous than human ones: genetic variability is minimized, and diet and living conditions are made identical for all the subjects regardless of the level of exposure. Human beings, willful and disorderly as they are, marry whom they please, choose their own lifestyles and diets, work in various occupations, and live in various kinds of houses, any of which may influence their risk of a particular disease. The diversity of risk factors in human populations makes it more difficult to isolate the effect of the exposure we are interested in.

One drawback of animal studies is the necessity to extrapolate from usually high exposures in the laboratory to the lower ones to which humans are exposed. We need large exposures, especially with rare diseases; otherwise, the numbers of animals needed to establish a risk would be very large, and the experiment enormously expensive (see chapter 3 for a fuller discussion). A major drawback is the uncertainty of applying results from one species of animal to another.

That we can use controlled exposures, large numbers, and homogeneous populations in animal experiments suggests that the results of such experiments should be more reliable—at least as far as animals are concerned—than observations on human populations. This is in the main true, but we will also see that even under such ideal conditions living things are complex enough that we cannot always duplicate the results of experiments. The outcome often differs from one laboratory to another, from one scientist to another, and from one time to another, for reasons hard to discern.

Do Magnetic Fields Cause Cancer in Animals?

In laboratory experiments to test the possibility that fields cause cancer, animals were exposed for a number of hours a day over long periods of time to 50- or 60-hertz magnetic fields, with strengths as high as 1000 microtesla. No increase in any form of cancer was found in a number of different species of animals.

There is, however, another, less direct, way that fields might have caused cancers. It was not expected that the fields could act as directly as ionizing radiation does, in damaging the DNA molecules in the chromosomes, thus initiating the process eventually leading to malignant cells. (For more details on carcinogenesis and ionizing radiation, see chapters 2 and 7.) Because 60-hertz electric and magnetic fields do not carry energy in anything like the concentrated bursts (photons) of ionizing radiation, they cannot cause mutations directly. However, the process by which cancer begins in an animal or a human being is more complex and less well understood than just the initiating damage to DNA. Another step, called *promotion*, may also be needed to further transform the damaged cell toward a cancerous state. There are specific chemicals known that do not initiate cancer, but are necessary to promote its future development; for example, hormones such as estrogen are believed to act as promoters in the development of breast cancer (see chapters 5 and 6).

Do Magnetic Fields Promote Cancer?

To test if magnetic fields act as promoters, initiation was first carried out either by exposing animals or cells to carcinogenic chemicals or to ionizing radiation, or by directly implanting cancerous cells from other animals. Then the animals were exposed to magnetic fields of known strenghts (usually considerably higher than human residential exposures). Other experiments were done on species of animals genetically prone to leukemia. The animals or cells were exposed to magnetic fields of known strengths and compared with animals or cells also exposed to initiating factors but not to magnetic fields. In most such experiments magnetic fields did not promote cancer. The types of cancer studied in these experiments included leukemia and mammary, skin, and liver cancers.

Exposure to radiation or to carcinogenic chemicals produces not only cancers but usually birth defects or miscarriages as well. A number of studies on mice and rats did not find that magnetic fields had any such effects.

Melatonin, the Pineal Gland, and Breast Cancer

A number of experiments on laboratory animals have shown effects of electric and magnetic fields on the production of a hormone called melatonin, produced in the pineal gland, a small gland located below the brain and apparently associated with vision. Melatonin can be purchased in health food stores, and had been claimed to reduce jet lag, a claim recently disproved. There is some evidence that levels of melatonin could have an indirect effect on the development of cancer and on the immune system: animals that have had their pineal glands removed are more susceptible to cancer when exposed to carcinogenic chemicals, but the susceptibility is reduced if they are then given melatonin. Melatonin synthesis in the body is diminished by exposure to daylight, and levels in the bloodstream are many times higher at night than in the daytime.

There have been two speculative theories as to how a decrease in melatonin could be carcinogenic. A decrease of melatonin level in the body is known to increase the activity of certain reproductive hormones. In turn, it is thought that an increase in these hormones could lead to an increase in cell proliferation in hormone-sensitive cells such as are found in breast and prostate tissue, leading eventually to cancer in these organs. Another theory is that melatonin helps destroy certain oxidizing substances, known as "free radicals," in the body and might decrease their known ability to damage DNA and initiate cancer. If either speculative theory is correct, and if magnetic fields really do decrease melatonin production, then a plausible biological mechanism for an effect of magnetic fields on cancer would be established.

The influence of electric and magnetic fields on melatonin production in the pineal gland and on melatonin concentration in the bloodstream have been studied in a number of laboratories and on a variety of animals: rats, hamsters, sheep, and baboons. Not all studies have shown an effect of electric or magnetic fields, but those that do have usually found that fields decrease the production of melatonin or its levels in blood, similar to the effect of light.

Studies on human beings have been inconclusive. The NIEHS report concluded that they "provide little support that exposure [to electromagnetic fields] is altering melatonin levels in humans."

Epidemiological studies of the relation of breast cancer to magnetic field exposure have shown mixed results, the majority showing no effect (see chapters 5 and 6). Studies on cultures of breast cancer cells have indeed shown that relatively low magnetic fields, comparable to residential fields, do counteract the effects of melatonin or tamoxifen in regulating cell growth. The effects are small, so what bearing they have on breast cancer is not clear, but the finding does suggest that more research on melatonin levels and cancer are needed, as well as evidence on whether magnetic fields do reduce melatonin levels in humans.

Bone Healing

One striking and well-reproduced effect of electric or magnetic fields is that they help heal bone fractures. The fields needed are much larger than residential fields. The effect of magnetic fields on fracture healing is universally attributed to the electric currents they induce. Electrical effects on bone growth are not surprising; bones are known to show such electrical properties as piezoelectricity, the production of electric currents by certain crystalline substances when they are placed under elastic stress. There is no obvious connection between this well-established fact and the possibility that much weaker fields may cause cancer, but it is important to be aware that electric or magnetic fields can have effects on living organisms.

Cells, Signals, Membranes, and Heat Stress

Living cells suspended in water solutions of salts and nutrients are simpler systems than whole animals and have also been studied. No observable effects have been found when cell suspensions have been exposed to magnetic fields at strengths comparable to those of residential fields, but under higher field strengths—100 to 1,000 times residential levels—some interesting and reproducible effects have been demonstrated. A cell is enclosed in a membrane, through which it interacts with its environment. Sometimes the interaction is accomplished by a molecule penetrating through the membrane, and sometimes a molecule arriving at the outside surface causes a signal to be transmitted through the membrane. Cells produce a substance called ornithine decarboxylase (ODC) that plays a role in this transmission of signals. The activity of ODC can be measured in the medium surrounding the cell. It has been demonstrated in more than one laboratory that ODC activity is increased by exposure to 60-hertz fields of 10–100 microteslas, about 100 or more times average residential levels (which are typically a few tenths of a microtesla). Interestingly, ODC activity is also increased by tumor-producing agents. In the range of fields between 50 and 500 microtesla, the increase of ODC activity has so far been one of the few reproducible effects of magnetic fields. However, one report that fields of 10 microtesla (higher than average residential fields but not higher than those produced by current surges) increased ODC activity in mouse lymphoma (cancer) cells could not be duplicated in other laboratories.

Is the Case for Excess Cancers Biologically Plausible?

How well have the laboratory experiments on animals, cells, and tissues supported the relation between magnetic fields and cancer found in epidemiological studies? There are some clear-cut biological effects of magnetic fields at higher strengths than residential fields, but the relation of these effects to disease, and specifically cancer, are highly speculative. So far no cancer-producing effects have been demonstrated at field strengths comparable to those in homes.

The conclusions of the 1997 National Research Council Report on this question were as follows:

> The data at different biological complexities, taken in total, do not provide convincing evidence that electric and magnetic fields experienced in residential environments are carcinogenic. No tests or studies can prove that an agent is not carcinogenic at some dose level, in combination with some other biologic agent or for some sensitive populations of

humans. All that can be stated is that under the exact experimental conditions of an extremely large number of studies exposure to power frequency electric and magnetic fields at environmental strengths does not produce patterns of data similar to those found for other agents that have been shown to be carcinogenic.

The more recent NIEHS report comes to a similar conclusion: the studies on animals and cell lines "fail to demonstrate any consistent pattern across studies, although sporadic findings of biological effects [of magnetic fields] have been reported."

The contrast with studies of ionizing radiation is worth repeating: in spite of many gaps in knowledge of the mechanism of carcinogenesis, such radiation, shown in epidemiological studies to be associated with cancer in humans, produces cancers in laboratory animals and malignant changes in individual cells at exposures and rates quite consistent with the epidemiological studies. Further, much more is known about the biological and chemical steps by which ionizing radiation produces malignancies.

Coherence with the Laws of Physics?

Some physicists have questioned the plausibility of harm from magnetic and electric fields, on the grounds that the fields produced within the body by residential sources are much weaker than fields produced within the body from its own nature and functioning. Transitory fields result from the electrical activity of nerve cells and muscles. Further, other transitory fields result from the fact that living tissue, like all other forms of matter at ordinary temperatures, is made up of molecules that contain electrical charges and are in constant motion and collision. As a result of this constant motion, at any point in the body, say at the surface of a cell, there are constantly changing magnetic and electric fields. The magnitudes of these fields, both those that arise from electrical activity of living tissue and those that arise from the nature of matter itself, are known to be as much as 100 or 1,000 times greater than fields associated with electrical wiring in or near the home. They can be thought of as a kind of noise that would drown out any effect of the residential fields. Under these circumstances, ask the skeptics, how could residential fields produce any harmful or other biological effects at all?

A few physicists do not agree. They have speculated that residential fields are more uniform in space and time than the fluctuating fields from processes within the body even though they are usually weaker, and that cells may be able to respond to this spatial and temporal uniformity. This hypothesis has had some experimental support.

SUMMARY

As of this writing, a large number of the epidemiological studies have found an association of childhood leukemia with at least the highest levels of magnetic fields known to occur in homes. How best to estimate average fields to which subjects have been exposed many years in the past, or even whether average fields are the things to measure, are matters of controversy. So is the possibility that the important fields are much higher short-term transient ones, arising from surges in current when appliances are turned on or off.

Attempts to explain the association as fortuitous, a result of factors such as social class, population density, age of home, or anything else that may independently affect leukemia risk and at the same time be accidentally correlated with the residential magnetic fields, have not been successful. It may be that some as yet uninvestigated accidental factor will turn out to explain the association, and it could also turn out that the association really reflects a causal relation between some aspect of magnetic fields and leukemia.

Is such a causal relation coherent with other fields of science, such as biology and physics? Biological studies of magnetic fields have not yet provided much support. Those biological effects that, on the one hand, can be reproduced from laboratory to laboratory almost always involve field strengths much higher than residential fields, and, on the other, have not yet been shown to play a role in the development of cancer. The questions raised by some physicists about the swamping of residential magnetic fields within the body by fluctuating fields from body processes and from molecular motion have not been answered to everyone's satisfaction. Biology and physics have not proved that magnetic fields cannot possibly cause cancer, but neither have they yet made a plausible case for a cause-and-effect relation.

The 1999 report of the NIEHS gave its conclusion in the following words:

The National Institute of Environmental Health and Safety believes that the probability that electromagnetic field exposure is truly a health hazard is currently small. The weak epidemiologic associations and lack of any laboratory support for these associations provide only marginal scientific support that exposure to this agent is causing any degree of harm. . . .

Virtually all the laboratory evidence in animals and humans and most of the mechanistic studies in cells fail to support a causal relationship.

What to Do?

The fact that we do not yet know for sure whether magnetic fields in homes are harmless or confer some cancer risk does not necessarily mean we should do nothing to avoid them. The NIEHS, as well as a number of individual scientists, have made an argument for prudence: magnetic fields may ultimately be shown to do harm, and perhaps out of caution we should take measures to minimize exposure, provided they are not too expensive or disruptive. Some suggested measures include siting power lines to reduce exposure, exploring safe ways to reduce magnetic fields around transmission and distribution lines, repositioning certain appliances known to produce high fields in their immediate vicinities, or avoiding close proximity to them, and measuring fields within the home to look for local "hot spots."

Environmental agencies often regulate exposure to chemicals when the risk of serious harm is 1 per 100,000 people. If the association between childhood leukemia and some aspect of residential magnetic fields should turn out to be a cause-and-effect one, it would meet this criterion. This, however, does not tell us the cost to society of the regulation. The problem with electricity is that it is everywhere in the modern world, and the cost of reducing exposure to the magnetic fields associated with it is hard to calculate and might be very high indeed. Matters are made worse by the fact that we do not know what aspect of electromagnetic fields we should be concerned with. In any event, distribution lines would have to be buried underground, and wiring in homes in general and in specific appliances would have to be redesigned.

A report on electromagnetic fields and human health by the Harvard Center for Risk Analysis stated as follows:

The potential economic costs of mitigating the possible health effects associated with [electromagnetic fields] are substantial. For example, concern over high voltage power lines has led to delays and cancellations of new projects constructing these lines. Not only can this lead to higher costs from having to find alternative sites for the lines, but it also may increase the frequency of brownouts and power outages to consumers. Concern over power lines may also decrease property values along transmission routes or induce power companies to move or redesign existing lines at considerable expense to the public. The cost to the average consumer of changes such as these may be significant, not only in the size of citizens' electric bills, but also in the potential availability of electricity for heat, air conditioning, and other household necessities.

If it were only a question of money, one might be tempted to balance the cost against the possible suffering and lives of the children, and decide to move or redesign the power lines. Unfortunately, higher utility bills have health consequences also. In the summer of 1998 a prolonged heat spell caused the deaths of several hundred elderly people in various areas of the United States, most of them because they could not afford air conditioning. An electric power shortage and a consequent dramatic increase in cost in California is front-page news in 2001. There are always what are called "unintended consequences" of any course of action, no matter how beneficial it seems when proposed.

We must hope that further studies, both epidemiological and in the laboratory, will answer the question one way or another before long. Until then, what should be done? Should we wait for a definitive scientific answer, or should we take precautionary measures now, and if we want to take precautions, what should they be? There is a sense of urgency from the fact that electric power use is increasing both in the developed and developing world, and many more millions of people are being exposed.

On the other hand many scientists believe that the case for harm from magnetic fields is too weak to merit much additional expensive research, even though the excess of childhood leukemia has not been explained, and that the problem should be put aside for the time being instead of making strenuous efforts to solve it, on the ground that there are more promising and more pressing ones to spend our research dollars on. The NIEHS for example has concluded that no new epidemiological studies are warranted unless they differ from existing ones in some unique way and test new hypotheses. Perhaps new developments in molecular biology will suggest such hypotheses. It is not a happy situation, but science does not always provide clear answers to the questions we ask at the time we ask them, and its limitations must be accepted. In any event, we think it unlikely that we will again need an ice-man to lead a donkey car loaded with blocks of ice through our neighborhoods.

A CLOSER LOOK: WHAT ARE ELECTRIC AND MAGNETIC FIELDS?

What Almost Everybody Knows about Electricity

One does not need to know all that much about the basic science of electromagnetism to follow our discussion. Our goal is to explain a little about the concepts, which we will attempt by building on some common knowledge.

If a metal wire is connected between the positive and negative terminals of a battery, a current of electrons will flow through the wire until the battery is discharged, as happens when a flashlight is left on. The electrons, which bear a negative electric charge, flow from the negative terminal to the positive terminal. A historical note on terminology: before the electron and the proton were discovered, it was realized that there were two different kinds of electricity: if two bodies both are charged with the same kind, they repel each other. If each of the two is charged with a different kind, they attract each other, and if they come into contact tend to neutralize each other. In effect the two equal and opposite charges cancel out. The choice of the terms "negative" and "positive" for the two kinds reflects this neutralizing tendency, but the electron could as easily have been called "positive," and the proton "negative."

The current from a battery flows through the wire in one direction only and is called a direct current (D.C.). Household electric current in the United States alternates in direction (A.C.), the electrons flowing back and forth in the wires, changing direction at a frequency of 60 times a second (in Europe current alternates 50 times a second). The scientific unit of frequency is the hertz, and a current alternating at a frequency of 60 times a second is said to alternate at 60 hertz. The reason A.C. is commonly used is that the electrical energy can be transmitted from the power plant to the home with smaller losses in the transmission lines, using very high voltages.

Fields

We say there is a "field" in some region of space if we find that there is a force exerted on a body placed anywhere in that region. The gravitational field of the earth exerts a force on any body in its neighborhood: the force exerted by the earth's gravity on a body is what we mean by the "weight" of the body. An electric field exerts a force on an electrically charged body such as an electron and makes it move; that is how we know that there is an electric field. A magnetic field exerts forces on a magnet, attracting one of its poles and repelling the other. The two forces are equal and opposite; the net effect is that the magnetic field makes the magnet point in a particular direction: it orients, rather than drags the magnet.

When a current flows in an electric wire it produces a magnetic field in the space around the wires. This is how electromagnets are made. If the electric current is changing direction in the wire at 60 hertz, the magnetic field of the electromagnet also changes direction at 60 hertz.

What Do Fields Do to Us?

Because human bodies are good electrical conductors (the fluids of the body, such as blood and cellular fluids, contain dissolved salts), electrical fields cause currents to flow in their outer surfaces, but do not penetrate them. However, magnetic fields do, and could produce effects inside.

We may think we encounter magnetism less often than electricity, but this is a misconception. Where there are electric currents, there are always magnetic fields. Magnets commonly come to our attention as children's toys, minor gadgets like those used to hold notes on the doors of refrigerators, and compass needles, though many of us also know that an electromagnet can be made by running an electric current through a coil of wire. The common doorbell uses (or once used) an electromagnet, but a more important industrial application is to lift heavy chunks of iron. The compass needle, opposite ends of which are marked with the letters N and S, or painted different colors, tells direction because the earth itself is a magnet with a "north" pole and a "south" pole.

Visualizing the Magnetic Field

We use a compass to tell direction on the earth's surface, but another way to think about a compass is as a device to visualize the earth's magnetic field. Everywhere on the earth we place the compass, the needle will point toward what is called the earth's North Magnetic Pole. If turned away from that direction, it swings back. If we imagine drawing on a map of the earth a little arrow pointing the way the compass does at that spot, and doing this at a sufficiently large number of places, we will end up with a map full of arrows showing at each point the direction of the earth's magnetic field. As we move into outer space, the earth's magnetic field becomes weaker, but cannot be considered to end at some definite place. The strength of the magnetic field as well as its direction in space therefore varies from one place to another.

Another way to map a magnetic field is by the use of iron filings, elongated particles of metallic iron, which line up in the direction of the field (fig. 7-6).

Static Fields and Time-Varying Fields

We have mentioned two particular examples of a magnetic field: the first that of the earth itself, which stays essentially constant in strength and direction, at least over short periods of time, and the field around wires carrying 60-Hertz alternating electric current, which alters in direction and strength also at 60 hertz. Magnetic fields that stay the same in strength and direction are called

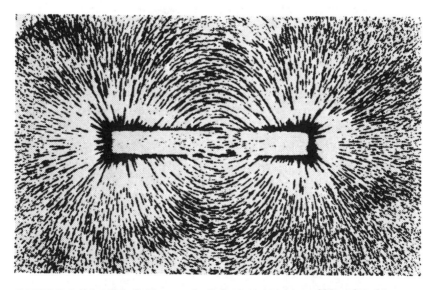

FIGURE 7-6 Magnetic field around a bar magnet. An iron filing placed in a magnetic field becomes a magnet itself, with a north and a south pole, and then aligns itself with the magnetic field. Each filing acts just like a compass needle would, if placed in the same position, and shows the direction of the field at that position. From the book, *PSSC Physics*, and reproduced with the permission of the Educational Development Center, Inc., Newton, MA.

"static" fields, and do not produce any electrical currents in near-by metal wires that are not moving, but magnetic fields that are changing with time cause electric currents to flow in wires. Alternatively, if metal wires are moved in a static magnetic field, electric currents are induced in them. This is how electric power is produced, using either fuels or falling water to rotate coils of metal wires in a magnetic field. We can measure low-frequency alternating magnetic fields by the electric currents they produce in an electric circuit.

Magnetic field strengths are expressed in one of two units: the older unit is called the gauss (abbreviated G) and has recently officially been replaced by the tesla (T). However, the gauss is still often used. One tesla is equal to 10,000 gauss; in words, a magnetic field of one tesla is ten thousand times stronger than a field of one gauss. The strength of the earth's static field is about 0.5 G or about fifty-millionths of a tesla. A millionth of a tesla is called a microtesla. The alternating magnetic fields measured inside homes range up to about 5 milligauss (thousandths of a gauss, abbreviated mG) or 0.5 microtesla.

One important property of magnetic fields is that they decrease rapidly with distance from their sources (see fig. 7-2, p. 207).

8

CANCER FROM THE LANDFILL?

THE LANDFILL AT PELHAM BAY

How It Began

In the first chapter we described several clusters of childhood cancers discovered by concerned residents of Woburn, Massachusetts, of Toms River, New Jersey, and of the Pelham Bay section of the Bronx, New York City. The residents in Pelham Bay blamed the cluster on a landfill nearby, in which hundreds of thousands of gallons of toxic chemicals, including waste oil sludges, metal plating wastes, lacquer, cyanides, ethyl benzene, toluene, and other organic solvents had been illegally dumped (fig. 8-1). This had been reported by an employee of the chemical company responsible, in testimony before a Congressional investigation of crime, and was never directly confirmed. Residents of the community had obtained a court order that stopped dumping in 1978, before the testimony about toxic wastes had been given.

The story of this cancer cluster—both how it was discovered and what conclusions were reached about its causes—is typical of thousands of clusters reported each year to health authorities throughout the United States.

After the alarm in Pelham Bay was sounded by the mother of a child with leukemia, ten years after dumping ceased, the New York City Department of Environmental Protection (NYCDEP) made measurements of

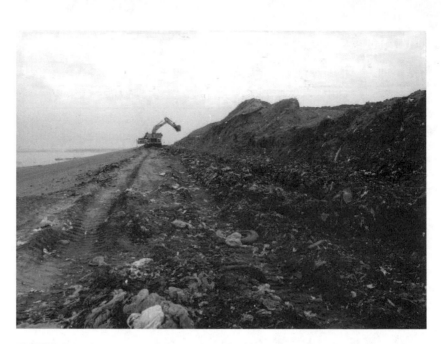

FIGURE 8-1   One corner of the mountain of garbage, with Pelham Bay in the background. Courtesy of the New York City Department of Environmental Protection.

hazardous chemicals in the air around the landfill, but found no significant amounts. The drinking water of the community came from the general New York City water supply system, so seepage from the landfill into the groundwater was not a possible route of exposure. It was concluded that by the time the measurements were made the landfill was no longer a threat to health. What the situation may have been in the past, during the time of dumping and just after, could no longer be known.

After dumping had been stopped in 1978, the NYCDEP had covered the 150-foot-high mound of garbage, refuse, street sweepings, construction debris, and household and commercial waste, along with whatever may have been illegally dumped there, with a thin layer of soil. It was a hasty job, and it did not last. The soil cover cracked and eroded, washing away all the faster because of the steep slopes of the mound. Rain fell on the mound, some running off the surface and some seeping through to form ponds around the base, in which the concentrations of heavy metals and toxic organic compounds exceeded safety standards for surface water. The groundwater in the vicinity of the mound, its level rising and falling with the tides, carried metals and organic contaminants to the waters of the bay.

After the community charged that toxic chemicals from the landfill were causing high rates of cancer, the NYCDEP made a comprehensive effort to seal off the landfill and prevent any further exposure to hazardous substances. Drainage systems were installed so that water seeping through the mound could be regularly collected and disposed of safely elsewhere. Gases, mainly non-toxic methane, produced by chemical and biological degradation of garbage, are now collected and burned. The mound has been given what is hoped to be a permanent covering: a layer of impermeable plastic, covered with a layer of soil stabilized against erosion by the planting of vegetation. Someday, if the cover lasts and the concentrations of hazardous substances in the vicinity of the mound are found to be safe, the site may once again be part of the surrounding park.

The New York City Department of Health (DOH) began a health study in response to the concerns of the community and reported on its progress at frequent intervals to residents at community meetings. In the course of the study, the DOH issued a number of written reports on its findings, the most comprehensive one in 1994, which were distributed to the residents.

One of this book's authors, Inge, served on a scientific advisory committee established by the NYCDEP to serve as a liaison between the department and the community. A considerable part of her time was spent helping the community residents understand how the DOH assessed the health consequences of the landfill. It required her to find ways to explain to them some of the basics of cancer epidemiology, the meaning of certain technical terms such as statistical significance, power, and confidence interval, and to enable them to make sense of tables of data that initially they found intimidating.

In what follows we use this study as an example of how the health hazards from toxic wastes are evaluated scientifically, and as a further opportunity, even at the risk of repetition, to clarify the meaning of some of the statistical concepts discussed in other chapters.

THE DEPARTMENT OF HEALTH STUDY

What the DOH Looked For

The feeling in the community was that not only leukemia but many other forms of cancer were elevated. The DOH, responding to these concerns, investigated a number of types of cancer in addition to childhood leukemia, specifically those cancers which there was some reason to believe might be caused by exposure to toxic chemicals.

An important scientific fact about cancer was noted in the DOH report: most human cancers take on the average from twenty to fifty years to develop from the time of exposure to cancer-causing agents to the time a case of cancer is diagnosed. Since the most likely time period of high exposure to possible cancer-causing substances from the Pelham Bay Landfill was in the *late 1970s*, when the greatest amount of illegal dumping is believed to have occurred, and the investigation initially had data only on cancers diagnosed between 1978 and 1987, it is not likely that exposure from the landfill could have caused any excess. Sufficient time had not elapsed.

This is not true, however, for those cancers of the blood system called the leukemias. These have been shown to occur as little as five years after exposure to agents such as benzene or ionizing radiation. Thus, in contrast to most other types of cancer, sufficient time would have elapsed to observe an increase in leukemia associated with landfill exposure—if such an increase has in fact occurred.

While the DOH made these points in its report, the impression in the community that other cancer rates were also high needed to be addressed. In addition, these rates for the period 1978–1987 would be needed to provide a reference point for some future study to determine if there really are increases in cancer rates due to exposures from the landfill after the lapse of sufficient time.

What Were They Exposed to, and How Much?

There was one major obstacle to deciding if there were health effects of past exposures to the Pelham Bay Landfill: we do not know the amounts or the chemical nature of substances emanating from the landfill when dumping was going on. We only know that the exposures measured at the start of the study, years after the closure of the landfill in 1978 and after constant tidal washing and flushing of the site, were too low to cause any significant adverse health effects.

Could unknown *past* exposures to the landfill have been responsible for any excesses in leukemia or other cancer rates? If one knew what these past exposures were, one could attempt to answer that question more confidently. Since they were not known, the best the DOH could do was to see if the numbers of specific cancers that occurred in the Pelham Bay community were higher than the numbers that one would expect to occur. The rates of the same cancers in the population of the rest of New York City, not exposed to emissions from the landfill, were used for the comparison. The time period for the study was from 1978, both the year of maximum dumping of toxic wastes and the year dumping stopped, to 1987, the most recent year at that time for which cancer data was available. Later, data on leukemia was extended through 1991. If the rates of various cancers were found to be about the same in the community as in the rest of the city, we could reasonably conclude that any exposures from the landfill had not been great enough to cause a significant increase in the disease by the time of the study. If, on the other hand, increases in the cancer rates in the community had been found, we could at least consider exposures from the landfill as an explanation, though we would want stronger evidence, including cancer rates for a longer period of time, before we consider it probable, given how long it usually takes for such cancers to develop after exposure.

What the DOH Concluded

The conclusions from these studies, as given in the DOH reports, can briefly be summarized as follows:

The rates of cancers of selected individual sites in the body (e.g., liver cancer, stomach cancer, leukemia) and of cancers of all sites combined in the Pelham Bay area in the period 1978–1987 are generally similar to the rates of such cancers that occur in the other health districts of New York City for the same time period. In particular, this was the case for childhood leukemia, which was the type of cancer that had first aroused concern. Where differences occurred, it was concluded that the cancers were not likely to have resulted from exposures to the landfill. Typical results on a number of types of cancer are given in table 8-1, extracted and condensed from tables (2a, 2b, 2c, 2d) in one of the DOH reports, "Cancer Incidence in the Pelham Bay Area," published in January 1994. How does one interpret such a table, and how did the DOH use the data to reach its conclusion?

How the DOH Went about It

The DOH compared the numbers of various types of cancer over a ten-year period in the Pelham Bay community to the numbers expected from the rates in New York City as a whole.

TABLE 8-1   Observed and Expected Numbers of Cancer Cases of Various
Types in the Pelham Bay Community, 1978–1987

Type of Cancer	Observed	Expected	Ratio of Observed to Expected	95% Confidence Interval for Ratio
Adult Males				
Pharynx	397	460	0.86	0.78–0.95
Colon	1358	1254	1.08	1.03–1.14[a]
Pancreas	375	347	1.08	0.97–1.19
Lung	2178	2119	1.03	0.98–1.07
Prostate	1756	1833	0.96	0.91–1.00
Lymphoma	436	476	0.92	0.83–1.00
Leukemias	318	279	1.14	1.01–1.26[a]
All Sites	11,006	11,067	0.99	0.98–1.01
Adult Females				
Pharynx	224	220	1.02	0.88–1.15
Colon	1,522	1,477	1.03	0.92–1.12
Pancreas	380	411	0.92	0.83–1.02
Lung	1,093	1,159	0.94	0.89–0.99[a]
Breast	3,125	3,203	0.98	0.94–1.01
Lymphoma	484	469	1.03	0.94–1.12
Leukemias	288	270	1.07	0.94–1.19
All Sites	12,883	12,997	0.99	0.97–1.01
Male Children				
Lymphoma	17	10.3	1.65	0.87–2.44
Leukemias	25	23.3	1.07	0.65–1.49
All Sites	75	72.2	1.04	0.80–1.27
Female Children				
Lymphoma	6	4.8	1.25	0.25–2.25
Leukemias	18	16.8	1.07	0.58–1.57
All Sites	61	58.5	1.04	0.78–1.30

[a]Ratios whose 95% confidence interval does not include 1.00.

The "rate" of a disease is the number of cases occurring in a specified time period (such as a year) per 100,000 people (the use of 100,000 people as the reference is arbitrary, but it is a common choice). It is obvious that the number of cases of cancer (or for that matter, of measles) will be larger in New York City with its 6 million people than in the Pelham Bay community, which has a population of about half a million. Thus a rate of

50 cancers per 100,000 people per year corresponds to 3,000 cases in New York City as a whole, and 250 in Pelham Bay.

In comparing rates in two different communities, we need to take into account other characteristics of the two populations. Most types of cancer are more common among older people, and if there are more older people in one community than the other, more cancers are to be expected there, so it is necessary to correct for age differences, if they exist.

But the rate of any specific type of cancer varies not only with age but with such other factors as sex, ethnicity, occupation, dietary habits, and smoking. Such characteristics that are correlated with an increased rate of cancer—whether or not we know why—are known as "risk factors" (see discussion of risk factors and age adjustment in chapter 5). Ideally, the comparison population should be similar in all these factors to the Pelham Bay population, or else they should be corrected for. However, the DOH did not have enough information to make all such corrections, but only for the differences in age, sex, and race distribution between the local community and the city as a whole. The DOH used these corrected rates to calculate the numbers of cases expected in the Pelham Bay area. The assumption for the purposes of the study is that on the average, exposures to any cancer-causing substances except for possible emanations from the landfill are the same in New York City as a whole as in Pelham Bay. Thus, if more cancers are observed than expected in the Pelham Bay community in subsequent years, this excess, in the absence of any other plausible explanation, would tend to support the hypothesis that emissions from the landfill are responsible.

HOW WE DEAL WITH CHANCE

How Much of an Increase in Disease Can We Detect?

There is a problem that affects all epidemiological studies: the number of cases of disease that actually occur in any single year will vary from one year to the next in an unpredictable way because of factors of which we are ignorant or which we cannot control. These random or chance variations make it more difficult to answer the questions we want answered. Certainly, the community does not want even one additional child to get cancer, but our methods of study may not be sensitive enough to distinguish one extra case of cancer caused by the landfill from one extra case due to random variation. How many additional cancers must occur before we rule out random variation as responsible? Is it two cancers, or five? Must the rate of cancer double or triple in Pelham Bay before we conclude that there really is an excess of cancer that might have been caused by exposure to the landfill? The answer for childhood leukemia in Pelham Bay is, unfortunately, that the rate of the disease would have to double before we can detect the increase, and we will explain why in what follows.

To answer questions like these, certain concepts have been developed by statisticians, such as "statistical significance," "confidence interval," and "power." To explain these concepts here we will use the data and analyses of the DOH. They are also discussed in chapters 3 and 4.

Why Statistics?

Most cancer clusters involve small numbers of cases, and the smaller the number of cases, the harder it is to rule out chance. The number of cases of any disease we find in a community depends on two things: the size of the population and whether the disease is common or rare. Childhood leukemia is a relatively rare disease. In New York City, on the average about 4 children per year per 100,000 children and approximately 13 adults per year per 100,000 adults develop leukemia. There were approximately 406,700 adults and 97,000 children in the Pelham Bay community (at the time of the DOH study); thus, if the leukemia rates were similar to the rate in New York City we could expect about four children and about fifty-two adults in the community to get leukemia each year. However, the number of children getting leukemia each year varies by chance from year to year: there might be two one year and five the next. Among adults, although the average per year is fifty-two, anything between forty-five and sixty cases in a given year would not be surprising.

Why does "chance" play a role? Certainly, each individual case of cancer bears with it a burden of suffering and tragedy, for the victim, for the family, and for the community. Cannot the actual cause of each case be identified?

It is a natural human trait, when misfortune occurs, to want to know why. If our child catches a cold, we wonder whom she was playing with or if she went outside too soon after a bath. When we hear of someone dying of lung cancer, we wonder if he was a heavy smoker. Indeed, with many illnesses we can find a cause: we often know what we ate that caused a stomach upset, or whom we caught an infectious disease from. When the disease is serious and life threatening, like cancer, we feel all the more strongly that there must be a reason for it. We ask, why me? why my child?

Although we know much about the biological mechanisms involved in cancer, and something about factors that increase the individual's risk of cancer, such as age, exposure to certain toxic chemicals, smoking, and radiation, we still cannot predict which person will get cancer and when, nor can we usually tell, once the disease has manifested itself, what specifically caused it. This may change: methods of molecular biology may yet distinguish different patterns of genetic changes that provide clues to exposure. But we are not there yet.

It is like asking who, in the coming year, will be injured in an auto accident. Statistics show that very young drivers have a greater risk and so do very old ones, as well as drivers who drink. But which individuals will have an accident this year depends on too many other factors we never know in advance, such as emotional upsets, road conditions and weather, the behavior of other drivers, defects in the car. As far as predicting accidents, we can do no better than treat it as a kind of lottery, in which names are drawn at random out of a hat or by spinning a numbered wheel. For the most part, who the individual victims will be next year is a matter of chance.

Raisin Cakes and Chance

To develop some feeling for how chance operates, let us use the example of a raisin cake, which is to contain 200 raisins, and which after being cut into 20 slices will be eaten by the children in a family. These children, being normal children, like to count the raisins in the slices they get, rejoice when they get more than another child, and complain that it is unfair when they get less. Their father, who is going to bake the cake, wants to ensure that each slice has the same number of raisins, ten per slice. The first time he bakes he finds to his annoyance that a few of the slices have from thirty to fifty raisins, and most of the others none. He concludes that he did not mix the raisins in the dough long enough, and the next time he bakes he uses the mixer for a good five minutes. This time, again to his annoyance, the raisins come out unevenly distributed, though not as badly as before. He finds about as many slices with nine raisins as with ten, and only slightly fewer with eleven. There is even one slice with fourteen! In fact, there are only two ten-raisin slices, even though he expected most of them to have ten. The children squabble, and the irritated father decides next time to use the mixer for fifteen minutes instead of five. When he does so, the results come out much the same. Slices with ten raisins, even with careful and prolonged mixing of the dough, remain relatively rare. If we took an average over many cakes, we would find only 2.5 slices with ten raisins per cake.

What is wrong? Nothing, except the baker's preconceived idea that careful mixing of a dough should produce a perfectly uniform distribution of the raisins. In fact, results exactly equal to the average occur rarely. Chance produces uneven results, and can be described as "lumpy."

Given that chance alone determines how the raisins are distributed (i.e., assuming that the dough was well mixed, that the raisins do not stick together, etc.), the theory of probability enables us to predict such behavior quantitatively, telling us just how many ten-raisin slices will occur on the average (12.5% of the slices, or 2.5 slices out of twenty), how often slices with sixteen or more raisins occur on the average (5% of the slices), and how often a cake will come out with exactly ten raisins in each slice (much less often than one cake out of a trillion baked). The theory of probability has not been tested on one trillion raisin cakes, but it has been tested repeatedly in similar situations, those where chance alone determines the outcome, and it has been found to agree excellently with experience. (See the discussion in chapter 4 on chance and the Poisson distribution. Table 4-1 on p. 117 applies to raisin cakes with an average of five raisins per slice.)

Sometimes chance does not account for everything, as in the first not-too-well mixed cake the baker baked, and sometimes plays no role at all, as would be the case if the baker were patient enough, once the cake is in the baking pan, to insert exactly ten raisins by hand at twenty regular intervals, thus producing, at the expense of some work, a perfect raisin cake.

Chance and the Twenty-eight Additional Pancreatic Cancers

Members of the Pelham Bay community had the impression that other forms of cancer than leukemia were also elevated and had asked that this be looked into. The discussion of raisin cakes should suggest that by chance alone, some kinds of cancer would appear elevated, and others would appear to occur at lower than expected rates.

Let us consider one particular form of cancer that actually was elevated in the Pelham Bay community. During the ten-year period of the study, 375 cases of cancer of the pancreas in adult men (see table 8-1) occurred, while only 347 cases were expected from the rates in New York City as a whole. Is this excess of 28 cases a real increase of the disease, or could it be a result of chance?

This is actually a bad way to word the question. Any difference *could* be a result of chance variation; we can never be 100% sure, no matter how great the difference, that chance could not possibly have caused it. However, we can ask the question in another way. We first calculate what the probability is that the difference observed could be attributed to chance alone. This probability will lie between 0%, meaning that it is "impossible" that it is due to chance, and 100%, meaning that it is "absolutely certain" that it is due to chance. If that probability is high enough, we assume that the rate of this cancer in the community is higher only by chance and is really the same as that in the rest of New York City. If that probability is low enough, we assume that the difference between the two cancer rates is not due to chance and take more seriously the possibility that some exposures to toxic chemicals might be responsible. We call such a result "statistically significant."

How Much Is "High Enough"?

"High enough" and "low enough" are too vague: the question is where to draw the line. The practice the scientific community has chosen to follow in studies of this type is to draw the line at 5%: we call a difference "statistically significant" if the probability that it is due to chance alone is 5% or less. This is equivalent to saying that the probability that the difference is not due to chance is 95% or more. This may strike many people as an unreasonably strict rule. In ordinary life we are used to making decisions on the basis of much lower odds: if we have to choose between two courses of action to gain a desired goal, and if the first course were only slightly more likely to be successful than the second, we would without hesitation choose the first. But in scientific research, before we accept an increased rate as real rather than a result of chance, we demand that the probability that it is not due to chance should be at least 95%. Why do we set such a strict standard?

False Positives and False Negatives

Whatever rule we use to distinguish real increases from chance increases, we will inevitably make some mistakes. At times we will mistakenly disregard small real increases because we conclude by the standard we have chosen that they are due to chance. Such a mistake is called a "false negative." At other times we will mistakenly conclude that increases due only to chance are real, because even a large enough increase to meet our standard will sometimes occur by chance alone. Such a mistake is called a "false positive." When we use a strict standard, like 5%, we will make the false negative mistake more often (attributing real increases to chance), and the false positive mistake less often (accepting a chance increase as real), than if we use a more lenient standard.

If both kinds of mistakes were equally harmful, there would be no reason to be so strict. Scientists, however, do not regard the two mistakes as equally harmful. Experience has taught them that there is more harm done by making a false positive mistake than by making a false negative one. We look for an increase in disease because we are testing some hypothesis about the cause, in this case that chemicals from the landfill have caused cancer. If we do really find an increase, it does not mean we have proved the hypothesis, but at least we think it is now more likely. Centuries of experience in science show that many more hypotheses turn out to be false than turn out to be true: put briefly, scientists throughout history have been wrong more often than they have been right, and they know it. Further, the consequences of believing a new hypothesis are significant: new research projects are begun, new courses of treatment or new drug therapies are adopted by physicians, people are advised to eat foods they do not enjoy or give up foods they do. For all these reason, scientists have learned to demand that evidence for belief in a new hypothesis be very strong.

As one of the DOH reports pointed out, the use of a strict standard is like the criterion used in Western legal practice for a finding of guilt in a criminal trial: guilt must be proved "beyond a reasonable doubt." Our practice favors the defendant: confessions may not be coerced, the defendant is free to refuse to testify if he chooses, the jury must convict by a unanimous vote, and so on. We have chosen these safeguards because the thought of an innocent person found guilty and going to prison or being executed (a false positive) is more offensive to our moral sense than the thought of a guilty one going free (a false negative).

Back to the Twenty-eight Cases of Pancreatic Cancer

Let us test the data on pancreatic cancer in Pelham Bay, using this standard. We first calculate the probability that by chance alone 375 cases or more occurred in this particular ten-year period, in this particular area of New York City, even though the expected number is 347. Direct calculation, using the same mathematics used in the raisin cake problem, shows that this probability is about 7%, a result that is not statistically significant (being greater than the 5% standard). This means, in the absence of any other evidence, that the apparently higher pancreatic cancer rate is to be considered a chance variation.

Of course, if we could get more data on pancreatic cancer in an exposed population, either for an additional time period or possibly a different area in which the population has been exposed to the same substances, and if we find that the number of cases continues to be high, the increase might then become statistically significant, and be taken more seriously.

Still More Tricks of Chance

Even if the exposures to chemicals from the landfill did not cause any increase of any type of cancer in Pelham Bay, if we compare the rates of twenty different types of cancer using a 5% significance test, it is a better than even chance that at least one will appear to be "statistically significant." Why should this be so?

We have said that the 5% criterion is a strict one, designed to rule out increases that might be due to chance, but we must recognize that even events with only a 5% chance of occurring do occur. In fact, the term "5% chance" means that on the average they occur 5% of the time. To see why, imagine a large jar full of small beads, 5% of which are red and the rest white. If we draw one bead at random from the jar, the chance of its being red is only 5%, but if we keep drawing we will get red beads occasionally. If we draw twenty beads, it is a better than even chance that at least one will be red.

In the DOH report, thirteen types of adult cancer and four types of childhood cancer—chosen because there is some evidence that they can be caused by exposures to toxic substances—were studied, a total of seventeen types in all. Further, they were classified by the sex of the victim, making a total of thirty-four separate comparisons between expected and observed rates. A 5% probability for an event means that on the average that event will occur 5% of the time, or once out of twenty times. Five percent of thirty-four is about one and a half, implying that even if there were no harmful effects of toxic substances in the community, so that the cancer rate should not be elevated, one or two rates of the thirty-four compared are likely by chance alone to appear elevated to a "statistically significant" extent. We use quotation marks to make the point that it is a misuse of the term, which correctly used implies something unlikely to have been a result of chance. Of course, these kinds of "statistically significant" results are quite likely to result from chance. This is the whole point. Indeed, two cancers did show "statistically significant" excess rates among adult men: colon cancers and leukemias. The DOH report concluded that these two excess cancer rates, even though they met the 5% rule when considered in isolation, are likely to occur by chance alone because of the large number of comparisons that were made.

It should be noted that "statistically significant" *lower* rates of pharynx cancer among men and lung cancer among women in Pelham Bay were found in the study. No one would suggest that exposure to toxic chemicals actually protects people against these forms of cancer; it makes no biological sense. These lower rates are almost certainly chance variations, again expected because of the multiple comparisons.

Confidence Interval: How Wrong Can We Go?

The leukemias, cancers of the blood-cell-producing system of the body, were especially important to the people of Pelham Bay. They are also one type of cancer that takes less time to develop after an exposure, and there had been sufficient time since the dumping of the toxic wastes in the landfill. Over the ten-year period from 1978 to 1987 the number of cases observed was greater than the number expected for all four categories of age and sex: boys, girls, men, and women (see table 8-2).

TABLE 8-2   Leukemia in Pelham Bay

Group Studied	Ratio, Observed to Expected Numbers of Leukemia Cases	95% Confidence Interval
Boys	1.07	0.65 to 1.49
Girls	1.07	0.58 to 1.57
Men	1.14	1.01 to 1.26
Women	1.07	0.94 to 1.19

Note that the ranges of the confidence intervals are wider for children than for adults. This is because the numbers of cases of leukemia among children are less, and therefore are somewhat more affected by random variations.

In the DOH reports the question of the statistical significance of these results was dealt with in a different but equivalent way. The ratios of observed to expected numbers of cases in Pelham Bay were calculated. If any of these ratios is greater than 1.0, it means that there are more cases than expected. Then what is called a "confidence interval" for the ratios was calculated (table 8-2).

Any measurement, even of the area of a room or the weight of a package, is subject to error: our measuring instruments are never of perfect accuracy, and they are used by fallible human beings. Whenever we repeat a measurement, we usually get a slightly different answer. Like numbers of cases of a disease, any measurement is subject to random variations. All we should expect when we measure something is a number we believe to be more or less close to some "true" value. The confidence interval tells us how close we are likely to be.

Here we are concerned with the ratios of observed to expected numbers of cases of various types of cancer. If the observed and expected numbers happen to be equal, the ratio of observed to expected cases is 1.0. If the observed number of cases exceeds the expected, the ratio will be greater than 1.0, which is the case here. Ratios of observed to expected leukemias were tabulated in the DOH report (see table 8-1) and are summarized again in table 8-2. (The ratio of 1.07 for boys means that the number of cases of leukemia is 7% greater than expected. All the ratios are greater than 1.0, but do they represent real increases or could they be the result of chance variation? How much confidence may we have in the numerical values given?

Even if the leukemia rates were really identical in Pelham Bay and New York City, in any short period of time the number of cases in Pelham Bay would be small, and chance alone could make the ratios observed either less than 1.0 or greater than 1.0. We could minimize the effect of chance if we could study very large populations similarly exposed. Since this is not usually possible when the exposure is from toxic waste dumps, the most we can say is that the real value of each ratio, which we are trying to estimate, probably lies within some more or less narrow range about the value we actually observed.

Target Practice

Suppose a number of soldiers in training were to shoot at a paper target bearing the usual bull's eye and fastened to a concrete wall. Suppose further that after the target practice the paper target were removed, and we were shown only the bullet-scarred concrete wall and asked to guess where the bull's eye had been located. We would guess, of course, that the spot where the bullet marks are closest together is likely to have been where the bull's eye was, but we could not pinpoint its location exactly. We would instead draw a circle around the area where the bullet marks are most dense, and say it probably was somewhere inside the circle. Now the larger the circle we draw, the greater the probability that we capture the true location of the bull's eye within it. The confidence interval is defined as the circle just large enough to give us a 95% chance of including the bull's eye, and thus a 5% chance of leaving it outside.

The confidence interval tells us how much confidence we can have in the result of a measurement of any quantity. In particular here it provides us with an alternative way to evaluate whether the difference between an observed and an expected value of the number of cases of a disease is statistically significant. If the expected number of cases lies within the 95% confidence interval around the observed number, we can conclude that the difference is not statistically significant. If it lies outside that interval, we can conclude that the difference is too great to be a likely result of chance, and is thus significant. When it is applied to the ratios of observed to expected cases, as in table 8-2, a ratio of 1.0 is equivalent to no difference between expected and observed rates, so if 1.0 lies within the confidence interval, the difference is not significant. In other words, the difference between observed and expected values is most likely a result of chance (see fig. 8-2).

Leukemia in Pelham Bay

It follows from the confidence intervals given in table 8-2 that the slightly elevated rates of leukemia among children of either sex and among female adults are not statistically significant, probably a result of chance. The excess among male adults, on the other hand, is not so likely to be a result of chance since the confidence interval does not include the value 1.0. This excess rate should be followed in the future. It is a possible consequence of exposure to benzene and perhaps of other organic solvents, and unlike the solid tumor cancers there has been sufficient time for leukemia to develop.

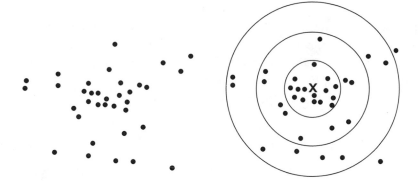

FIGURE 8-2 Schematic representation of a *95% confidence interval*. Bullets have been fired at a target with a bull's eye. The target is then removed, but the bullet marks on the wall remain, and the idea is to guess where the bull's eye was located when the shots were fired. The most likely location is at the center of density of the bullet holes, a point calculated mathematically from the locations of the holes and shown by an X. However the bull's eye might not have been exactly where the X was found to be. If we draw a small circle about the X we are making a more realistic guess—somewhere in the small circle is more likely than exactly on the X, but if the circle is too small, the probability that the bull's eye is outside the circle is correspondingly large. If we make the circle very large we can be almost certain we have captured the bull's eye, but we have not pinned down its location at all precisely. We choose a compromise: a circle large enough to capture the bull's eye 95% of the time, but small enough to give us some real sense of where the bull's eye actually was (the medium-sized circle).

Power: How Small an Increase Can We Detect?

The DOH report shows that while the numbers of cases of childhood leukemia observed in the Pelham Bay community is greater than the number expected, the 95% confidence intervals show that the excesses could very likely be the result of chance; although the ratios for both girls and boys is greater than 1.0, the confidence intervals are quite large: 0.65 to 1.49 for boys and 0.58 to 1.57 for girls. These large confidence intervals are results of the small number of cases of leukemia among children expected in a population this size.

The upper limits of the confidence intervals, 1.49 for boys and 1.58 for girls, are both about one and a half times the expected rate, or a 50% increase. This suggests something distressing: there could have been a real increase of about 50% in leukemia in children, and our 5% criterion would require us to attribute this increase to chance! This shows how hard it is to detect real increases of a rare disease like childhood leukemia in a population the size of Pelham Bay. How large an increase in leukemia would have to occur, before we rule out chance as responsible? This is the question that the concept of "power" was designed to answer.

"I've Got the Horse Right Here . . ."

Suppose we have a friend who likes to bet on horse races. He is not tremendously successful in spite of having an elaborate system to pick the horses, winning about one time in ten. This is not as bad as it sounds because the payoff can be at odds of 5 to 1 or 10 to 1, but over time he loses money. He figures out a new system that he believes will win two out of ten times and with which he will do a little better than break even. He tries his new system, and on the first ten races he bets on he actually wins twice and tells us with great pride that his new system works.

We would tend to be skeptical. We know that by chance alone his old system, although it averaged only one win in ten races, often gave him two wins out of ten (and of course gave him bad days on which he did not win any). So we challenge him to keep trying his new system longer, for 100 races rather than ten, to see if he really can win 20% of the time with it. Intuitively we feel that 100 races provide a real test of his claim, while ten races do not. In the language of statistics, an experiment involving only ten races does not have the *power* to establish the difference between an average of one win out of ten and an average of two wins out of ten, while a test involving 100 races does.

On the other hand, suppose our gambler had claimed to discover a system so good that it would pick winners 70% of the time. Then, on the first ten races he bets on he actually picks winners in six of the races. This time we would not be so skeptical. We feel that there is only a very small probability that if his new system were no better than his old one he would happen to pick six winners in one set of ten races, so we conclude that he has made a pretty good case for his claim of 70% success. In technical language, his experiment on ten races has the "power" to distinguish a 70% success rate from a 10% success rate, but not the "power" to distinguish a 20% success rate from a 10% success rate.

How Large an Increase in Leukemia Rates Can We Detect?

As with the gambler and the horse races, so it is with our ability to detect an increase in cancer rates. The smaller the number of expected cases, the greater the relative importance of chance variations, and the less our power to detect an effect. Thus, it is easier to detect a large increase than a small one, an increase in a common disease than in a rare one, and an increase of a rare disease in a large population than a small one. In discussing power in chapter 3, we used the metaphor of detecting a radio signal above a noisy background. As we noted there, the weaker the signal compared to the noisy background, the harder it is to detect.

The DOH reports showed that there has been no statistically significant increase in childhood leukemia in Pelham Bay. This, however, does not necessarily satisfy the concerns of the community, which has a right to ask the question, could there have been an increase that the study failed to detect? This is a question of power, and the DOH showed that, given the number of cases expected in the ten-year time period of the study, only if there had been at least a doubling of the rate of leukemia—a 100% increase—would the study have had the power to detect it. The size of the population, combined with the fact that leukemia in children is a rare disease to begin with, means that the study could not distinguish between a smaller real increase and a chance variation. The observed increase among girls and boys was 7%, and for the small numbers of cases involved, well within the range of chance variation. This is an unfortunate limitation of the epidemiological method, but it was the best the DOH could do with the information available.

Specificity versus Power

The comparisons between expected and observed cancer rates have been made for adults and children separately, and for the two sexes separately, and for a number of different types of cancer. This subdivision into age and sex categories makes epidemiological and biological sense: the different sexes have different susceptibilities, and different types of cancer are known to be caused by different chemical toxins. By subdividing, we make our comparisons more specific. On the other hand, any subdivision necessarily reduces the number of cases considered in each comparison and therefore reduces the power of the comparison to detect a difference.

There is thus a trade-off: a gain in specificity means a loss in power, and it is a question of scientific judgment how to weigh these conflicting goals.

In the DOH study, trends of cancer cases with time were searched for, on the assumption that if toxic chemicals were causing cancers, the numbers of cases would increase as time went on. This, however, means subdividing the numbers of cases over the total ten-year period into numbers of cases by each year, with a consequent poor power to detect any increase of cancer rate with time. A similar consideration applies to a study made by the DOH of the dependence of cancer rates on distance of homes from the landfill: the subdivision of cases into categories of greater or lesser distance from the landfill was found to have too little power to show much of anything.

What Statistical Analysis Cannot Tell Us

The primary question considered in the DOH report is: has cancer increased in the Pelham Bay area due to exposure to toxic chemicals from the landfill? Suppose we find, as in fact we did, that there is an excess rate of leukemia among adult men in Pelham Bay that is statistically significant at the 5% level. Does this mean that the probability that the excess rate is due to toxic chemicals is more than 95%? The answer is a firm no: it means nothing of the sort.

All we show by the test of significance is that it is a result unlikely to have occurred by chance, and that is absolutely all we may conclude. There are too many reasons that a statistically significant result might be found because of factors other than the one—here, exposure to toxic chemicals from the landfill—that we are testing for. We have mentioned that in using the population of New York City as a comparison group, we were only able to correct for a few of the risk factors that might have a bearing on the cancer rates. An excess in Pelham Bay may reflect a risk factor we did not have enough information on to correct for, rather than exposure to chemicals from the landfill. For example, suppose a group of men living in the community worked in a dry cleaning plant in which they were not properly protected from the organic solvents used, and a few of them developed leukemia as a result. It would not take many cases of this rare disease to create a statistically significant excess.

As another example, the excess of childhood leukemia cases around the Sellafield nuclear plant described in chapter 4 were even more unlikely to have occurred by chance, but this of itself did not prove that radioactivity from the plant caused them, and in fact another explanation appears more likely.

JUDGMENT ON PELHAM BAY

Finally, after the statistical analysis has been done and the statistically significant effects noted, our work is not yet done. We may have found some excess of disease needing an explanation, but there might be other reasons for it than the one factor we were suspicious of when we began. We must always ask if the hypothesis we are testing is in accord with what is known biologically and medically about the disease. For example, we have mentioned earlier that, with the exception of the leukemias, cancer caused by exposure to toxic chemicals usually takes twenty or more years to develop. In the DOH study, it was found that colon cancer among adult men in Pelham Bay was higher than in the rest of New York City by a statistically significant extent. But our knowledge of the long delay time for cancer to appear after exposure makes it unlikely that it was caused by exposure less than ten or so years earlier. The report further reasoned that it is not plausible that only adult men and not adult women should have been affected by toxic substances and concluded finally that the observation of one or two "statistically significant" results out of over thirty comparisons is highly likely, and the colon cancer excess among men may well be one of them. So for that matter may the excess leukemia among adult men.

There has been sufficient time since the possible exposure to expect the increase in leukemia among adult men, but the DOH report suggested that it would be surprising, if exposure were responsible, that it should affect men but not women. Perhaps there could be a reason why it should, but before assuming that exposure really is the cause, one would want to explain why there is this difference, or at least see if it persists through the next five or ten years.

Certainly, the leukemia data suggest that there is one thing worth doing: continue to observe the rates for an additional period of time. If it continues significantly high among men, or is found to be high also among women and children, the possibility that exposure to the landfill was responsible can be taken more seriously. In fact, in a more recent DOH report, additional data on childhood leukemia for four more years has been analyzed, and still no statistically significant increase was found.

Even if a statistically significant increase had been found, it would not have been the end of the scientific investigation, but a basis for looking further.

The DOH study concluded, we think correctly, that so far cancer rates in the Pelham Bay community, either for leukemia or for other cancers, are not elevated enough to suggest that the health of the community has been affected by chemicals from the landfill. This does not, however, close the book on the issue. Solid tumor cancers, the most common types of the disease, have not yet had time since the presumed period of highest exposure in the late 1970s to show themselves, but may yet appear in the decade beginning in 2000. This would parallel the increasing rate of solid tumor cancers in the Japanese survivor study found thirty years or more after the exposure. The data gathered by the DOH for the period through 1987 would then serve as a baseline, with which future cancer rates might be compared. Additional data on both leukemia and solid tumor cancers are being collected by the New York State Cancer Registry, but the results have not yet been reported. As far as childhood leukemia is concerned, all we can say is the small increases above expected rates seen so far are less than we have the power to distinguish from chance variations. Additional data for more years may allow a different conclusion.

Unlike in an American courtroom where the possible verdicts are either "guilty" or "innocent," the DOH report suggested that we must allow also for the Scotch verdict, "not proven."

This may not satisfy the people who live in Pelham Bay. The only clear-cut finding of all the efforts in research and remediation that they can find comfort in is that the landfill poses no danger to anyone today. A high mound in the center of the park, surrounded by a relatively flat area, it affords a pleasant view of the park and the bay.

After the Reports

There is one further question about Pelham Bay: if there was no appreciable increase in the childhood leukemia rate in the Pelham Bay area, why did the members of the community, who patiently collected a list of victims, think there was? In fact, the DOH, having better access to medical records, not only confirmed the number of cases found by the concerned citizens but located two additional cases not on their list. In spite of this, the analysis showed that the observed number of cases was close to the number expected.

The sad truth is that when disease strikes our own family or in our own circle of acquaintances, it has a disproportionate impact on how we think and what we notice. When we have not suffered some particular kind of misfortune ourselves, we pay less attention to it when we hear of some stranger suffering it. But when someone close to us is the victim, every additional case we hear of strikes us with considerable force. Break a leg and suddenly casts appear on all sides around us; sneeze and everybody has the flu. Another reason we notice misfortunes like our own more is that being sick, we seek treatment in clinics or hospitals, where we meet other victims. Still another reason is that when there is an obvious source of contamination, like the odorous, unsightly landfill in Pelham Bay, or a nearby nuclear facility, we expect illness, and we find it.

The people of Pelham Bay had to put up with smells, the sight of a mountain of garbage, filthy water oozing from that mountain, the sense that their neighborhood and the waters of the bay that made it a pleasant place to live were being contaminated; they put up with this for ten years before they managed to stop it. They cannot be blamed for their frustration, their suspicions, and their fury when they learned, on top of the ugly mess and bad smells they had borne for so long, they had been exposed without knowing it to chemicals that might have caused cancers.

OTHER CLUSTERS

In Pelham Bay so far, there does not seem to have been a real excess of cancer in spite of the perceptions of the residents. However, in many reported clusters there really was more cancer or other illness than expected: this was clearly so for the childhood leukemia clusters in Woburn, Massachusetts, near the Sellafield nuclear facility (see chapter 4), and in Toms River, New Jersey, where there was an excess of both childhood leukemia and of brain and nervous system cancers. What has been discovered about the causes of these clusters? How can they be explained?

Clusters and Chance

In chapter 4 we have described what we called the "lumpiness" of chance: the way in which events occurring purely by chance may occur so close together in space or in time as to fool us into thinking that they have some common cause. It is often difficult to rule chance out as an explanation for clusters of disease.

We have discussed the 5% standard used as the definitive test for statistical significance, but noted that events with a 5% probability do occur 5% of the time. Suppose we ask how many "statistically significant" cancer clusters would occur by chance alone, if environmental and genetic factors causing cancer were the same everywhere. Such a calculation was done by Dr. R. R. Neutra, an epidemiologist at the State Department of Health in California. To make his point forcefully he used a stricter standard for statistical significance: 1% rather than 5%. He noted that there are 5,000 census tracts in California, so that in any given time period 1% of them will have by chance alone a "statistically significant" excess of any one type of cancer, giving a total of fifty "clusters." But this is for only one type of cancer at a time. There are in fact eighty different types of cancer, most of which occur independently, so that we might expect 50×80, or 4,000, clusters of cancer of one type or another among the 5,000 census tracts. This is another example of the fact that when multiple comparisons are made, "improbable" results will probably occur. If Dr. Neutra had used the 5% standard in his analysis, it is easy to see that given eighty different forms of cancer, most census tracts in California would have more than one cancer cluster.

Fortunately for local health departments, not all such clusters attract attention, but whether they do or not is often itself a matter of chance: the chance that some member of the community notices the quite real high rate of one type of cancer, having noticed it thinks of a plausible source of contamination in the area, and has the energy and rapport with neighbors to arouse the concern of the community as a whole. In fact, thousands of clusters are reported by concerned citizens each year in the United States, and state health departments do their best to explain to them the often fuzzy distinction between clusters caused by chance variation and clusters requiring more intensive investigation.

Put another way, it is a question of the proper and improper use of the test of statistical significance. We use it properly when we start with a hypothesis about the cause of some disease and then test it by looking for higher rates in an exposed group. We use it improperly when we start by noticing higher rates of disease in some group and then look for a hypothesis about what exposure might have caused them.

As an example of proper use: suppose we have evidence that some particular chemical used in industrial processes is a carcinogen, based on experiments in which it caused leukemia in laboratory animals. We learn that a chemical plant using this chemical in a certain community has been careless in controlling emissions from the plant, thus exposing the community. We decide to see if the rate of leukemia is elevated in this community. Let us suppose that indeed we find it is elevated. Then we ask, could this elevation have occurred by chance? This is where the usual test for statistical significance is properly applied: we picked the community because of its exposure, knowing nothing in advance about its rate of leukemia. If we find the elevation of leukemia statistically significant, we have made our hypothesis that emissions from the plant caused it more plausible.

Contrast this with what often happens in cluster investigations: a high rate of leukemia is observed in a certain community, which at the start was not known to be exposed to a carcinogen. The community was picked for study only because of its high leukemia rate. Can we then ask what the probability is that this high rate occurred by chance? It is like asking what the probability is that our next door neighbor will win the million dollar jackpot in the state lottery. Yesterday, before the drawing, his chance was one in 10 million; today, after the winning ticket has been drawn, with his picture spread out over the front pages of the evening newspapers and his interview aired on the local television station, the probability of his winning is much, much greater than one in 10 million. Asking that question after the fact is doing what the Texas sharpshooter does when he paints the bull's eye around the bullet hole (see discussion of the Texas sharpshooter in relation to investigations of clusters in chapter 4).

Exposures in the Dim Past

The Pelham Bay story also illustrates why the study of cancer clusters is so difficult. As was noted, cancer is a disease that usually takes decades to develop after an initial carcinogenic exposure. Even after the initiating step, each individual case of cancer represents one of a number of possible sequences of mutations, so that the development of the disease in a number of individuals who may have been exposed originally at the same time occurs not only decades later, but also spread out in time rather than all at once. Also, because the exposure took place decades before, it is unlikely that we can tell anymore how much anyone was exposed. In the Japanese bomb survivor studies on the other hand, information about exposure was obtained shortly after the bombing, when people's memories about where they were and whether they were shielded by clothing or buildings were still fresh. Also, it was known where the exposure came from and to what and how much the victims were exposed.

In the modern complex world, all of us are exposed to many different agents, most of which have not been shown to be human carcinogens, though many of them may be. Only a small fraction of industrial chemicals have been tested for carcinogenicity on animals. In Woburn, most chemicals found in the water supply were not even on the list of known or suspected human carcinogens. One chemical found in the well water, and known to have been carelessly disposed of by one of the chemical plants in the area, was only "suspected" to be a human carcinogen.

The Woburn Cluster

We will omit most of those details of this famous cluster that were adequately covered in the popular book *A Civil Action* and the film made from it, and summarize only the most recent results of the various studies. Again, an alert mother of a child with leukemia sounded the alarm. Between the years 1969 and 1979 there had been twelve cases of childhood leukemia in the town, slightly more than double the expected rate. Most strikingly, six of the cases were in one small area of six blocks, where the drinking water had come from wells known to have been contaminated with organochlorines and which had been closed shortly before the discovery of the cluster. The Massachusetts Department of Public Health continued to monitor the area, and up to 1986 a total of twenty-one cases had occurred in Woburn, the additional ones no longer predominantly from the small area of six blocks. The town had been a center of industry for more than one hundred years, and waste products contaminating the ground and water included arsenic and other metals, and organochlorines such as trichlorethylene (TCE), perchlorethylene (PCE), and chloroform.

The small area where the six cases of leukemia were concentrated got some of its drinking water from two wells dug in the 1960s into an aquifer already known to be polluted. Complaints about the taste, smell, and color of the water began almost immediately, but it was only in 1979 that the Massachusetts Department of Public Health (DPH) tested the water and found concentrations of TCE and PCE that exceeded drinking water guidelines. The wells were then closed off. Ironically, that was the year the leukemia cluster was first reported.

The Massachusetts DPH, as well as universities in the Boston area, began studies of the leukemia cases, but have not yet reached any firm conclusions about what caused them. The DPH issued a summarizing document in 1997 in which it reported one statistically significant finding: children born to mothers who drank the water from the two contaminated wells during pregnancy were at a higher risk of leukemia. The children who drank this water were not found to be at higher risk.

This finding has not yet been published in the peer-reviewed scientific literature, where its method and conclusions will receive the scrutiny of other scientists. The implication that chemicals ingested by pregnant mothers may be carcinogenic to their children is new and has not yet been observed in other studies. Further, a plausible candidate for carcinogenicity in the drinking water has not been identified. TCE and PCE have not been proven to be human carcinogens, even in occupational settings where exposures are much higher than in Woburn; on the other hand, a fetus may be far more sensitive than an adult. The leukemia cluster in Woburn, tragic for its victims and their families, remains unexplained.

The Toms River Cluster

As in Pelham Bay, an alert mother sounded the alarm in this southern New Jersey town: her child had a painful and disfiguring type of cancer of the nervous system. Several types of childhood cancer were found to be significantly elevated, both in Toms River and in Dover Township in which Toms River is located: brain and central nervous system cancers, and leukemia. There were two abandoned industrial sites in the area, and there had been leakage of toxic chemicals, including the possible human carcinogen TCE, also suspected in the Woburn cluster, into the ground water that supplied some of the town's wells. This route of exposure was absent in Pelham Bay, where the drinking water came from the New York City water supply. The New Jersey Department of Health has begun a study of the relation to childhood cancers in Dover Township to exposure to chemicals from the sites through air and drinking water. Other suspected risk factors for childhood cancers will also be studied, including parent's occupation, medicines taken by the mothers during pregnancy, electromagnetic fields from appliances, radiation, use of pesticides, and ionizing radiation. It is hoped that some thirty to forty children who suffered cancer in a roughly fifteen-year time period will be studied. It is unfortunately not too likely, given the small number of cases combined with the uncertain estimates of past exposures to substances not known to be human carcinogens, that a cause of the excess cancers will be identified.

Clusters, Residential and Occupational

The sad fact is that investigations of clusters of disease, particularly of cancer, occurring in communities and discovered by alert residents, have almost never resulted in a clear identification of a cause. Most can be explained as very likely the result of chance, an explanation that never satisfies a perturbed community; for others, ignorance of what people were exposed to, and to how much, and when, has defeated attempts to find a cause.

There are only a few exceptions. One was a cluster of thirty-five cases of cancer of the lining of the lung cavity (mesothelioma) in a Turkish village of fewer than 600 people, brought to the attention of an epidemiologist at a Turkish university, Dr. Y. Baris, by the headman of the village. Dr. Baris's investigation found that the extraordinary rate of the disease, several hundred times its rate elsewhere, could be attributed to a mineral related to asbestos in the stones the villagers built their homes from. The story ended sadly for the villagers and for the scientist: the Turkish government refused to help the villagers relocate, and they have been ostracized by neighboring communities as coming from a "cancer village." In turn, they blame Dr Baris for their problems. Meanwhile, new cases of the disease add to the cluster.

Occupational Clusters

In contrast, clusters in the workplace have often led to important discoveries. It is unlikely that Dr. Baris in Turkey would have thought of the mineral content of the stones as a cause of mesothelioma if it had not been for the earlier observation by Dr. I. Selikoff of an extraordinary number of cases of the same rare disease among asbestos workers in a plant in Passaic, New Jersey. Benzene has been identified repeatedly as a cause of leukemia clusters among workers in shoe factories and other industries that use it. Both melanoma, a particularly aggressive skin cancer, and leukemia were common among radiologists practicing in the early years of the specialty, before lead shielding and other protective measures were widely used.

Why have investigations of occupational clusters often identified a cause, while residential ones have gone unexplained? There are a number of important differences in the two situations. Workplace exposures are usually much higher than residential ones, so that the number of cases of disease is much greater than expected, and chance can more easily be ruled out. This does not of itself make finding a cause easier, but it does ensure that such clusters get more serious attention by scientists. Once a cluster is recognized as worth taking seriously, the task of finding a cause is made simpler by the fact that there are usually only a few possible agents in any one workplace that might cause disease. Often there are records of the extent of exposures in the workplace, and when particular employees were exposed. In contrast, in residential area clusters, neither the agent, nor the time of exposure, nor the amount of exposure, is usually known.

This is not to say that every example of a workplace cluster has been explained. At the time of writing, twenty cases of brain cancer have occurred among employees of a research laboratory of a major oil company, eight times the expected number. The cluster is being studied closely, but its cause is not yet known.

Toxic Chemical Exposure: The Danger from Within

Concern with chemicals in the environment has focused on such sources as the factories of chemical industry, automobile traffic, toxic waste dumps, and large-scale aerial spraying of pesticides. Exposure from such sources is most usually through the air, but sometimes through the contamination of water supplies. These sources of exposure are now closely regulated by law, and by and large the levels of chemical agents from them have been reduced to a satisfactorily low level. Unfortunately, there are many toxic dumps from before regulation still around, polluting their immediate neighborhoods.

Some recent research gives a radically different perspective on environmental exposures to chemicals. In the 1980s the U.S. Environmental Protection Agency performed a series of studies to determine precisely how and where people are actually exposed to environmental agents known or suspected to have harmful effects on health. The studies were given the acronym TEAM, standing for Total Exposure Assessment Methodology, this name being chosen almost surely because it made a nice acronym. They were made possible by two technological advances: the invention of small easily portable personal monitors of exposure, and the development of analytical methods for identifying and accurately measuring very low concentrations of a number of hazardous substances in both air and water. Both outdoor and indoor air were monitored and in addition personal monitors were worn by individual subjects for a twenty-four hour period, during which time the subjects kept records of where they were each hour of the day. For some of the substances, concentrations in the exhaled breath was also measured. This combination of measurements meant that the exposure of each subject could be reliably determined.

The substances studied included volatile organic compounds (VOCs), polyaromatic hydrocarbons, respirable particles, which were analyzed for heavy metals like lead and for pesticides, and some other pollutants. The VOCs are a broad class of substances that includes some hydrocarbons like benzene, a known human carcinogen, and some organochlorines such as TCE, implicated in the Woburn leukemia cluster, and tetrachlorethane, a dry-cleaning fluid. Both these organochlorines are carcinogenic in animals, though their effects on humans are not definitely known. Pesticides and polyaromatic hydrocarbons are described at more length in chapter 5.

The results of the studies were startling. The main sources of the exposures in almost all cases were not from the factories of chemical industries polluting the outside air, but mostly within the home itself, including cigarettes, chemical products like deodorants, household cleaners, paints, sprays, even the furniture itself and the fabrics that cover it, which when new give off significant amounts of volatile organics.

The results for benzene are an example. As we have noted, benzene is a human carcinogen, known to cause leukemia in adults. It is a common raw material for making various commercially important products and occurs as a contaminant in other organic liquids such as gasoline. Of the benzene in outdoor air, 85% comes from gasoline-powered vehicles, and 15% from chemical industry. Benzene is also a contaminant of cigarette smoke, but this source contributes only 0.1% of the benzene in outdoor air, a seemingly trivial share. However, most of the actual exposure of individuals to benzene comes from cigarettes, both among smokers and among those who share a house with them. Smokers, as measured from their breath, have six to ten times as much benzene in their blood as nonsmokers. Even nonsmokers exposed to the cigarettes of others get 10% of their exposure by this route, and another 50% of their total exposure is from other indoor sources. Forty percent is from outdoor sources, most of it from gasoline. Only 3% of the total exposure is from chemical plants and other industrial sources. The exposure of smokers to benzene is much greater than would be expected even from the benzene concentration in the air of their homes: cigarette smoke directly drawn from the cigarette is a more concentrated source of benzene than the air of a room hazy with cigarette smoke (fig. 8-3).

The story is similar with other hazardous substances. Studies of about twenty-five volatile organic compounds in northern New Jersey, a center of chemical industry, showed that measured concentrations were no greater for people living within one kilometer of chemical industries than for people living further away. Their exposures to the most prevalent

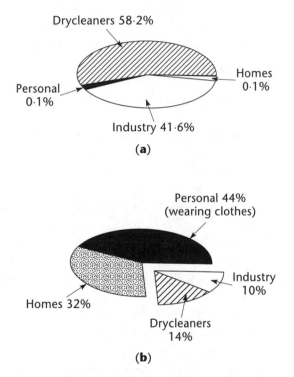

FIGURE 8-3 Results of the TEAM study for the suspected carcinogen tetrachloroethylene (TCE). The diagram (a) shows outdoor concentrations of TCE; more than 99% is from dry-cleaning establishments and industrial plants. The diagram (b) shows the sources of actual human exposures, as determined from personal monitors. Only *24%* comes from industrial sources and dry-cleaning establishments; 32% comes from clothes hung in closets in the home, and 44% from wearing clothes recently dry-cleaned. Courtesy of Dr Lance Wallace of the Environmental Protection Agency.

volatile organics, as measured by personal monitors, were three times higher than what would have been predicted from the outdoor air concentrations polluted by nearby chemical industries. The indoor concentrations came primarily from indoor sources: cigarette smoke, clothes fresh from the dry cleaner, toilet deodorants, air fresheners, and even tap water. Paradichlorobenzene, a moth repellant and a known animal carcinogen, is also used in bathroom deodorants and other household products. Chloroform, a volatile organic and an animal carcinogen, is present in tap water as a result of chlorination of water contaminated with hydrocarbons, and people are exposed to it not only when they drink water but also when they take a shower or bath or do the laundry. Its concentration in bottled soft drinks is almost the same as in tap water. Pesticide exposures in homes was found to be five to ten times greater than outdoor exposures. One way pesticides get indoors is being tracked in on shoes; another way is if they are stored in the home. Rugs and carpets trap dust and particles; ordinary vacuuming is not an efficient way to remove such trapped dust, and the authors of the study suggest bare floors might be healthier (fig. 8-4).

One of the most striking results was that personal exposures in this highly industrialized area of northern New Jersey were no greater than personal exposures in a rural town in the southern United States with no chemical industries: in both areas indoor sources were the main ones.

Most of the industrial chemicals that people in the United States are exposed to are not yet known to be human carcinogens. What proportion of all cancers is caused by such chemicals is uncertain, but is believed to be only a few percent or so. The TEAM scientist estimated that 85% of that imprecisely known "few percent or so" is due to indoor exposures.

Even if most exposures to known and regulated hazardous chemicals come more from household sources than from industrial sources or motor vehicles, it does not imply that we should ignore the threats from toxic waste dumps and does not imply that cancer clusters should not be a cause for concern. It should, however, make us realize the importance of measuring exposures to suspected hazards from all sources and to know which of the sources of any exposure are the most significant.

Limitations and How We May Yet Get Around Them

To summarize: We fail to find causes for clusters of disease far more often than we succeed. Among the reasons is that we do not usually know past

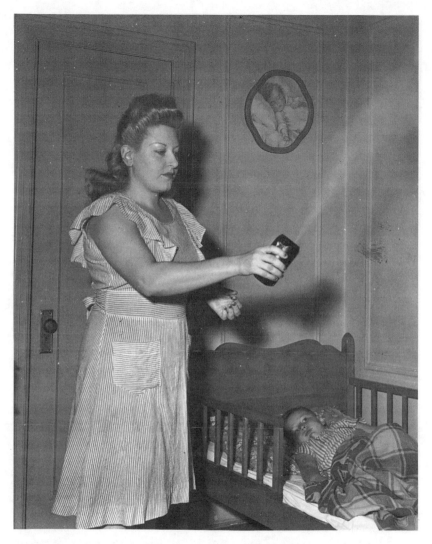

FIGURE 8-4   The caption on this photograph provided by the U.S. Army, whose photographers took it shortly after World War II, deserves to be quoted verbatim: "Mrs. Gee Goldstein of Brooklyn, shown using the army's DDT 'bomb' to spray her bedroom and so kill all insects. Her son Robert, 5, watches from bed, and illustrates the fact that the spray is not harmful, except to winged pests." Copyright Bettman/Corbis.

exposures, and that the number of cases in most reported clusters is too small to rule out chance as responsible. Another important reason is that cases of disease caused by exposures to specific chemicals cannot yet be distinguished from cases that occur for other reasons. This is not yet possible, but it may become so if we learn how to identify the particular pattern of mutations in individual cases of cancer. Research on the complete sequence of all human genes has just been completed. Methods of identifying which genes are abnormal or mutated in a sample of tissue or blood are being rapidly developed and will be used increasingly in environmental health studies. It is believed that six or so genes are involved in any particular case of cancer (in childhood cancers like childhood leukemia, fewer are involved). These may be predisposing genes that the individual inherited, or genes that have undergone a mutation during the lifetime of the individual. These six or so genes need not be identical in two different individuals, even if the type of cancer is the same. At least some of the mutated genes may reflect particular exposures and provide us with a more precise answer to the question, what caused this particular case of cancer? Epidemiology, the study of diseases in human populations, will have greater statistical power and discrimination as a result. We may hope that our present helplessness in the face of such episodes as Pelham Bay, Woburn, and Toms River will be a thing of the past.

Going Beyond Science

Whatever is ultimately concluded about Pelham Bay and the other communities exposed to toxic wastes, there is surely no excuse for dumping toxic chemicals or even household garbage in close proximity to homes. It is not just a question of scientifically proven health hazards but of freedom of anxiety about health, and also of other values: freedom from bad smells and the unsightliness of a hill of garbage in the midst of a park. Dumping of toxic chemicals by industrial plants is finally closely regulated by law, as it should be, and many known sites of such dumping are being cleaned up. "Not In My Backyard" is sometimes a perfectly reasonable demand.

9

ASTHMA, ALLERGY, AND AIR POLLUTION

ASTHMA: SUFFERING AND DEATH

One night in early October 1997, Felipe G., a nine-year-old child of Do-
minican immigrants to New York City living in East Harlem, woke up
struggling for breath. Felipe had had asthma attacks before, and his parents knew, or thought they knew, what to do: they called for an ambu-
lance, which rushed him to the emergency room of Harlem Hospital
nearby. But this time he stopped breathing on the way to the hospital,
and could not be revived there. His younger sister Ana also has asthma,
but so far has never had to go to the emergency room.

The tenement building in which Felipe's family lives is three blocks
from the Harlem River Drive, a highway on which thousands of cars travel
each workday, emitting, in spite of their catalytic converters, large quantities of oxides of nitrogen, carbon monoxide, and incompletely com-
busted gasoline. Several blocks north is a parking garage for the diesel
trucks of the New York City Department of Sanitation. The drivers of the
trucks that use the lot often keep their motors idling, so that great quantities of diesel exhaust particles are emitted to the surrounding area. The
Harlem district of New York City, inhabited mainly by African-Americans
and Hispanics, is shielded to a large extent from the prevailing west winds
by higher areas on the west side of Manhattan. Hence, air pollution pro-

duced within Harlem—for example, by cars, diesel trucks, and buses, and by an electric power generating plant located there—tends to remain longer than in other areas of the city. The New York City Department of Environmental Protection operated a network of air monitoring stations from the 1940s to the 1970s, during which time Harlem was consistently found to be the most polluted area in the city. It had then, and still has, one of the highest rates of hospitalization for asthma in the city.

In most countries, asthma is more common among children of higher social class. In the United States this pattern is reversed: people living in the inner cities of the United States, mostly low-income minorities, have higher rates of asthma than other Americans. Why do they? What role does air pollution play in these higher rates? Are there other factors besides air pollution? How many children are at risk of dying as Felipe died? What can be done to prevent such deaths?

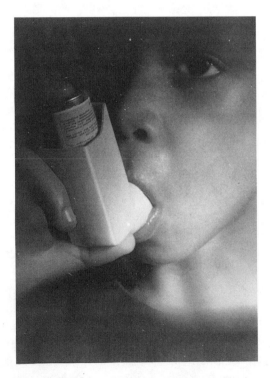

FIGURE 9-1   Asthmatic child using respirator. Photograph courtesy of West Harlem Environmental Action (WEACT, a community organization concerned with the environment).

What Asthma Is Like

Asthma is a disease characterized by intermittent attacks of wheezing (a characteristic whistling sound in the chest while breathing) and breathlessness. Between attacks there are often long symptom-free periods. The difficulty in breathing comes when the airways in the lungs are narrowed in response to different stimuli, which happens too easily and too often. The victim finds it difficult to exhale, and feels like he is choking. In an article in the magazine *Newsweek*, the mother of an asthmatic child vividly described what an attack is like: "Run in place for two minutes, then hold your nose and try to breathe through a straw!" Medications, often dispensed through inhalers, alleviate attacks, and other medications, such as steroids, taken regularly, help prevent them. Death is a possible outcome of an attack, but rare with the available medications and the training now given asthmatics and their families in how to manage their condition. Although severe asthma can be debilitating, with proper treatment its victims can live a normal life, as evidenced by the number of Olympic medalists who have suffered from it.

The Human and the Social Cost

Approximately one child out of eight in the United States and one out of five in the United Kingdom suffers from asthma, and it is the second largest cause of hospitalization of children (after accidents). Two million school days a year in the United States are lost because of it. It is not only a disease of children; workdays lost by asthmatics cost the U.S. economy about $4.6 billion a year, and the medical costs of treating it are estimated as another $8.1 billion in 2000 (The National Heart Lung and Blood Institute, National Instiues of Health).

Asthma has been rising dramatically all over the world in the last several decades. In the United States there were 7 million asthmatics in the early 1980s, and less than two decades later, in 1998, there were 17 million. If this trend continues for another two decades, there will be 30 million. The reason for this rise is not yet known (figs. 9-2, 9-3). Although asthma runs in families, implying a role for genetics, environmental agents are known to precipitate attacks, but few such agents have been identified. What role such agents play in causing the disease initially is not yet clear.

While there now are effective medications for managing the disease, it would be better to prevent attacks, and still better if people did

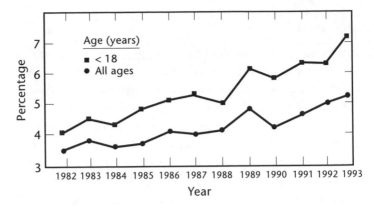

FIGURE 9-2 Rise in asthma prevalence over time, in both children and in the general population. "Prevalence" is the proportion of people suffering from the disease at any one point in time. There has been almost a doubling in the course of one decade. From an article in *Environmental Health Perspectives*, based on data of the National Heart, Lung, and Blood Institute, National Institutes of Health.

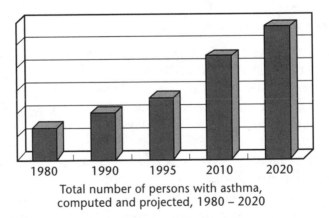

Total number of persons with asthma, computed and projected, 1980 – 2020

FIGURE 9-3 The prevalence of asthma, past and predicted. If present trends continue, it will be twice as prevalent in 2020, compared to 1995. Reproduced with the permission of the Pew Environmental Health Commission.

not become asthmatics in the first place. For these goals we need to answer two questions. How do environmental factors interact with genetic ones to cause asthma in the first place? And second, which environmental factors trigger attacks of asthma in people who already have the disease? These are different, but related, questions, and we will begin with the second: what triggers attacks in those who suffer from asthma? What do we now know, and what clues do we have to what is yet unknown?

WHAT TRIGGERS ASTHMA ATTACKS?

Where to Look

Many of the environmental agents that trigger attacks are airborne, not surprising for a chronic respiratory disease associated with sensitive airways. Even when we cannot identify the specific agent responsible, there is often no doubt about the route by which it reaches the victim. A primary focus of research on triggers, therefore, is on what is in the air we breathe.

Clusters of Asthma

In the center of New Orleans on October 26, 1964, 206 adults with severe asthma attacks were rushed to the emergency room of Charity Hospital, which usually saw twenty or thirty asthma patients a day. Such a cluster of attacks, with the patients coming in at six to ten times the usual rate in a short period of time, might also be called an "epidemic." The epidemic in October of 1964 was not the only one in New Orleans: similar ones had been observed earlier, and they continued for more than a decade in that city.

On January 23, 1986, about one hundred adults showed up with severe asthma attacks in emergency rooms in several hospitals in Barcelona, Spain, all located in one small section of the city, an area near the port, with a number of industrial facilities. The usual number of asthmatic patients at these hospitals was five or six per day. There were several similar epidemics in the years following.

Why did so many asthmatics have severe attacks in New Orleans and Barcelona on those particular days?

Known Environmental Triggers

Among the environmental agents known to precipitate asthma attacks are pets in general and cats in particular, mice, rats, the pollen of certain plants and molds, insects such as cockroaches and a widespread but almost invisible one, the house dust mite. The house dust mite is a tiny insect, difficult to see, that feeds on flakes of human skin and lives mostly in warm moist bedding, mattresses, furniture upholstery, rugs, and carpets (fig. 9-4).

Asthmatics differ in their sensitivities, which depend partly on genetic differences and partly on what they have been exposed to during

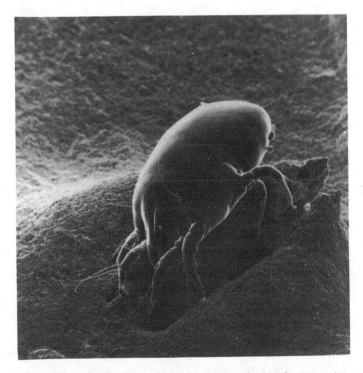

FIGURE 9-4 The house-dust mite, as viewed through the electron microscope, which gives a more powerful magnification than ordinary microscopes.
Reproduced from an article by J. E. M. H. van Bronswijk, in *Acta Allergica*, v. 28, p. 180 (1973), with the permission of Munksgard International Publishers, inc., Copenhagen, Denmark.

their lifetimes and when. No asthmatics are sensitive to every allergen that triggers attacks in other victims of the disease; each has her own repertoire of sensitivities.

Not all factors triggering attacks or asthma symptoms need be allergens; certain gases that are common pollutants (sulfur dioxide, ozone, and oxides of nitrogen) are irritants rather than allergens. Some asthmatics have symptoms or attacks when they exercise, others when exposed to very cold dry air. Butchers, who in the course of their daily work go in and out of cold rooms frequently, suffer from "occupational" asthma.

The environmental agents known to trigger asthma attacks do not account for the majority of such attacks, and one goal of current research is to identify those that are as yet unknown. We shall show in the following discussion how some of these questions are addressed (fig. 9-5).

EPIDEMICS

Asthma Clusters or Epidemics

Asthma attacks occur intermittently; the asthmatic is not undergoing an attack most of the time. It is a remarkable feature of this disease that sometimes large numbers of asthmatics in a particular geographical area suffer attacks almost simultaneously, within a period of a few hours. In addition to New Orleans and Barcelona, other such episodes have occurred and still occur in Brisbane, Australia; Yokohama, Japan; Baran, Brazil; Birmingham, United Kingdom; Toledo, Ohio, and New York City. We have used the term "cluster" in chapter 4 to describe a situation where the rate of a disease in a local area or in a short time interval is greater than its expected or average rate. The often used term "asthma epidemic" is not meant to imply that asthma is contagious, only that a large number of asthmatic individuals suffered attacks within a short time, probably because they were exposed to some airborne environmental agent. These asthma clusters are not like cancer clusters described in chapters 4 and 8, in which long periods of latency are involved and in which the cases appear one at a time over a longer time period, and usually involve no more than a dozen cases. Asthma epidemics often involve tens or hundreds of victims and are concentrated in a brief period of time, often a few hours, and in a small area. No subtle statistical tests are needed to rule out chance as an explanation.

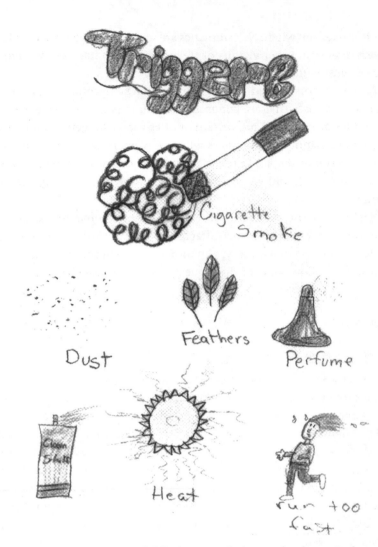

FIGURE 9-5 Prize-winning child's drawing of triggers of asthma attacks.
Courtesy of the National Heart, Lung, and Blood Institute, National Institutes
of Health.

Asthma Clusters in the Emergency Room

Gathering the data for studies of asthma clusters is less difficult than with
many other diseases, because attacks, when they occur, are severe enough
for the victims or their families to have to seek medical assistance almost
immediately. The quickest way to get that assistance, not only for the poor

who may not have a personal physician, but even for the well-to-do, is to go to the nearest hospital emergency room. This makes hospital emergency room records an invaluable resource. From them we can learn where patients lived, where they were when they got sick, how severe the attack was, and how quickly they recovered. Asthma attacks usually occur minutes or hours after exposure to the triggering agent, which makes it easier to pinpoint the time and location of the exposure.

Although identifying these striking medical events is relatively easy, and although they occur often and in many places in the world, it has not been so easy to discover what environmental agents are responsible. Most remain unexplained.

What Caused the New Orleans Epidemic?

A number of polluting industries were operating in New Orleans at the time of the epidemics. However, the air pollutants measured on those days were no higher than on other days. There was a large underground waste dump in the area that occasionally caught fire and emitted quantities of smoke, which was long suspected to be responsible. However, closing the dump did not stop the epidemics. Over time, they gradually waned, and by the 1970s were no longer taking place, but what caused them and why they stopped remained mysterious.

The victims of attacks during the New Orleans epidemics showed some evidence of allergic sensitivity in blood tests, but the specific agents to which they were allergic could not be identified at that time.

Barcelona: A Detective Story

In Barcelona, Spain, one of the epidemics involved a forty-fold abrupt increase in asthma visits at several hospital clinics within a four-hour period. The probability that this could have happened by chance alone was calculated by one of the physicians who studied it to be 1.5×10^{-17}, smaller than the chance that the earth will be hit by a comet or asteroid in the next 100 years. Again it was clear that there must have been some environmental factor responsible, but what was it? A map recording the locations where the attacks took place showed that most of them started when the individual affected was near the port area of the city. An examination of emergency room records identified twelve other asthma epidemics during a two-year period that had not drawn much attention at the time. All of them took place within a one- to four-hour period on the day in question, and all were localized either in the port area or in those parts of the city in which the wind direction was from the port area on the day of the epidemic (fig. 9-6). While this pinpointed the port itself or the industrial area nearby as the source of the agent responsible, no additional leads emerged. The local police and fire departments had not recorded anything unusual about those days. During the two year period of the epidemics there had been several air pollution episodes—periods of a day or two on which levels of the measured air pollutants were unusually high—but these days did not coincide with the epidemic days, nor did asthma patients recall any unusual symptoms on them.

Finally, two Barcelona physicians, Drs. J. Anto and P. Sunyer, found a clue by a search of the records of the harbor administration: on two

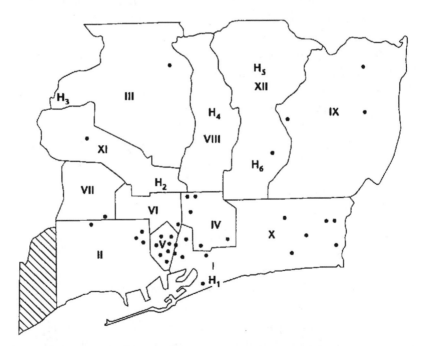

FIGURE 9-6   The asthma epidemic in Barcelona on November 26, 1984. The heavy concentration of cases in the area of the port is apparent. From the chapter "Soya Bean as a Risk Factor for Epidemic Asthma," by J. M. Anto and J. Sunyer, in *Geographical and Environmental Epidemiology: Methods for Small-area Studies*, by P. Elliott et al., Oxford University Press, 1996.

of the epidemic days cargoes of soybeans had been unloaded at the port. Following this up, Anto and Sunyer investigated just when two dozen different products handled at the port were unloaded during the two year period (730 days) on which thirteen asthma epidemics ocurred. They found that only soybean cargoes coincided with all the epidemic days, while no epidemics occurred unless soybeans were unloaded (table 9-1).

Soybeans were loaded from the ships into two silos in the port area, designated Silo A and Silo B. The close relation between the epidemics and the unloading of soybeans was almost all due to unloading into Silo A, which unlike Silo B was not equipped with special filters installed in the dust collection system. In the absence of filters, soybean dust was released into the air. Once filters were installed in Silo A, the epidemics ceased, further confirming the conclusion that soybean dust was the triggering agent. Soybeans were also unloaded on 249 days on which there were no epidemics. This might seem to count against the idea that soybeans caused the epidemics, but other conditions than just unloading soybeans had to be met to cause an epidemic: the wind direction had to be such as to blow the dust toward the port area rather than out to sea, and the wind should not have been blowing so strongly as to quickly disperse the dust.

Subsequently blood tests for allergic sensitivity to soybeans done on asthmatics who had had attacks during the epidemics were compared

TABLE 9-1   Cargoes Unloaded and Asthma Epidemic Days

Cargo	Number of Days Each Cargo Was Unloaded		Number of Days Each Cargo Was not Unloading	
	Number of Days of No Epidemics	Number of Epidemic Days	Number of Days of No Epidemics	Number of Epidemic Days
Coal	196	4	521	9
Fuel oil	150	3	567	10
Gasoline	180	2	537	11
Cotton	399	7	318	6
Coffee	300	5	417	8
Corn	135	1	582	12
Soybeans	249	13	468	0
Butane	140	1	577	12

to tests done on a control group of asthmatics who had not had such attacks. The great majority of attack victims showed sensitivity, compared to a small fraction in the control group. Sensitivity to soybeans had already been recognized by physicians specializing in allergy, and a commercial preparation of soybean extract had been prepared by a pharmaceutical company for use in testing patients. Ironically, the asthma victims in Barcelona showed less sensitivity to the commercial preparation than to samples of soybean dust collected during the Barcelona epidemics.

Back to Charity Hospital

Once soybeans were shown to be the agent responsible for the Barcelona epidemics, researchers at the Centers for Disease Control in Atlanta, together with one of the authors of this book, reinvestigated the notorious New Orleans epidemics, which had gradually waned after the 1960s but had remained a mystery. New Orleans is also a seaport, handling all sorts of cargoes, including chemicals and grains. The records kept by the shipping industry during the period of the asthma epidemics were examined to determine what cargoes were unloaded in the harbor. These records, unfortunately, did not show the specific days on which the ships were unloaded, but did give the days the ships bearing cargoes of soybeans and other suspected agents had been docked in the port. The specific day of unloading would have to have been one of those days. What cargoes had been on ships in the port on the day of each asthma epidemic? The answer was clear-cut: soybeans again. The previously unexplained decline of the epidemics in the 1960's and after was attributed to a general upgrading at just that time of industrial hygiene practices at all grain facilities, including the installation of dust filters.

Soybeans have also been implicated in another asthma epidemic in Cartagena, in southeastern Spain.

Why Thunderstorms?

People who suffer from arthritis, most of them old, often complain that the weather makes their joints hurt: that weather can do this has often been dismissed as an old wives' tale, though old husbands also complain. Other conditions that, according to their victims, are influenced by weather include migraine headaches and pain in healed broken bones and old war wounds. An influence of weather and climate on disease was first claimed by Hippocrates, in ancient Greece. In 1711, Joseph Addison wrote: "A cloudy day, or a little sunshine, have as great an influence on many constitutions as the most real blessings or misfortunes." Scientists today are taking weather more seriously than they used to.

Some dramatic asthma epidemics in Australia and the United Kingdom have occurred during or just after severe thunderstorms. Only a few of the known epidemics around the world have been associated with thunderstorms, and most thunderstorms do not give rise to them. What distinguishes those few thunderstorms that trigger attacks from all others is not yet fully understood. It has been suggested that the sudden strong rainstorms that often go with thunderstorms release large quantities of certain pollens into the air, to which asthmatics are sensitive. This would imply that specific weather and seasonal factors must accompany the thunderstorms to trigger the epidemics.

In Australia on one spring night, just after a thunderstorm accompanied by heavy rains, almost three hundred patients with asthma attacks came to one clinic where the daily average was about twenty-five. During and just before this episode there were no changes in measured levels of air pollutants. An unusual concentration of a certain rye-grass pollen was in the air before the epidemic, but it was assumed that the grass pollen grains were much too large to enter the lung. Since then, however, it has been shown that heavy rains cause the pollen grains to swell and rupture, releasing hundreds of small starch granules that contain the rye-grass allergen. Once released, the granules are small enough to enter deep into the lung and remain there. The concentration of such starch granules in the air has been found to increase fiftyfold during rainfall, and to much higher levels during some thunderstorms. This provides a plausible explanation for at least some of the epidemics associated with thunderstorms.

A sharp increase of asthma attacks consistently occurs around the world every fall season, particularly in children and younger adults. This sharp increase persists for a period of a few weeks and then the number gradually decreases to a lower rate in the winter. The same phenomenon is observed in the fall season in the Southern Hemisphere, for example, in Australia and South America. The reason is unknown, but it has been suggested that it has something to do with the greater frequency of respiratory infections once the school year begins, or alternatively that there is a seasonal increase in some as yet unidentified mold spores.

ASTHMA ATTACKS AND AIR POLLUTION

London Smog

The most notorious air pollution episode of all time, "The Great London Smog Episode," took place in December 1952 in London. A weather inversion—conditions under which air near the ground is trapped under a blanket of warmer air—lasting four or five days caused air pollutants, mainly from home heating systems and power plants, to accumulate to levels more than ten times those usually seen at that time, and about one hundred times the levels seen in the United States today (fig. 9-7). Cattle dropped dead while being brought to the city slaughterhouses, and movie theaters had to close because the image projected from the back of the theater did not reach the screen. In those few days there were 4,000 excess deaths, mainly among those elderly suffering from chronic bronchitis, emphysema, and cardiac problems. Asthmatics suffered somewhat, but less than expected (fig. 9-8).

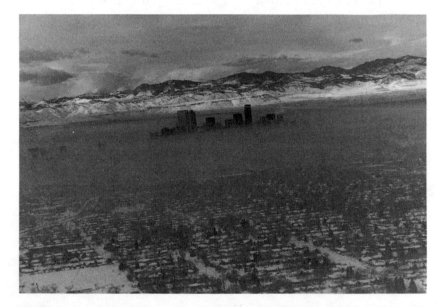

FIGURE 9-7   Inversion in Denver, Colorado, in December 1983. A pollution alert was issued because of a brown cloud of pollution hanging over the city. Above a certain level visible in the photograph the air is relatively clear. Copyright Bettman/Corbis.

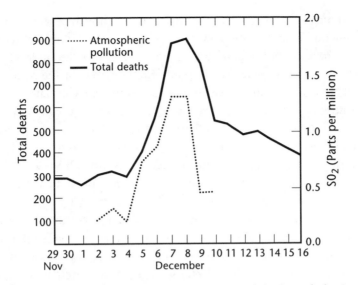

FIGURE 9-8   The London Smog Episode. Shown are total deaths each day in December 1952, as well as the sulfur dioxide concentration on each day. Reproduced from *Epidemiology: Principles and Methods*, by Brian MacMahon and Thomas F. Pugh, Little, Brown and Company, Boston, 1970, and reproduced with the permission of Professor MacMahon and of Lippincott, Williams and Wilkins.

The United States has had only a few lethal episodes. One of them took place in Donora, Pennsylvania, in 1948, in which about twenty people died and hundreds were made ill.

The Setting of Air Pollution Standards

These episodes marked the beginning of intensive research on the health effects of air pollution, in particular on the relations between various respiratory conditions and pollution levels. Asthmatics, clearly a sensitive population that responded quickly to environmental triggers, were considered an ideal population to study.

Regulation of emissions of pollutants and the adoption of air pollution standards around the world followed the London Smog episode. The standards were set to reduce illnesses and deaths caused by pollution to negligible rates. There is much evidence that their goals were reached: in the United Kingdom prior to the reductions in air pollution that followed the setting of standards, individuals with chronic bronchitis had been asked to keep diaries in which they recorded coughing and other respiratory symptoms on a daily basis, and comparison of their diaries with measured daily air pollution showed a close relationship. However, after the reduction in air pollution levels, coughs and other symptoms recorded in the diaries no longer showed a relationship with pollution levels, even though those levels varied considerably from one day to the next. In the United States, acceptable levels to protect health were calculated from extrapolation of the rates of deaths and illness caused by the high pollution in such episodes as the London Smog. Extrapolation is necessary because at the low levels current in the Western industrialized countries, where for the most part strict standards are enforced, it is difficult to detect health effects with accuracy. Extrapolation is necessary for much the same reasons as it is in setting health standards for low-dose ionizing radiation from experience at high doses (see chapters 2 and 3). In 1997 the U.S. air quality standards were made even stricter, to reduce exposure to very minute particles (which had not been measured in the earlier studies and are likely to reach and remain in the lungs) and gaseous ozone. There is still controversy about whether these current standards need to be tightened further.

The standards are designed not only to protect the health of the population but also to prevent materials exposed to air from being damaged. Historic marble sculptures have suffered damage in Italy, Greece, and elsewhere from acidic sulfur dioxide in the ambient air.

What Pollutes the Air?

The air we breathe contains thousands of substances, both of natural origin and by-products of human activity. Only a few of these are regulated under the standards and measured in a more or less systematic fashion. Their concentrations in the air are greatly influenced by weather conditions: wind, rain, sun, and atmospheric inversions. High winds and upward convection of air tend to disperse pollutants, while still air and inversions favor accumulation, sometimes to very high levels. When those pollutants we measure are at high levels, trapped by specific meteorological conditions, other pollutants that we do not measure, if emitted at the same time, are also likely to be trapped as well. One might expect that the few pollutants that are monitored serve as indicators of the presence of the others that we do not yet measure. This is only an assumption, supported by direct experiment for a few common pollutants, but not for all of them, and not under all conditions. There has been relatively little research on possible harmful pollutants other than the regulated ones.

Polluting Gases

The regulated gaseous air pollutants include sulfur dioxide (emitted by combustion of sulfur-containing fuels), nitrogen dioxide (most of which comes from automobile emissions), and ozone (formed by the action of ultraviolet radiation on such substances as oxides of nitrogen). The latter two are responsible for eye and nose irritation in smoggy areas, and ozone in particular has been linked to damage to the respiratory system in humans and animals.

Measurement of the concentrations of these regulated gaseous pollutants in the ambient air is a relatively straightforward application of chemical analysis and can be done with high accuracy.

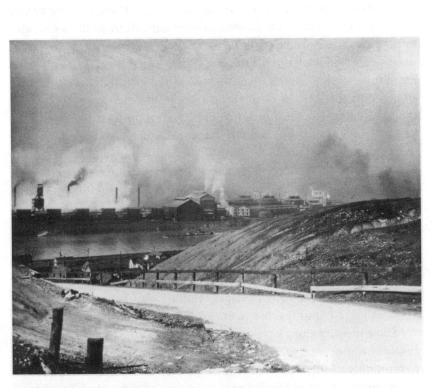

FIGURE 9-9   Air pollution from the area of Pittsburgh, Pennsylvania, in the period before regulation. Courtesy National Library for the History of Medicine, Nation Institutes of Health.

Particulates

Small solid and liquid particles, referred to together as "particulates," are what make air pollution visible and unsightly. Their chemical makeup depends on their source: sulfur dioxide in the air gradually combines with oxygen, water vapor, and metals to form droplets of sulphuric acid and solid sulfates; the combustion of diesel fuel produces solid and liquid hydrocarbons, some of which are known carcinogens. Some particulate pollution is "natural," formed when sunlight and oxygen convert gaseous organic substances emitted by plants into liquid or solid particles.

Unlike the measurement of gas concentrations, the measurement of particulates is much more complicated and has undergone a number of modifications in recent years. In the past, measurements were quite undiscriminating, lumping together particles of all sizes and all chemical compositions under the terms "smoke" or "haze." These were measured either by their effect on the transmission of light through the air, or else by filtering the air to collect all the particulates and measuring their total weight per cubic meter of air (termed "total suspended particles"). This has not been very informative, because whether inhaled particles are absorbed in the surfaces of the lung ("respirable" particles), trapped in the nasal passages, or just breathed out depends on their size (see chapter 3). The particles of the size most responsible for haze are too large to reach the lung, and are instead absorbed in the nose and trachea. It is particles less than 10 microns in size that reach the lungs (10 microns is four ten-thousandths of an inch). In recent years more refined methods of measuring particle concentrations of particular size ranges have been developed and their effects on exposed populations are currently being determined. Recent studies have reported that it is not all respirable particles (those below 10 microns in size) that are important in health studies, but mainly the smaller ones, below 2.5 microns, which penetrate more deeply into the lung passages, and are also believed to be composed of more harmful substances.

Some investigations have suggested that exposure to irritant particles and to irritant gases, such as ozone and nitrogen dioxide, increase the susceptibility of the lung to allergens, perhaps by causing inflammation of the lung tissues or by increasing their permeability to inhaled allergens. Attempts are being made to distinguish exactly where in the lung and respiratory system damage occurs.

Particles from Diesel Fuel

The particles from burning diesel fuel are usually smaller than 2.5 microns. They have been shown to increase the response of asthmatics to a number of allergens they are sensitive to. It is possible that these allergens are absorbed on the surface of these tiny particles and then carried into the lungs, and also possible that diesel particles produce some direct response of the immune system on their own. They are also known carcinogens. They are composed of a complicated mix of chemicals including polyaromatic hydrocarbons, discussed in chapter 5 (fig. 9-10).

Exposure, Indoors and Out

To determine the health effects of air pollution on humans, we need to know the exposures of the population we are studying, and the health effects, usually respiratory or cardiovascular. The problems of determining exposures are particularly difficult. Thousands of substances are emitted into the air in modern industrial societies, and we cannot possibly measure them all. As noted earlier, the best we can do is measure a few, either because they are easy to measure, or because they are known to have direct effects on health. We know also that people move between various indoor environments and various outdoor environments in the course of a day or a week, so that their exposures change all the time. Unless we monitor them continuously, we could not estimate their total exposure to air pollution accurately.

To most people "air pollution" means outdoor air polluted by factories and automobiles. However people in temperate climates do most of their breathing, along with most of their other activities, indoors. For many, 90 to 95% of the air they breathe is indoor air, which may therefore be more important than outdoor air for asthma and other respiratory diseases. In many current asthma studies, indoor air is being monitored for allergens, some regulated outdoor air pollutants, tobacco smoke, and chemical contaminants from products used in the home such as solvents, spray propellants, and insecticides. Surprisingly, levels of chemical contaminants have been found to be higher indoors than in the outdoor air even in the vicinity of polluting chemical factories (see TEAM studies described later in this chapter and in chapter 8).

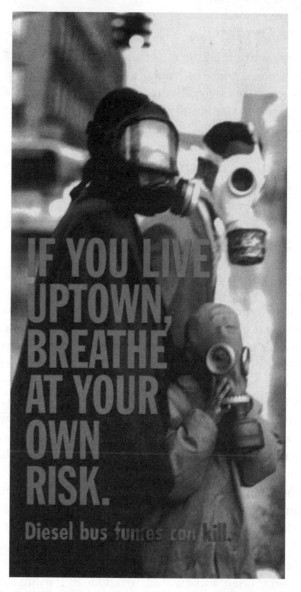

FIGURE 9-10   Poster warning people in Harlem, New York City, of diesel
fumes, courtesy of West Harlem Environmental Action (WEACT). As part of a
"Dump Dirty Diesel" campaign, WEACT used imagery of community members
in gas masks to drive home its message against the continuing siting of diesel
bus depots in upper Manhattan. Diesel pollution has been linked to increased
asthma attacks. Upper Manhattan is home to some of the highest hospitalization rates in the country, as well as six diesel bus depots. Photo by Marc
Baptiste.

Chamber Studies

Studies on asthmatics have been performed in sealed chambers in which they were exposed to known concentrations of pollutants for specified periods of time. In addition to recording symptoms such as shortness of breath, the investigators also measured changes in the subjects' lung function, for example, the quantity of air the subject can rapidly expel after inhaling as deeply as possible. Lung function is a useful diagnostic tool for a variety of lung diseases or breathing disorders, being a more objective and reliable measure than asking people what symptoms they feel. In chamber experiments lung function has been measured both in asthmatic and nonasthmatic subjects before, during, and after exposure to air pollutants such as sulfur dioxide or ozone. High levels of pollutants were found to cause temporary decreases in lung function even in nonasthmatic subjects. In addition, relatively low levels of sulfur dioxide, comparable to what is sometimes found today in ambient air, caused decreases in lung function in some of the asthmatics, while other asthmatics as well as nonasthmatic subjects did not appear to be specially sensitive.

Such experiments, comparing the response of asthmatic and nonasthmatic subjects to one or two air pollutants, have been useful in setting air pollution standards, and also in designing studies on populations of people with and without asthma to see how they respond to air pollutants while carrying on their normal daily activities.

There are, of course, differences between the exposure of large populations carrying on their day-to-day activities to whatever complex mixture of substances is out there and the carefully controlled conditions of a chamber study in which one or two substances are studied at a time, and in which the subject either does nothing or else rides an exercise bicycle at a fixed speed.

Epidemics and Air Pollution

Major asthma epidemics, like those in New Orleans, Barcelona, New York, and elsewhere, have not occurred on days when the commonly measured air pollutant concentrations have been high. Further, on days on which air pollution has been high, for the most part no excess numbers of asthma attacks have been observed. We have mentioned that in the London Smog episode of 1952, asthmatics did not suffer as much as might have been expected. In London today, severe asthma epidemics occur, and so do air pollution episodes in which specific air pollutants reach especially high levels. However, none of the more severe episodes of air pollution have been accompanied by unusually high numbers of asthma attacks; none of the asthma epidemics have been accompanied by an increase in the levels of the commonly measured pollutants.

Figure 9-11 shows the courses of both daily hospital admissions for asthma and daily levels of nitrogen dioxide, an irritant gaseous pollutant, in London in November and December of 1991. There was a major air pollution episode on December 13, and several minor episodes in mid-November and mid-January. During this particular period other monitored pollutants were also high, so the nitrogen dioxide level then was an indicator of air pollution in general. On almost all these days, most noteworthy in the December 13 episode, asthma hospital admissions were no higher than usual.

New York City has had several asthma epidemics every year somewhat less dramatic than those in Barcelona and New Orleans, but in which a sudden large surge of asthma attacks occurred simultaneously all over the city. Unlike the epidemics in Barcelona, which were localized in a small

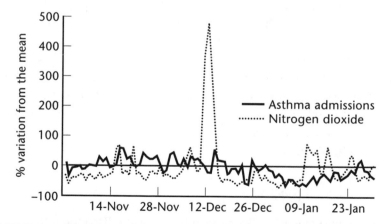

FIGURE 9-11 Comparison of daily asthma admissions to hospitals in London and daily nitrogen dioxide levels. On December 12, 1991, there was an unusually high nitrogen dioxide concentration, and no obvious increase in asthma admissions on that day or subsequently. Reproduced from an article by Ross Anderson, *British Medical Journal*, v. 312, pp. 1606–1607 (1996), with permission of the BMJ Publishing Group.

section of the city around Silo A, the so-far unidentified environmental trigger responsible must have been such as to expose the whole city at one time. Just as in London, there was no particular excess of the regulated air pollutants on these epidemic days, nor was there any increase in numbers of asthma attacks on days on which air pollution was high.

Many studies have compared the day-to-day variation of asthma symptoms, asthma attacks, or hospital visits to the day-to-day variation of the commonly monitored air pollutants over a period of a few years, and have found a weak relation between asthma symptoms and pollution levels, particularly if the pollution remains high for a period of at least three or four days. Other studies have failed to confirm this. Since high air pollution concentrations occur only under special weather conditions, and because weather itself may influence asthma attacks, it is often difficult to separate the possible effects of all aspects of weather on asthma from those of air pollution.

Indoor versus Outdoor

A number of studies carried out by the U.S. Environmental Protection Agency in the 1980s and 1990s have clearly demonstrated how unrepresentative of total personal exposure outdoor measurements are, both for some of the regulated pollutants and for other unregulated but known toxic chemicals.

In these studies (called the TEAM studies, described also in chapter 8) people carried personal monitors that measured the concentrations of a number of pollutants in their vicinity, and had samples of breath or saliva taken to determine their total exposures, usually over a twenty-four hour period. Exposures measured this way were compared with indoor and outdoor monitoring measurements. The results were unexpected. The major sources of the exposures were indoors, where levels of many pollutants were much higher than outdoors. Nitrogen dioxide is often higher indoors than outdoors because of emissions from gas stoves or other combustion appliances. Many volatile organic compounds—some of them known carcinogens—have important sources indoors, for example, from deodorant sprays, pesticides, mothballs, paints and paint solvents, furniture coverings, and so on. For some pollutants the personal exposures were higher than would have been expected even from the measured indoor concentrations. For example, smoking cigarettes exposes the smoker through inhalation of the concentrated direct smoke to higher levels of benzene than is found inside a room where the smoke from cigarettes has been allowed to spread. Exposures from hair sprays and deodorants is also greater for the user than would be inferred from measurements of average indoor concentrations. Accurate assessment of such exposures requires monitoring of the individuals involved rather than just monitoring the air in the room.

In summary: environmental causes have been found for only a few of the dramatic asthma epidemics, but the measured levels of air pollution appear to play no role in them. Studies of the day-to-day variations in asthma attacks or symptoms have found that air pollution might explain only a small part of them. Many of the exposures we associate with emissions from industry and traffic contribute only a small portion of a person's total exposure to many chemical agents; most exposure to them is indoors through commercial products used in homes. This is not to say that emissions to the outdoor air should be left uncontrolled nor that all health hazards are indoors, but it does demonstrate the importance of monitoring total exposure from all sources before assessing any health effects. We have already pointed out that most people in Western countries spend 90–95% of their time indoors; current studies of how asthma develops and why it is increasing are focused more on the indoor environment.

WHAT CAUSES ASTHMA?

Who Becomes Asthmatic?

So far we have discussed what is known about environmental factors that trigger asthma attacks in people who already suffer from asthma. We now turn to the second important question: what causes a child or adult to become asthmatic in the first place? Is it exposure to the same factors that trigger attacks in the already susceptible, or is it more complicated than that? It is certainly plausible that a disease of the breathing system and exacerbated by airborne agents could also be caused by exposure to these agents. On the other hand, some scientists have suggested a different origin. Before we examine the evidence for and against the different views, we will review briefly some of what is known about the condition.

History of Asthma

The disease has been known since the ancient Greeks. Hippocrates described it and coined the name "asthma" after a Greek word meaning "panting." Maimonides, writing in the 12th century, asserted that death from asthma could occur "should the rules of management go unheeded and one's desires and habits be followed indiscriminately." He recommended that sufferers from asthma avoid stress and move to a better climate. In 1660 a German physician, Konrad Schneider, proposed that asthma is caused by exposure to irritants, including dust.

In 1713, Bernardino Ramazzini published his classic "Diseases of Workers" (in Latin), in which occupational diseases were first recognized as a distinct entity. In the index under "asthma" we find among the victims miners, gilders, tinsmiths, glassblowers, tanners, bakers, millers, grain sifters, stone cutters, carders, ragmen, runners, riders, porters, farmers, and professors at the University of Padua.

As we noted earlier, the disease has more than doubled in the developed countries in the last few decades. In the United States there has been a steep increase in hospital admissions and deaths, especially in, but not limited to, the inner city. This recent increase cannot be attributed to any change in genetic factors: it has taken place too rapidly, and the children of immigrants from less developed countries, where asthma is low, suffer asthma at the high rates typical of Western developed countries. Changes in environmental factors, in the broadest sense of the word "environmental," must be responsible.

Asthma and Allergy

About 80% of asthmatics are known to also suffer from allergies. In other words, like other victims of allergy, they show skin sensitivity—rashes, eczema, hives, itching—or other reactions to certain substances applied to the skin or ingested. This skin sensitivity is the basis of "patch" tests for allergy: measured amounts of suspected allergens—grass pollen extract, for example—are applied to the skin of a patient, and the size of the inflamed area gives a measure of sensitivity.

Allergy results from an excessive response of the immune system, that system that serves to guard against harmful foreign organisms and substances. Among the ways the immune system defends the body is by making protein molecules designed to react with and neutralize foreign organisms and the toxins they produce. These molecules are called antibodies, and the ability of the body to tailor them to fit foreign material never previously encountered by the individual is remarkable. Sometimes the immune system overreacts in susceptible individuals to the presence of foreign substances that do not cause disease or discomfort in most people. Such substances are called "allergens." There is a wide variety of them that can act this way, either breathed in, eaten, or placed on the skin, among them plants and plant pollen, drugs, foreign proteins, and some metals. On first exposures to an allergen, the immune system of a susceptible person produces a specific type of antibody, called an immunoglobulin E (IgE, for short), which binds to the allergen on subsequent exposure and triggers the release of histamines and other chemicals. These are thought to cause the narrowing and inflammation of the airways associated with an asthma attack. In a hay-fever victim who is not asthmatic the release of histamines causes the sneezing, runny nose, and burning eyes characteristic of that disease.

Often the specific immunoglobulin produced in response to an allergen can be detected in the blood. For example, individuals sensitive to the German cockroach or to the house-dust mite and who have recently been exposed will have an immunoglobulin (IgE) specific to that cockroach or mite antigen in their blood. This not only makes it possible to show that the individual is sensitive to the allergen but also how recently he has been exposed to it. It thus serves as a "biological marker" of the exposure.

It is interesting to note that allergy has increased in the Western world in the last few decades even more rapidly than asthma.

Genetics or Environment?

Often several members of a single family will have asthma. This is consistent with, but does not prove, that there is a genetic predisposition to asthma: after all, members of a family also share a common environment and a common lifestyle. Studies of twins can distinguish genetic from environmental factors. If asthma were caused only by environmental agents, identical twins, who share identical genetic makeups, would be no more likely to simultaneously suffer from the disease than nonidentical twins or ordinary brothers or sisters (nonidentical twins are no more alike genetically than siblings generally). The frequency with which pairs of identical twins both suffer from asthma—known as the "concordance" of the disease—supports the idea of a genetic predisposition. Both twins of an identical pair are in fact found to suffer from asthma more often than nonidentical twins, suggesting an interaction between genetic and environmental factors. Scientists are now trying to identify the specific genes involved in asthma. Current views are that there are many genes that affect both the likelihood of developing the disease and the susceptibility to a variety of environmental agents.

Sufferers from asthma throughout the United States used to be advised by their doctors to move to the dry, hot climate of Arizona. On doing so, they found their asthma improving for a while, only to have it come back as they became sensitized to local allergens, for example, from plants indigenous to Arizona, such as cacti. The long-term result was that the number of asthma sufferers in Arizona has increased, partly because of the large influx of asthmatics and partly because they began to marry each other and have children. Tucson, Arizona, now has one of the highest rates of childhood asthma in the United States.

Genetics and Environment Both

Given that there is a genetic predisposition, not everyone with that predisposition need get the disease. Presumably some environmental factors must activate it, perhaps an exposure to an allergen or to other air pollutants interacting with something in the individual's medical history, such as an infection.

Asthma among rural villagers in Papua-New Guinea had been relatively rare. But after they moved to towns in the Eastern highlands of that country the prevalence of asthma among them increased from less than 1% to more than 7% in a very short period of time. Researchers have suggested that this dramatic rise came from the fortuitous combination of two factors: a previously unexpressed genetic susceptibility to allergens from the house-dust mite, followed by exposure to the mite only after their move to the towns. Their new lifestyle included the use of blankets and other bedding, and the use of soap. The first provided a warm, moist environment for the house-dust mite; the second caused drier skin that flaked off more readily, providing the mites with their food. The house-dust mite is found all over the world, and its allergens are one of the most common triggers of attacks.

Asthma behind the Iron Curtain

Some scientists have suggested that exposure to allergens, perhaps at an early age, can turn a genetic predisposition into a case of asthma. Studies are under way in which exposures of newborns and children to various known allergens are monitored, and related to any subsequent development of asthma. But it is also possible that whatever in the air triggers attacks in the already asthmatic person may not necessarily cause the disease in the first place. Could exposure to any of the common air pollutants cause asthma, possibly by causing inflammation and thus sensitization of lung tissue even though they are not allergens and have not been shown to be important triggers of attacks? If so, the geographical distribution of asthma should vary with the concentrations of these pollutants (ozone, NO_2, particles, and sulfur dioxide). Most studies have found that high rates of asthma in a region are not related to high levels of outdoor air pollution there. The experience of Eastern Europe offers a striking example.

In recent years the setting of air pollution standards has led to a marked reduction in most of the commonly measured pollutants in the industrialized countries. The use of low-sulfur fuels increased, scrubbers to reduce emissions from smokestacks were installed, the smokestacks were made taller to reduce exposure in communities immediately surrounding the power stations and factories, and traffic restrictions were imposed when weather conditions led to dangerous pollution buildup. All these changes are to the good, but one consequence is that it is now much harder, in Western countries, to determine if air pollution harms people.

When the Iron Curtain was lifted in 1989 from the socialist countries of Eastern Europe, it was found that pollution of the environment there was comparable to that during the worst years of the industrial revolution in the nineteenth century. Exposures unheard of in the West for many decades were common. Cheap high-sulfur fuels such as brown coal were used, and no efforts were made to control pollution from industries and power plants. Many of the radiators in the apartments in large communal apartment houses lacked shutoff valves or otherwise malfunctioned, so to avoid overheating in the winter many of the residents were forced to keep their windows open. This not only wastefully used more fuel but also exposed the residents even while indoors to high levels of sulfur dioxide and particulates from the outside air.

We have described in chapter 3 the working conditions of miners in the uranium mines of Czechoslovakia and the German Democratic Republic. In both cases the governments of the socialist countries showed an extreme indifference to the risk to the health of their citizens from environmental hazards. It is interesting to note that these countries had fairly good state-run comprehensive health care systems.

Surprise!

When Eastern Europe was opened up, not only business entrepreneurs rushed in, but so also did eager epidemiologists, recognizing an opportunity to study the health effects of high air pollution levels. They found, as they expected, that indeed many respiratory disorders, such as emphysema and bronchitis, were much more common than in Western Europe. But, to their great surprise, in the more polluted cities of the East bloc countries asthma, rather than being more prevalent than in the West, was significantly less so. Allergies, too, which are often associated with asthma, were about half as common as in the West.

When different rates of a disease are observed in different countries, one possible explanation is that doctors in the two countries diagnose the disease differently. To avoid this possible error in comparing the rates, the same teams of doctors made the diagnoses of asthma and other respiratory diseases in both Eastern and Western Europe.

There were many differences in lifestyle and exposures between the two regions of Europe. Western products and processes that introduce chemicals indoors, such as household cleansers and sprays, many synthetic fabrics used for clothing and furniture, paints, and pesticides, which were scarce in Eastern Europe prior to 1989, are now becoming more common there. Investigators have conjectured that as the Eastern European countries catch up to the Western lifestyle, the rate of asthma may also catch up.

Asthma and War in the Middle East

Although asthma is increasing around the world, particularly in the more developed countries, the levels of most regulated air pollutants have declined in the United States and Western Europe over this time period. No reason for the increase has yet been established, but speculation has focused on certain lifestyle changes in recent decades.

The 1973 Middle East war led to a sudden jump in fuel prices in the West, and in response energy conservation measures were introduced in homes, businesses, and means of transportation. Home and workplace heat losses were reduced by eliminating air leaks, replacing old windows with tightly fitting ones, and generally increasing insulation. These measures reduced fuel consumption, in part by reducing air exchange with the outside air, thus also retaining air pollutants whose sources are indoors. This includes tobacco smoke (which has been shown to both exacerbate asthma symptoms and to increase the risk of a child becoming asthmatic), the combustion products of gas stoves, insecticides, household cleanser sprays, solvents and other chemicals emitted from synthetic fabrics, paint, and furniture (such as formaldehyde). Reduced air exchange also insures that allergens from cockroaches, rodents, and pets will remain indoors. In addition, the decrease of air exchange led to an increase in home humidity, which favored the growth of molds and fungi known to exacerbate asthma, and provided more congenial conditions for the house-dust mite. Incidentally, it also increased the retention of radon (chapter 3). Meanwhile, many new chemical agents are constantly being introduced into the home environment, faster than their possible effects on asthma can be studied. These changes in the indoor environment may very well contribute to the increasing prevalence of asthma in the developed world.

Infections, Hygiene, Pigs

Meanwhile, ideas about the causes of asthma other than exposures to airborne agents are being explored. Some of these ideas have to do with the immune system and the effect on it of infectious diseases. The social-ist countries of Eastern Europe had a different and more comprehensive child care system than the West, with a higher proportion of children in day-care centers at an earlier age, and for longer hours. The children were therefore exposed to various infectious diseases at an earlier age, and it is possible that infections at an early age, because they stimulate the proper development of the immune system, may protect against asthma and allergy. Recent studies in Western countries showed less asthma among children who were in day-care centers during their first six months of life. One such report, in the *New England Journal of Medicine*, was accompanied by an editorial with the title, "Day Care, Siblings, and Asthma: Please Sneeze on My Child." A similar hypothesis about childhood leukemia has been discussed in chapter 4. Studies of the effect of immunization in early childhood against childhood diseases on asthma are also under way, but no clear answer has yet emerged.

It is interesting that studies of farming communities have repeatedly found a lower incidence of asthma than in rural but nonfarming com-munities. Living on a farm exposes infants and children to a great variety of both allergens and infectious agents: bacterial toxins, animal dander, mice, rats, cockroaches, grain, dust, fungi, and mold; is it possible that early exposure to them is protective against asthma, rather than a cause of it? In particular, it has been shown that keeping pigs in the house protects against asthma. This might be considered further evidence that too much hygiene is unhealthy. Of course, farming families differ from nonfarming ones in other ways than their exposure to a variety of allergens and infections: their diet is different, they spend more time outdoors and get more exercise, they usually have more children, and the mothers smoke less. Any of these factors may also explain some of their lower asthma incidence.

There is some evidence that to get the benefit of the unsanitary environment on a farm, one must spend the first year of one's life there. If one moves to a farm later in life, one is more, not less, likely to get asthma or suffer from allergies.

The Chicken or the Egg?

Another factor that has changed in the United States and other Western countries at about the same time as the increase in asthma is obesity. The average weights of both children and adults has increased significantly, perhaps as a result of too much time spent watching television and eating the foods advertised there. Obesity in the United States is considered an epidemic by nutritionists. Hispanic and African-American low-income children, even as young as four years old, show a higher rate of obesity compared to other American children, and this disparity is increasing each year.

Many studies have shown that obesity in children and asthma go together: they are "associated." Why there should be such a relation—is it lack of exercise or a result of diet?—is currently being investigated. Exercise often causes symptoms in asthmatics, and some parents of asthmatic children therefore restrict their physical activity. Lack of exercise may cause them to gain weight, or perhaps obese children just exercise less. In any event, without the deep breathing and stretching of the bronchial muscles that go with exercise, the airways tend to narrow. The "association" between asthma and obesity could reflect the possibility that asthma causes obesity, and equally well the possibility that obesity causes asthma.

The role of obesity in childhood on other diseases later on in life, such as cardiovascular disease, high blood pressure, and diabetes, is under study, together with efforts to reduce it. Certainly, reducing obesity in both adults and children will be good for their health in general; whether it will be good for asthma in particular is yet to be seen.

Conclusions about Causes

Asthma, a disease of extreme sensitivity to a variety of specific environmental agents, has risen dramatically in the developed world, and has been shown to increase when people move from developing countries to Western societies, and from rural villages to urban areas within developing countries. Neither the reasons for the dramatic rise in the disease nor the agents triggering attacks have all been identified. Some of the known triggering agents are related to industrialization and lifestyle: while soybean dust and other allergens from grains are natural substances, exposure to them occurs as a result of modern production and distribution methods developed over the past century. Other triggers, like those associated with thunderstorms, are most likely caused by exposures to natural allergens. Lifestyle factors govern exposure to a number of indoor triggers of asthma, such as the house-dust mite, cockroach, and pet allergens, while exposure to certain pollutants such as ozone and diesel particles may increase the asthmatic response to them.

What causes asthma is not yet understood. Some scientists have looked at exposure to airborne agents. Industrialization has not only introduced new chemicals into the outdoor and indoor environment but also changed the way chemicals and other goods are handled, stored, and distributed. It has led to changes in lifestyle—for example, in the amount of time spent indoors (influenced both by television and by fear of crime in the inner city) and the sealing of the indoor environment to save energy, increasing our exposure to pollutants from indoor sources, including other people's cigarettes. Other scientists are now looking at the elimination or reduction of exposures to certain infectious diseases at early ages, by better sanitation, by immunization, and by new drugs, which have saved and are still saving lives. If such measures are found to increase asthma, some way will have to be found to prevent this and still retain their benefits. Nutritional and other factors related to the rise in obesity (such as lack of exercise) have also changed in the last few decades. To detect which specific factors might be affecting asthma will require some imaginative detective work. The rapidly developing knowledge and techniques of molecular biology are expected to speed up the process of identifying them.

The increase in the rate of the disease, the amount of suffering it causes, particularly among inner-city minorities, and the high economic cost has led to a commensurate increase of research into the causes. The old adage "An ounce of prevention is worth a pound of cure" still applies. Unfortunately, which prevention we need an ounce of is not yet known.

Intervention Programs in the Inner Cities

Even though we do not yet understand which environmental factors cause a person to become asthmatic and have not identified most of the substances that trigger attacks, efforts are being made to eliminate or at least reduce exposure to some of the more plausible candidates. At present in the United States there are a number of large-scale asthma "intervention programs" in progress, focused on poor inner-city minority populations who often live in substandard housing conditions and have been most heavily affected by asthma attacks and deaths. Their asthmatic children are often too sick to attend schools. Emergency rooms and hospitals in their areas are overburdened with caring for them. They do not have adequate access to medical care or the means to comply with asthma treatment regimes. Their homes often have high levels of allergens from house dust mites, cockroaches, rats, mice, and molds, and in turn the residents, particularly those with asthma, have been shown to be highly sensitive to these allergens by immunological tests.

The programs attempt to reduce these exposures by teaching people how to seal and repair cracks in walls, eliminate moisture problems, improve garbage handling in buildings and apartments to control the cockroach and rat populations, and cover bedding and mattresses so as to make life less congenial for the house-dust mite. The researchers are measuring allergens in the homes, first to see if such measures reduce allergen levels, and then to see if any reduction in both immunological sensitivity and the asthma attacks and symptoms follow. If so, the intervention programs will have served a double purpose: minimize the suffering of the people involved and perhaps enlighten us about the causes of the high rates of asthma in inner-city communities in the United States. They might have saved Felipe G., and may yet make his sister Ana's life easier.

10

SUMMARY: LESSONS FROM A DISASTER

THE DRINKING WATER OF BANGLADESH

We have told a number of stories in this book about environmental health hazards. To summarize the main messages, we will briefly tell another.

There is one common pollutant, a product of human activity, that is responsible for many millions of deaths each year, most of them among small children. Human feces contaminating the water supply is the means by which cholera, dysentery, typhoid fever, and a number of parasitic diseases are spread. These diseases were killing people even in Western economically advanced countries throughout most of the nineteenth century, and are still among the most serious threats to the health of the majority of the people of the world. They can be prevented, as they are in the industrialized world, by rather simple measures, but measures that are beyond the economic resources of many of the less developed countries. Recently the United Nations has been providing funds and technological help in controlling them by improving access to uncontaminated drinking water. One such program in Bangladesh involved digging tube wells to get access to deep groundwater sources, so that the people would no longer have to drink surface water from ponds and streams contaminated by human and animal wastes.

Some Recent History

Bangladesh has had more than its share of misfortune. It is a low-lying country subject to floods and other natural disasters, which has not been spared disasters of human making as well. Originally part of Pakistan when British India was partitioned, it is cut off from the rest of Pakistan by a thousand miles of Indian territory. The people of Bangladesh, although Muslim in religion, were ethnically distinct and spoke a different language from the rest of Pakistan. Their attempts to gain greater autonomy for their region led to a brutal suppression by the Pakistan army in 1971, in which over 1 million people were killed. Indian military intervention led to the defeat of Pakistan and the creation of an independent country of about 150 million people, with the highest population density in the world and one of the lowest per capita incomes, under $300 a year.

The Problem Solved

Use of contaminated surface water for drinking and cooking was responsible for one of the world's highest infant and child mortality rates from diarrheal diseases and for epidemics of cholera during periods of severe flooding, which happened often. The country did not have the financial resources to develop a cleaner water supply, but in the 1960s and 1970s UNICEF (United Nations Children's Fund) and other U.N. agencies began a program of sinking tube wells, cylinders sunk into deep fresh water aquifers. Several million of these were dug, serving almost every village in Bangladesh, so that 97% of the population now has access to water free of fecal contamination. The result, as hoped, was a large drop in the mortality rate from diarrhea. A similar program had been adopted by the government of India, in the province of West Bengal, across the border from Bangladesh (fig. 10-1).

A New and Big Problem

An Indian analytical chemist, Dipankar Chakraborty, on a visit to West Bengal, learned that people living in villages there had an unusually high rate of precancerous and cancerous skin lesions, which he recognized were conditions that had been attributed to arsenic in the drinking water in other parts of the world. He had samples of the local water analyzed for arsenic content and found the levels considerably exceeded health stan-

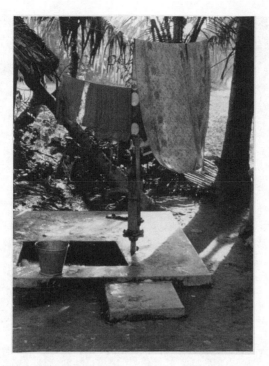

FIGURE 10-1   Pump for tube well in Bangladesh. Courtesy of Dr. Habibul Ahsan, Columbia University.

dards. His attempts to alert authorities, first in India and then across the border in Bangladesh, were initially either ignored or derided, and were taken seriously only when these symptoms of arsenic poisoning—nerve damage as well as skin lesions and skin cancers—were found to be widespread in the region (figs. 10-2, 10-3).

The arsenic levels in the water from each pump in each village depend on the mineral content of the underlying rock formations among other things, so that people living in different villages or even using different pumps in one village have been exposed to different amounts, not all of which are dangerous to health. The total number of people in Bangladesh and West Bengal at risk of cancer and other consequences of arsenic exposure might be more than 25 million, out of a total population of 125 million. It may be one of the worst environmental disasters of the modern era, sadly comparable in scale to the atomic bombing of Hiroshima and Nagasaki.

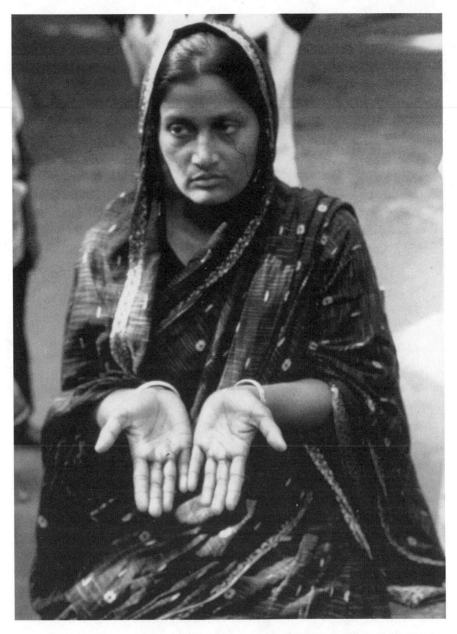

FIGURE 10-2 Bangladeshi woman showing lesions on her hands caused by arsenic exposure. Courtesy of Dr. Habibul Ahsan, Columbia University.

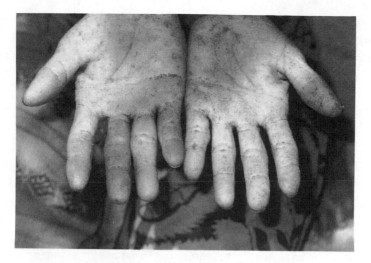

FIGURE 10-3 Close-up of the hands. Courtesy of Dr. Habibul Ahsan, Columbia University.

ARSENIC AND HEALTH

As everyone knows, arsenic in large quantities is a poison and kills quickly. Exposure to arsenic at lower levels but for long periods of time is carcinogenic. Exposure to arsenic-containing smoke from copper smelters causes lung cancer. Drinking water contaminated with arsenic from minerals has been associated with skin lesions and skin, bladder, lung, and liver cancers. Although almost all studies reported up to now have been ecological—an average exposure of the subjects estimated from measurements of arsenic in the water supply, with no direct information on individual exposure— the results from several different countries have been fairly consistent: greatly elevated rates of these cancers have been reported in areas of Argentina, Chile, and especially Taiwan. In the southwestern part of that island there was considerable arsenic in the water from deep wells, dug in the 1920s to avoid using water near the surface contaminated with human and animal wastes. The arsenic levels in the water found responsible for excess cancers in these studies, carried out in the 1980s and 1990s, usually exceeded 50 parts per billion. A recently published study by Taiwanese scientists is the first to use individual exposures to arsenic in water rather than ecological average exposures. The study was done in a region of northern Taiwan where the individual families each had their own wells, unlike in southeastern Taiwan where there were one or a few wells used by an entire village. This study gave results on cancers of the urinary tract consistent with the ecological studies, and provided some evidence of an increased cancer risk in the range 10 to 50 parts per billion, below the current U.S. standard.

Setting Standards

The U. S. standard for arsenic in drinking water, established in 1942, is 50 parts per billion. The standard in European countries is 10 parts per billion, in accord with a recommendation by the World Health Organization based on the studies described earlier. The U.S. Environmental Protection Agency, responsible for national standards in drinking water, asked the National Academy of Sciences to review the evidence on the health effects of arsenic. A comprehensive report, *Arsenic in Drinking Water,* issued by the Academy in 1999, strongly recommended a new standard be set lower than 50 parts per billion, but did not suggest a specific figure.

The Clinton administration, just before leaving office, lowered the standard to 10 parts per billion, in accord with the World Health Organization recommendation, to take effect in 2002. As we described in the preface, the Bush administration's Environmental Protection Agency administrator Whitman rescinded this decision, asserting: "It is clear that arsenic, while naturally occurring, is something that needs to be regulated. . . . [C]ertainly the standard should be less than 50 parts per billion, but the scientific indicators are not clear as to whether the standard needs to go as low as 10 parts per billion. . . . When we make a decision on arsenic, it will be based on sound science and solid analysis." Subsequently she promised that the new standard would be decided upon in time to meet the same deadline set by the Clinton administration.

What Do We Need to Know to Set a Standard?

Standards are set using a concept of "acceptable risk." The word "acceptable" is a matter of values, of weighing health consequences against other costs. "Risk" has to be estimated scientifically, and the process of doing so is the major topic of this book, and has been described in the case histories. It is a process fraught with problems: identifying hazards, characterizing their health effects, determining the exposures that cause them, extrapolating the harm observed at high exposures to the low exposures standards must be set at.

The U.S. Environmental Protection Agency considers as acceptable an upper-bound lifetime risk of cancer to an individual in the range of one chance in 10,000 to one chance in a million. The report of the National Academy of Sciences committee suggested on the basis of the ecological studies of arsenic in drinking water that the life-time cancer risk for people drinking water with 50 parts per billion of arsenic might be as high as 1 case per 100 people. A few members of the committee dissented from this conclusion, but if it is accepted it is clear that the present U.S. 50 parts per billion standard is far outside the range of "acceptable."

The Environmental Protection Agency, concerned about the safety of levels of arsenic in drinking water in parts of the United States—there are wells in New Jersey and Maine contaminated by arsenic-bearing wastes from pesticide and fungicide manufacture and in New Mexico from carelessly disposed mine waste, and water naturally contaminated by mineral deposits in some Western states—had funded a study beginning in the year 2000 of the consequences of arsenic ingestion for the people of Bangladesh.

That study, now underway, has been designed to cope with many of the problems that made determining the health effects of such hazards as low-level radiation, toxic chemicals from waste dumps or indiscriminate pesticide spraying, or electromagnetic fields so difficult and uncertain. We will compare and contrast it with those other studies to summarize the main lessons of this book.

Exposures Known and Unknown

We have described the tremendous effort that went into determining exposure for each victim of the Hiroshima and Nagasaki bombings—where she was standing, what she was wearing, whether indoors or out. It is in part because of this effort that the study of the survivors is a reliable standard for the health effects of radiation. In the Bangladesh study, the individual exposures will be known even better: the arsenic content of the water in the well used by each subject will be measured, and each subject will be asked how much water she and her family uses, for drinking and for cooking. Arsenic levels in the urine, blood, and hair will be determined. The content in urine is believed to reflect total arsenic in the person's body rather than only what that person has recently ingested.

In contrast, exposures were not known and could not be reconstructed in some of the studies we have described. The exposures from toxic waste dumps, as in Pelham Bay, Woburn, and Toms River, took place long before health problems were recognized, and which particular toxic agents might have caused the problems and how much of them reached the victims were unknown. Which property of residential electromagnetic fields might be relevant to childhood leukemia is uncertain. Even when average radon concentrations in a home over a person's lifetime can be reliably estimated, it is hard to estimate how much each individual's exposure has been influenced by such factors as home ventilation, time spent in and outdoors, and when spent indoors, in which rooms of the house. Little is known about the influence of exposure to most hazards at an early age: the greater risk of exposures early in life to such agents as X-rays or a woman's own hormones have been noted in chapters 2 and 6.

What Has the Exposure Caused?

Arsenic is a known human carcinogen, causing lung, skin, bladder, and liver cancer as well as nerve damage. Among the results of arsenic exposure so far found in Bangladesh are skin lesions, some of which are precancerous, and skin cancers. These appear as early as two years but sometimes as much as twenty years after exposure. Other consequences are stillbirths, miscarriages, birth defects, nerve damage, and kidney failure; lung and bladder cancers usually take longer to appear. In the 10,000 people to be studied in Bangladesh, it is expected that in the next five years about 500 subjects will develop skin lesions and some 400 skin cancers. These are large enough numbers to make the influence of chance variations minimal, in contrast to the small numbers of cases, five to ten usually, in typical leukemia clusters that make it so difficult to rule out chance as responsible. In other words, the study is expected to have the "power" to detect a dose-response relation between arsenic exposure and skin cancer incidence. It thus stands in contrast to the lack of power to detect increases of childhood leukemia of less than a doubling in Pelham Bay, a problem in many reported clusters of cancer and other diseases.

Biological Markers

One special problem in studing the health effects of arsenic is that it has not been found to cause cancer in laboratory animals or mutations in bacterial and mammalian cells, and how it causes cancer in humans is not well understood. Recently it has been shown to cause a type of mutation not easily detected in the usual assays, but the precise connection between this and its carcinogenic potential has not yet been clarified. It is hoped that the study will shed light on the biological mechanism of arsenic carcinogenesis.

The study will make good use of techniques of molecular biology. Variations in genetic susceptibilities will be looked for, in particular in the tumor suppressor genes known as p53 genes, which have been found to play a role in many kinds of cancer. There are also biological factors specific to arsenic exposure. The skin of the body is not a passive envelope we are packaged in, but a vital organ. A protein (abbreviated TGF-alpha) that plays a role in its functioning is produced in excess in people with various cancers, sometimes years in advance of the actual clinical diagnosis of cancer. People exposed to arsenic in particular and who have developed skin lesions or skin cancers show an excess of TGF-alpha in urine and blood, and the increase correlates well with the arsenic content of the urine. It is possible that TGF-alpha could serve as an early warning biomarker for cancer in susceptible individuals exposed to arsenic.

In most of the studies we described in this book, biological markers that might distinguish cancers caused by exposure to radiation or chemicals were not available.

Bangladesh and Hiroshima

The study in Bangladesh has features in common with the study of the effects of radiation on the survivors of the nuclear bombing of Japan. In both, a large number of people were exposed to an environmental agent known to cause many different types of cancer. In both, estimates of individual exposure are available. In both, a large population can be studied over a long period of time, so that cancers that develop only decades after exposure can be observed. In both, a wide range of exposures—arsenic levels in the water vary enormously from one pump to another, ranging from below 10 parts per billion (10 micrograms per liter), a level believed to have negligible effects, to 1,000 parts per billion—permit the precise relation between amount of exposure and amount of risk to be determined. While the number of people to be studied in Bangladesh is only 10,000, compared to nearly 100,000 in Japan, the rate of skin cancers and other health effects expected will unfortunately be quite large: as a result, uncertainty from chance variations will not be important. Just as the Japanese survivor study has provided a reliable standard for the effects of radiation on health, so the Bangladesh study is expected to provide a reliable standard for arsenic exposure.

An important difference is the extent to which techniques of molecular biology not available throughout most of the Japanese study will be used in the arsenic study. Biological markers of arsenic exposure and genes involved in cancer susceptibility that may be discovered in the study can be useful in the United States and elsewhere where there is concern about such exposure.

Another difference is that unfortunately nothing could be done in the Japanese study to protect survivors of the bombing from the consequences of their radiation exposure. In Bangladesh, vitamin supplements will be tested, initially with pregnant women, to see if they might help the body detoxify and excrete arsenic. One phase of the study will be a search for inexpensive methods of removing arsenic from drinking water, a problem many other scientists have been working on also. It is to be hoped that some alternative source of clean water or some economically feasible method of treating water to remove the arsenic contamination will be found.

The story of arsenic in Bangladesh has encapsulated many of the issues that arise in all studies of environmental hazards. It also permits us to draw the moral that not all environmental health problems are the result of greed or irresponsibility: they can be caused by actions taken with the best of intentions.

WHAT THIS BOOK HAS FAILED TO DO

We have probably disappointed some readers who wanted definite answers to such questions as: are electromagnetic fields responsible for leukemia in children? Are pesticides behind the epidemic of breast cancer? Is the cluster of brain cancer in my neighborhood caused by toxic wastes from an abandoned chemical plant? We could have chosen only those problems where the health risk of a given level of exposure has been clearly established: cigarette smoking and lung cancer; asbestos and cancer of the lung cavity lining; X-rays and leukemia. We concentrated on controversial ones partly because they have attracted much public attention, but mainly because there is more to be learned from them about science: how it is done, what its strengths and limitations are. We have not tried to turn our readers into environmental health scientists, but we do hope that they will be better able to understand such scientists when they tell what they have done, what they have learned from it, and what they do not yet know. We hope also they will get some sense for the distinction between good science and bad when they read newspaper stories or watch television shows about environmental hazards.

Scientific knowledge, specifically in fields relevant to health and disease, is growing rapidly, but there are certain basic principles that do not change: the appeal to experiment, the openness to new ideas, the obligation always to test what we think we know. In this book we tried to deal both with the recent advances, and with what will remain the same.

We may have surprised other readers, those for whom "environmental pollution" only refers to toxic chemicals from waste dumps or chemical factories or radioactive substances from nuclear facilities, and believe that they cause large numbers of cancers and other diseases such as asthma. There is no doubt that such agents have caused cancers and probably contribute to the suffering of asthmatics, no doubt that the regulations now in force to control them were long overdue, and reason to think that for some of them, stricter regulations are needed. But the chemicals that pollute the environment do not only come from factories and dumps. In the "TEAM" studies, sponsored by the EPA, which we have described in several places in this book, the investigators carefully monitored the immediate environment of individuals living near chemical industries known to emit large quantities of toxic organic chemicals. To their surprise, the greatest proportion of the exposure to these most feared industrial chemicals came not from the admittedly polluted outside air, but from sources in homes. The indoor pollutants included cigarette smoke, chlorinated tap water, pesticides and other chemicals stored in the home, and emissions from products like furniture, plastics, sprays, and deodorants. People living in rural towns with no industrial plants and hardly any pollution of the outdoor air were found to be exposed to the same toxic chemicals and to about the same extent as the people living near chemical industries. Again, the main exposures were from sources inside the homes.

THE DISEASES OF CIVILIZATION

We are now learning that some of the health problems of modernization come paradoxically from its health benefits: our success in reducing the rates of disease and death from infectious diseases, by sanitation, medication, and immunizations. There is some evidence that asthma and childhood leukemia may be related to modern hygienic practices that avoid or delay specific challenges to the developing immune system of children and leave them vulnerable to certain diseases later in life. Other health consequences follow from the freedom of modern lifestyle choices, in childbearing, smoking, living a sedentary life, eating too much, the ease of travel. Breast cancer may have more to do with freedom of reproductive choice than with pesticides. The pleasures of television and the Internet have their downside; there is mounting evidence that lack of exercise increases the risk of a number of chronic diseases: heart problems certainly, and possibly cancer and asthma. Radon has always been present in homes, but as we make homes more energy-efficient, surely a desirable goal, we increase its indoor concentration.

Environment—in the broad sense of the word, meaning everything other than what is genetically determined—includes all these factors of our modern lifestyle, not just the external well-recognized agents such as toxic chemicals, ionizing radiation, magnetic fields, or allergens. Sometimes these lifestyle factors influence the response of the individual to other exposures or pollutants, as is believed to be the case with asthma. Sometimes they account for diseases erroneously attributed to chemicals or radiation.

Some of these ideas are new and not yet firmly established, but are being taken very seriously. Already it has been suggested that, as a preventive for asthma, infants be exposed to bacterial toxins to "make up" for their too sanitary upbringing. It sounds like a risky remedy until one remembers that, after all, immunizations and vaccinations already expose children to weakened bacterial toxins and viruses, and the benefits so far outweigh the occasional side effects. Even if modernization creates new health problems in place of old ones, it does not follow that we must return to an earlier brutish and unsanitary existence to avoid them. More children have died of the diseases of poor sanitation than will die of asthma or leukemia; more women die in childbirth in less developed societies than of breast cancer in advanced ones. We need not go back to the life of hunters and gatherers, nor need we return to the hovel or the cave. If science indeed confirms these connections between the benefits of modern life and the diseases of modern life, one must hope it will find ways to cope with them also.

OUR LAST WORD

The rapid changes taking place in the environment, changes in urbanization, communications, transportation, industrialization, globalization, the loss of biological diversity and of the various habitats in which it flourishes, the possibilities of global warming and of depletion of the ozone layer, the problems of feeding and providing a decent standard of living for an ever-growing world population—all of these have direct or indirect impacts on human health. All of them involve both scientific and other questions; questions of economics, of politics, of ethics. Science alone is not sufficient to solve the problems they create, but it is a necessary component of the solutions.

Concern about the environment, hardly felt and barely expressed a half-century ago, has moved to center stage today and will remain there for the foreseeable future. This is a tremendous achievement of a multitude of activists of various kinds who have formed organizations, written letters to newspapers or appeared on television and radio shows, and petitioned legislative bodies.

Their energy and effort have already accomplished wonders. They could not have accomplished so much if they had not felt so strongly. Strong feelings are a spur to action, but no guarantee that a desired goal will be met. If the energy and effort of those concerned individuals are not to be frittered away on unimportant problems or unsolvable ones, they will need the perspective of science.

BIBLIOGRAPHY

INTRODUCTION

Useful websites for general information on health, disease, and the environment are maintained by the National Institutes of Health (*http://www.nih.gov*), the National Cancer Institute (*http://rex.nci.nih.gov*), and the Environmental Protection Agency (*http://www.epa.gov*).

On epidemiology: Paul Stolley and Tamar Lasky, *Investigating Disease Patterns*, W. H. Freeman, San Francisco, 1991.

Simple introductions to probability and statistics are given in another book by the authors of this one: Martin Goldstein and Inge F. Goldstein, *The Experience of Science*, Plenum, New York, 1984.

On cancer (molecular biology, epidemiology, etc.):

Robert A. Weinberg, *One Renegade Cell: How Cancer Begins*, Basic Books, New York, 1998.

John Cairns, *Matters of Life and Death: Perpectives on Public Health, Molecular Biology, Cancer, and the Prospects for the Human Race,* Princeton University Press, Princeton, 1997.

Mel Greaves, *Cancer: The Evolutionary Legacy*, Oxford University Press, New York, 2000.

ATOMIC BOMBS, NUCLEAR FALLOUT, AND DENTAL X-RAYS

Our main sources for information from the Life Span Study were as follows: William J. Schull, *Effects of Atomic Radiation: A Half-Century of Studies from*

Hiroshima and Nagasaki (Wiley-Liss, New York, 1995), not only describes the scientific methodology and results of the study but is also a compassionate history of the bombing and its aftermath.

The quotations from Dr. Hachiya are from *Hiroshima Diary: The Journal of a Japanese Physician, August 6–September 30, 1945*, by Michihiko Hachiya, translated by Warner Wells, M. D. Copyright 1955 by the University of North Carolina Press. Used by permission of the publisher. This work was reissued in 1995.

BEIR V: Health Effects of Exposure to Low Levels of Ionizing Radiation (National Academy Press, Washington, D.C., 1990) is a report of the National Research Council, prepared by a committee of seventeen experts, and not easy reading. The acronym BEIR stands for "Biological Effects of Ionizing Radiation." There have also been BEIR reports on radon in homes, which are cited in the next chapter.

The scientific article "Studies of the Mortality of Atomic Bomb Survivors. Report 12, Part 1. Cancer: 1950–1990," by D. A. Pierce and associates, published in the journal *Radiation Research*, vol. 146, pp. 1–27 (1996), is one of a series giving the most recent summary of the results of the study. Table 2-2 is adapted from data in this article with permission of *Radiation Research*.

Howard Ball, *Justice Downwind: America's Atomic Testing Program in the 1950s* (Oxford University Press, New York, 1986), is an excellent history of the impact of the nuclear test series of 1953–1961 on the people in the path of the fallout. Some of its conclusions about leukemia and other cancers attributed to the fallout are now out of date.

Estimates of the number of thyroid cancers that will result from the fallout of radioactive iodine were reported by Charles Land to the National Academy of Sciences Institute of Medicine Committee on Exposure of the American People from Nevada Atomic Bomb Tests on December 19, 1997. A summary was available on the National Cancer Institute website: *http://rex.nci.nih.gov/massmedia/falloutcalculation/html*. The study "Association of Nuclear Fallout with Leukemia in the U.S.," by V. Archer ("fallout" referring to both American and Soviet weapons tests), appeared in *Archives of Environmental Health*, vol. 42, pp. 263–271 (1987).

Current estimates of dose from natural background radiation are given in the chapter "Contribution of Natural Ionizing Radiation to Cancer Mortality in the U.S.," by Sarah Darby, in *Origins of Human Cancer: A Comprehensive Review*, edited by Joan Brugge et al., Cold Spring Harbor Laboratory Press, 1991.

An excellent book for the nonspecialist on radiation, its benefits and its hazards, is Eric J. Hall, *Radiation and Life*, 2nd edition, Pergamon Press, New York, 1984, from which we took the material on cancers caused by medical X-rays.

RADON IN YOUR BASEMENT

An excellent book on radon in homes, written for a lay readership, is *Radon: Risk and Remedy*, by David J. Brenner, W. H. Freeman, New York, 1989.

Our main source on the health studies of miners and the estimated lung cancer risk from radon in homes is the report of the National Research Council Committee on Health Risks of Exposure to Radon, *BEIR VI: Health Risks of Exposure to Radon*, National Academy Press, Washington, D.C., 1999.

Information on radon concentrations in U.S. homes is from the article by F. Marcinowski et al., in *Health Physics*, vol. 66, pp. 699–706 (1994).

Papers by T. K. Hei and associates on targeted alpha radiation on cells have appeared in *The Proceedings of the National Academy of Sciences (U.S.A.), Cell Biology Section*, vol. 94, pp. 3765–3770 (1997); vol. 96, pp. 4959–4964 (1999); and vol. 97, pp. 2099–2104 (2000).

The determination of twenty-five–year average radon exposures by examination of glass windows and mirrors and its effect on lung cancer risk is described by M. Alavanja and associates in the *American Journal of Public Health*, vol. 89, pp. 1042–1048 (1999).

CHILDHOOD LEUKEMIA NEAR NUCLEAR PLANTS

A description of the Windscale fire and its aftermath is given in *Windscale 1957: Anatomy of a Nuclear Accident*, by Lorna Arnold, St. Martin's Press, New York, 1992.

A summary of the evidence given at the trial and of the court's decision is given in the article "Childhood Leukemia and Sellafield: The Legal Cases," by R. Wakeford and E. J. Tawn, *Journal of Radiation Protection*, vol. 14, 293–316 (1994).

The epidemiology of leukemia is reviewed in chapter 40, "The Leukemias," by M. S. Linet and R. A. Cartwright, pp. 841–892, in *Cancer Epidemiology and Prevention*, 2nd edition, edited by D. Schottenfeld and J. F. Fraumeni, Oxford University Press, New York, 1996.

Articles on Clusters in General and Leukemia Clusters in Particular

"Historical Aspects of Leukaemia Clusters," by P. Boyle, A. M. Walker, and F. E. Alexander, chapter 1 in *Methods for Investigating Localized Clustering of Disease*, edited by F. E. Alexander and P. Boyle, International Agency for Research on Cancer, World Health Organization, Publication No. 135 (1996).

The Niles, Illinois, cluster: "Leukemia Among Children in a Suburban Community," by C. W. Heath and R. J. Hasterlik, *American Journal of Medicine*, vol. 34, pp. 796–812 (1963).

Leo Kinlen published a commentary on a report on the Sellafield cluster issued by the Committee on Medical Aspects of Radiation in the Environment (acronym: COMARE), in which he summarized research by himself and by others on the population mixing hypothesis. The article gives references to the published work to that date: "The Excess of Childhood Leukaemia Near Sellafield: A Commentary on the Fourth COMARE Report," *Journal of Radiation Protection*, vol. 17, pp. 63–71 (1997). The quantitative treatment of population mixing in Cumbria is given in H. Dickinson and L. Parker, "Quantifying the Effect of Population Mixing on Childhood Leukemia Risk: The Seascale Cluster," *British Journal of Cancer*, vol. 81, pp. 144–151 (1999). Sir Richard Doll's editorial appears on pp. 3–5 of the same issue of the journal. An article by Dr. Kinlen summarizing the evidence for his hypothesis in the light of the Dickinson-Parker article, entitled "Infection, Childhood Leukaemia, and the Seascale Cluster," has appeared in the journal, *Radiological Protection Bulletin*, No. 226, pp. 9–18 (2000).

Two general discussions of disease clusters are "A Sobering Start for the Cluster Busters' Conference," by K. J. Rothman, in the *American Journal of Epidemiology*, vol. 132, supplement 1, pp. S6–S13 (1990), and "Counterpoint from a Cluster Buster," by R. R. Neutra, in the same journal, vol. 132, pp. 1–8 (1990).

The study of the impact of improved sanitary conditions in Japan on the incidence of childhood leukemia there is given in the article "Evidence that Childhood Acute Lymphoblastic Leukemia Is Associated with an Infectious Agent . . . ," by Malcolm A. Smith et al., *Cancer Causes and Control*, vol. 9, pp. 285–299 (1998).

BREAST CANCER, PARTS 1 AND 2

Relevant Websites and Organizations

The leading activist organization, The National Breast Cancer Coalition, has a site: *www.stopbreastcancer.org*.

The Program on Breast Cancer and Environmental Risk Factors is based at Cornell University, Ithaca, New York. Its website, *www.cfe.cornell.edu/bcerf*, provides statistics on breast cancer in New York State, as well as very clearly written fact sheets for lay readers on many topics related to the disease. Silent Spring Institute, 29 Crafts St., Newton, MA 02458 (Phone 617-332-4288), has published two pamphlets on its program: "Investigating Breast Cancer and the Environment on Cape Cod: Research Protocol for the Cape Cod Breast Cancer and Environmental Study, Phase 2," in 1997, and "The Cape Cod Breast Cancer and Environmental Study: Results of the First Three Years of Study," in 1998.

Articles on the Epidemiology of Breast Cancer

B. E. Henderson, David Schottenfeld, and J. F. Fraumeni, "Breast Cancer," chapter 47, pp. 1022–1039, in *Cancer Epidemiology and Prevention*, 2nd Edition, edited by David Schottenfeld and J. F. Fraumeni, Oxford University Press, New York, 1996.

"Epidemiology and Prevention of Breast Cancer," by J. L. Kelsey and L. Bernstein, *Annual Review of Public Heath*, 1996, pp. 47–67.

The journal *Epidemiological Reviews* devoted a full issue, vol. 15, no. 1, of 1993, to the epidemiology of breast cancer, with review articles on molecular biology of the disease, reproductive and hormonal risk factors, diet, alcohol, cigarette smoking, and prevention.

The National Research Council's report is entitled "Hormonally Active Agents in the Environment." A preliminary version was published by the National Academy Press in 1999.

A strong statement of the hormone mimicking hypotheses is by Theo Colborn: "Pesticides—How Research Has Succeeded and Failed to Translate Science into Policy: Endocrinological Effects on Wildlife," *Environmental Health Perspectives*, vol. 103, Supplement 6, pp. 81–85 (1995).

Other Articles We Have Discussed at Some Length

M. R. Alavanja et al. "The Agricultural Health Study," Environmental Health Perspectives, vol. 104, pp. 362–369 (1996).

S. Shapiro, "Bias in the Evaluation of Low Magnitude Association: An Empirical Perspective," *American Journal of Epidemiology*, vol. 151, pp. 939–945 (2000).

A. S. Robbins et al., "Regional Differences in Known Risk Factors and the Higher Incidence of Breast Cancer in San Francisco," *Journal of the National Cancer Institute*, vol. 89, pp. 960–965 (1997).

D. J. Hunter et al., "Plasma Organochlorine Levels and the Risk of Breast Cancer," *New England Journal of Medicine*, vol. 337, pp. 1253–1258 (1997).

POWER LINES, MAGNETIC FIELDS, AND CANCER

Paul Brodeur's two books argue strongly that electromagnetic fields cause cancer: *Currents of Death: Power Lines, Computer Terminals, and the Attempt to Cover Up*

Their Threats to Your Health, Simon and Schuster, New York, 1989; *The Great Power Line Cover-up: How the Utilities and the Government Are Trying to Hide the Cancer Hazard Posed by Electromagnetic Fields*, Little, Brown and Co., Boston, 1993.

Exactly the opposite position is taken by Robert L. Park, a leading physicist, in *Voodoo Science: The Road from Foolishness to Fraud*, Oxford University Press, New York, 2000.

A more neutral evaluation, although accused of pro-utilities bias by one reviewer, is by Leonard Sagan, a scientist formerly employed by the Electric Power Research Institute: *Electric and Magnetic Fields: Invisible Risk?* Gordon and Breach, Amsterdam, 1996. The book covers the basic physics, as well as biological and epidemiological studies, and is written for a lay readership.

The article that started it all, "Electrical Wiring Configurations and Childhood Cancer," is by N. Wertheimer and E. Leeper, in the *American Journal of Epidemiology*, vol. 109, pp. 273–284 (1979).

The report by the National Research Council, *Possible Health Effects of Exposure to Residential Electric and Magnetic Fields*, was published by the National Academy Press in 1997.

Epidemiological studies published subsequently to this report which we discuss include: "Residential Exposure to Magnetic Fields and Acute Lymphoblastic Leukemia in Children," by M. S. Linet and colleagues, *New England Journal of Medicine*, vol. 337, pp. 1–7 (1997). "Exposure to Power-Frequency Magnetic Fields and the Risk of Childhood Leukemia," in the *Lancet*, vol. 354, pp. 1925–1931 (1999). The author is given as "U.K. Childhood Cancer Study Investigators."

The National Institute of Environmental Health Sciences report *Health Effects from Exposure to Power-Line Frequency Electric and Magnetic Fields"* is National Institutes of Health Publication No. 99-4493, and was available on the NIEHS website, *http://www.niehs.nih.gov*.

Booklets on electromagnetic fields and their health effects, written for nonspecialist readers, are available both from the Department of Engineering and Public Policy, Carnegie Mellon University, Pittsburgh, PA 15213, and from the Electric Power Research Institute, 3412 Hillview Avenue, P.O. Box 10412, Palo Alto, CA 94303.

CANCER FROM THE LANDFILL?

The New York City Department of Health, Environmental Epidemiology Unit, has published several reports on its study of the health effects of the landfill. The most comprehensive is "Cancer Incidence in the Pelham Bay Area of the

Bronx," by N. L. Jeffrey and S. Klitzman, in 1994. The address of the department is 125 Worth St., Box 34C, New York, NY 10013.

The Massachusetts Department of Public Health, Bureau of Environmental Health Assessment, 250 Washington St., Boston, MA 02108-4619, issued a final report in 1997, "Woburn Childhood Leukemia Follow-up Study," in two volumes.

A paper on the Woburn cluster, entitled "An Analysis of Contaminated Well Water in Woburn, Massachusetts," by S. W. Lagakos, B. J. Wessen, and M. Zelen, appeared in the *Journal of the American Statistical Association*, vol. 81, pp. 583–596 (1986). This paper was followed in the same issue of the journal by comments and criticisms by a number of epidemiologists and statisticians, pp. 597–614.

The Division of Epidemiology, Environmental and Occupational Health, of the New Jersey Department of Health and Senior Services, P.O. Box 360, Trenton, NJ 08625-0360, has not yet completed its study of the Toms River (Dover Township) clusters of childhood leukemia and nervous system cancers. An interim report describing how the study is to be carried out was issued in December 1999.

The cluster of cancer of the lining of the lung cavity (mesothelioma) in a Turkish village is described in Y. I. Baris et al., "Epidemiological and Environmental Evidence of the Health Effects of Erionite Fibers," *International Journal of Cancer*, vol. 39, pp. 10–17 (1987).

The *New York Times* of Tuesday, April 6, 1999, p. A18, reported the unusual number of brain cancers among employees of an oil company under the headline, "Oil Company Confronts Cluster of Brain Tumors."

The results of the TEAM study of chemical pollution indoors and out, done under the auspices of the Environmental Protection Agency, are described by W. R. Ott and J. W. Roberts in the article "Everyday Exposure to Toxic Pollutants," *Scientific American*, February 1998, pp. 86–91.

More references on disease clusters are given in the bibliographic notes to chapter 4.

ASTHMA, ALLERGY, AND AIR POLLLUTION

General Information on Asthma and Allergy is available on the following websites: American Lung Association *http://www.lungusa.org*; American Academy of Allergy, Asthma, and Immunology, *http://www.aaaai.org*; National Institute of Allergy and Infectious Diseases, *http://www.niaid.nih.gov*; National Heart, Lung, and Blood Institute, *http://www.nhlbi.nih.gov*.

The Barcelona story is told by Drs. J. Anto and J. Sunyer in several articles: "Soya Bean as a Risk Factor for Epidemic Asthma," in *Geographical and Environmental Epidemiology: Methods for Small-Area Studies*, P. Elliot et al., Oxford University Press, New York, 1996; "A Point Source Asthma Outbreak," in *Lancet*, vol. ii, pp. 900–903 (1986); and "Epidemiologic Studies of Asthma in Barcelona," in *Chest*, vol. 98(5), pp. 185S–190S (1990).

The long history of asthma in New Orleans is summarized in a paper M. White, R. Etzel, and I. F. Goldstein, "A Re-examination of Epidemic Asthma in New Orleans in Relation to the Presence of Soy at the Harbor," in the *American Journal of Epidemiology*, vol. 154, pp. 432–438 (1997).

Asthma in Eastern Europe: C. von Mutius, E. Fritzsch, et al.: "Prevalence of Asthma and Allergic Disorders in United Germany: A Descriptive Comparison," *British Medical Journal*, vol. 305, 1395–1399 (1992).

Cockroaches: "The Role of Cockroach Allergy and Exposure to Cockroach Allergens in Causing Morbidity in Inner-City Children with Asthma," by D. L. Rosenstreich et al. *New England Journal of Medicine*, vol. 336, 1356–1363 (1997).

Thunderstorms: "Thunderstorm Asthma Due to Grass Pollen," by C. Suphioglu, in the *International Archives of Allergy and Immunology*, vol. 116, 253–260 (1998).

An excellent popular article on asthma by Ellen R. Shell, "Does Civilization Cause Asthma?" appeared in the *Atlantic Monthly*, May 2000, p. 90.

SUMMARY: LESSONS FROM A DISASTER

The arsenic crisis in Bangladesh was the subject of an article in the *New York Times* on November 10, 1998, under the headline, "Arsenic Poses Threat to Millions in Bangladesh."

INDEX

"A Civil Action," 260
acute lymphoblastic leukemia (ALL).
    See childhood leukemia
Addison, Joseph, 281
age adjustment. *See* breast cancer risk
    factors
Agricola, Georgius (Georg Bauer), 67
air pollution
    allergen interaction with, 286
    carbon monoxide, 269
    diesel exhaust, 269, 287–88
    Donora smog episode, 283
    in Harlem, New York City, 269–70
    health effects (*see* asthma;
        bronchitis)
    indoor levels of, 287, 291–92
    indoor sources of, 264–66
    indoors and outdoors compared, 287
    industrial, 287
    London smog episode, 282
    natural particulates, 286
    nitrogen oxides indoors, 291
    nitrogen oxides, 269, 275, 283, 285,
        286, 296
    ozone, 275, 286, 296
    particulate size, 286
    particulates, 269, 286, 296
    polyaromatic hydrocarbons, 287
    regulated pollutants, 284–85
    respirable particulates, definition, 286
    standards, 283–84
    sulfur dioxide, 275, 285, 289, 296
    TEAM studies of indoor and
        outdoor air, 263–66, 287, 291–92,
        313–14
    from traffic, 269
    weather and levels of, 284, 291
allergens. *See also* asthma, triggers of
    cat, 274
    cockroach, 274, 294, 301
    exposure on farms, 298–99
    house dust mite, 274, 294, 295, 301
    molds, 274, 301
    rodent, 274, 301
    rye-grass pollen, 281
    soybeans, 279–80
allergy
    antibodies in, 294
    description of, 293–94
    in Eastern Europe, 297
    immunoglobulin E (IgE), 294
    life-style and, 297–98

alpha particles. *See* radioactive
elements, radioactivity; radiation,
types of; radon
alpha particle microbeam, 86–89
American Physical Society
statement on harm from magnetic
fields, 201–2
animal studies. *See also* cell studies
advantages and drawbacks of, 37,
221–22
breast cancer and, 148, 188–89, 196
extrapolation to humans from, 221
of magnetic fields and cancer, 222–23
of paternal irradiation and
leukemia, 112
of radiation, 36–37, 48
Anto, J., 278
Archer, V., 44
arsenic
Bangladesh study of cancer from,
309–12
in Bangladesh water, 305
Bangladesh, tragedy of, 305
carcinogenic mechanism of, 310–11
carcinogenicity of, 307, 310
copper smelters and, 307
in drinking water, 10
health effects (*see* cancer, lung
cancer, nerve damage, skin
lesions)
industrial sources of contamination,
309
as poison, 307
in Taiwan water, 307–8
in U.S. water, 308–9
in West Bengal (India) water, 304–5
association (statistical)
causation, distinction from, 219–20
definition of, 218–19
of magnetic fields and childhood
leukemia, 227–28
asthma
air exchange in homes and, 297
air pollution and, 10, 275, 286,
289–91, 292, 296
allergen exposure and, 298
allergy and, 293–94, 297
antibodies in, 294

biomarkers for, 294
causation of, summary, 300
causes, search for 292–301
chamber studies of, 289
climate and, 294
deaths from, 269, 271
energy conservation measures and,
297
environmental factors in, 294
exercise and, 299
in farming communities, 298–99
genetic factors in, 294–95
history of disease, 292–93
household products and, 297
in immune system development, 298
immunization and, 298
immunoglobulin E (IgE), 294
infections and, 298
in inner cities, 269
intervention programs, 301
lifestyle factors in, 297–98
modernization and, 10
nature of, 271
nutrition and, 299–300
and obesity in children, 299
in Papua-New Guinea, 294
prevalence, 271
respiratory infections and, 281
sanitation and, 298
social cost of, 271
socio-economic class and, 270
tobacco smoke and, 297
world-wide increase in, summary 300
asthma clusters. *See* asthma epidemics
asthma epidemics
air pollution and, 289–91, 292
allergic sensitivity in, 277
in Barcelona, 273, 275, 277–80
in Birmingham, U. K., 275
in Brisbane, Australia, 275
in Cartagena, Spain, 280
definition, 275
industrial pollution and, 277
in New Orleans, 273, 275, 280
in New York City, 275, 290–91
soybeans and, 279–80
waste dump fires and, 277
in Yokohama, Japan, 275

asthma rates
    in Eastern Europe, 295–296
    in fall seasons, 281
    in farming communities, 298–99
    immigration and, 293
    increase in U. S., 272
    increase world-wide, 271, 293
    in inner cities in U. S., 269–70
    in minorities in U. S., 270
    in minorities, 10
    in New York City, 269
    socio-economic class and, 270
asthma, triggers of. *See also* allergens
    allergens, 274–75
    cockroach, 274, 301
    cold air, 275
    environmental agents, 273–76
    exercise, 275
    house-dust mite in Papua-New
        Guinea, 294
    house-dust mite, 274, 294, 295,
        301
    irritants, 275
    moulds, 274
    pets, 274
    pollen, 274
    rodents, 274, 301
    rye-grass pollen, 281
    soy beans, 279–80
    thunderstorms, 280–81
atomic bombing of Japan, 8, 15, 17–
    20, 305 (*see also* Life Span Study)
Atomic Energy Commission (U.S.)
    (AEC)
    nuclear weapons tests, 21–23,
        29
atomic particles, 54

Bangladesh
    arsenic and cancer study, 309–12
    fecal contamination of drinking
        water, 303–304
    history, 304
Baris, Y., 262
beta particles. *See* radiation, types of;
    radioactivity
biomarkers, 294, 310–11 (*see also*
    molecular biology)

birth defects
    arsenic in Bangladesh and, 310
    radiation and, 24
bone fracture healing
    magnetic fields and, 224
breast cancer
    animal studies of, 148, 188–89, 196
    BRCA1 and BRCA2 genes in, 176
    Cape Cod studies, 188
    causes, 139
    chemical hazards and, 137, 185–86
    chemical industry employment and,
        180–81
    childbearing and, 139–40
    electromagnetic fields and, 9
    "epidemic" of, 162–63
    estrogen hypothesis, 146–49
    estrogen receptors in, 175
    evolution and 148–49
    genetic susceptibilities and, 176–78
    hormonally active agents and, 168–
        69
    hormone replacement therapy
        (HRT) and, 147, 181–82
    initiation and promotion of, 178–79
    lifestyle factors and, 183, 197–98
    Long Island studies, 188
    magnetic fields and, 194, 224
    melatonin and, 224
    menarche and, 142
    menstrual periods and, 139
    molecular biology of, 172–80
    oral contraceptives and, 161–62
    p450 genes in, 177
    pesticides and, 9, 137, 184–87
    plasticizers and, 151
    power lines and, 9, 137
    pregnancy and hormones, 140
    public concern about, 135–36
    radiation and, 137, 139
    radiation dose and, 30–31
    smoking and genetic susceptibility,
        177
    tamoxifen therapy and, 175
    toxic waste dumps and, 9, 152
    xenoestrogens and, 168
    X-ray fluoroscopy and, 36
    X-rays and, 139

breast cancer rates, 10
  in New York City areas, 135
  international differences in, 142–44,
    146, 148
  ethnic differences, 144
  migration and, 144
  socio-economic class, 146
  on Cape Cod, 152–53
  on Long Island, 152–53
  in San Francisco, 152
  increase over time, 162–63
  mammography effect on, 163–64
  origin of excess in, 164–66
  validation of excess in, 164–65
  risk factor adjustment of, 154–62
  in African-American women, 160
  in Caucasian-American women, 160
breast cancer risk factors, 141–44, 146
  adjustment for, reasons, 155–56
  adjustment of rates for, 157–58
  age adjustment, 156–58
  age at hazard exposure, 146
  age, 141
  alcohol, 146
  avoidable, 142–43
  body weight, 146
  in Jewish women, 142
  nutrition and, 142–43, 144, 146
  oral contraceptives, 161–62
  radiation, 146
  reproductive factors, 141–42
  sex, 141
  smoking, 146
  socio-economic class, 146
breast feeding
  effect on breast cancer risk, 177–78
Brodeur, Paul, 200
bronchitis, chronic
  London smog episode, 282
Bush, George W., 308

cancer. See also breast cancer; cancer
    clusters; carcinogenesis;
    childhood leukemia; leukemia;
    thyroid cancer
  arsenic and, 307
  atomic bomb and, 30–34
  Bangladesh arsenic study, 309–12

in bomb survivors, 30–32
brain, and cell phones, 201
delay time after exposure, 182, 238,
    286
in electrical workers, 211
magnetic fields and melatonin,
    223–24
magnetic fields and promotion of,
    222–23
non-Hodgkins lymphoma in
    Seascale, 106, 111
non-Hodgkins lymphoma, 123
pancreatic, in Pelham Bay, 244–45,
    246–47
in Pelham Bay, 5
in Pelham Bay, rates, 239–40
in Pelham Bay, risk factors in, 241
in Pelham Bay, summary 255–56
radiation and, 19–20, 24
risk at U.S. arsenic standard, 303
skin, from arsenic in Bangladesh,
    305
skin, from arsenic, 310
skin, in West Bengal, 304
solid tumors and radiation, 30–32
urinary tract, from arsenic, 308
cancer clusters. See also chance;
    childhood leukemia; random
    variation
  asbestos and, 262
  asbestos-like mineral, 262
  boundary determination in, 122–
    125
  brain, in chemical laboratory, 262
  definition, 113
  near Dounreay nuclear plant, 112,
    127, 132
  near electric power sub-station, 200
  explanation of, 262
  frequency of chance occurrence,
    258
  Niles, Illinois, 122, 127
  occupational 113, 262–63
  Pelham Bay, 235
  perception of community, 256–57
  in schools near power lines, 200
  Seascale, 101, 105–7, 110–12, 125–
    26, 131–33

Toms River, 6–7, 261–62
Woburn, 6, 260–61
carcinogenesis. *See also* DNA; genes;
   molecular biology
   arsenic, 307
   bystander effect in radiation, 87–88
   cytoplasm irradiation, 87
   estrogens as promoters, 178
   initiation of, 174
   initiation, definition, 178
   magnetic fields as promoters of,
      223–24
   magnetic fields, 218, 225–26
   microbeam studies and linear
      model, 87–88
   microbeam studies of, 86–89
   multi-step process of, 174–75
   promotion, definition, 178
   radiation and, 56–57, 85–89, 226
causation
   of cholera, theories, 219–21
   coherence and, 221–27
   criteria for, 220–21
cardiac disease
   London smog episode, 282
Carson, Rachel, 149–50
case-control studies
   breast cancer on Cape Cod, 189–90
   breast cancer on Long Island, 190–
      91, 193–94
   childhood leukemia and magnetic
      fields, 203–4
   control selection in, 204–5
   "nested" studies, 185–87
   of pesticides and breast cancer, 184–
      87
   questionnaires, use of, in, 189–90
   of radon in homes, 72
cell phones
   brain cancer and, 201
cell studies. *See also* animal studies
   alpha particle microbeam studies,
      86–89
   of breast cancer, 179, 182, 188, 189
   of magnetic fields 222–23, 224–25
   of radiation, 37
Centers for Disease Control
   asthma study, 280

Chakraborty, Dipankar, 304
chance. *See also* random variation
   lumpiness of, and clusters, 257–58
   lumpiness of, 115–16, 118, 244
   meaning of, 114–15, 241
   models of, 115–20
   non-random events, 121–22
   patterns perceived in, 125
   Poisson distribution, 116–17
   and probability theory, 116–17
   Seascale cluster and, 112–13, 125–26
   simple illustrative examples of, 116–
      18, 243–44
   "Texas sharpshooter" effect and,
      122–24
chemical hazards, 166–68. *See also* air
      pollutants; TEAM studies; toxic
      dumps
   alkyl phenols, 168
   benzene and leukemia, 109
   benzene from cigarettes, 264–65
   benzene, 264–65
   chlordane, 194
   DDT, 167, 194
   dioxins, 167, 182
   household products, 266, 287
   indoor sources, 287, 313
   industrial sources outdoors, 292
   industrial sources, 266, 268
   industrial vs. residential sources, 313
   organochlorines and breast cancer,
      185–86
   organochlorines in Toms River,
      261–62
   organochlorines in Woburn, 260
   organochlorines, 166–67
   outdoor vs. indoor sources, 263–66
   PBB's, 182
   PCB's, 167, 182, 194
   Pelham Bay exposures, 239
   from Pelham Bay landfill, 235
   pesticides indoors, 291
   pesticides, 266–67
   plasticizers, 168
   polyaromatic hydrocarbons (PAH's),
      167–68, 194
   Seveso accident, 182–83
   smoking, 291–92

chemical hazards (*continued*)
    TEAM studies, 263–66, 287, 291–92, 313–14
    volatile organics indoors, 291–92
    volatile organics, 264
childhood leukemia
    acute lymphoblastic (ALL), 109
    blood cells in, 107–8
    cluster in Seascale, 101
    clusters near power lines, 200
    coherence in magnetic field studies, 227
    Dounreay cluster, 112, 132
    electrical appliance use and, 209–10
    electromagnetic fields and, 10
    infections and, 128–30
    lawsuit over Seascale cluster, 106–8
    Linet study of magnetic fields and, 214–17
    magnetic fields and, 203–4
    magnetic fields and, summary, 207–8
    nature of, 107–8
    NIEHS report on electric and magnetic fields, 218
    Niles cluster, 127–28
    nuclear plants and, 8
    paternal irradiation and, 106, 110–11
    Pelham Bay cluster, 5, 235
    Pelham Bay DOH study, 237–38
    population mixing and, 131–33
    population mixing, quantitative measure of, 132–33
    radiation and, 32–33
    radioactive fallout and, 8, 44–45
    risk factors for, 204
    sanitation and, 128–30
    Seascale cluster and chance, 126
    Seascale cluster and population mixing, 132–33
    Seascale cluster and radiation, 105–6
    Seascale dose estimates and, 110
    U.K. study of magnetic fields and, 217
    Woburn cluster of, 6, 260–61
cholera
    fecal contamination of water and, 303

London epidemics, 219
    theories about causation, 219
civilization, diseases of, 128–30, 313
Clinton, William J., 308
Cohen, Morris R., 156
coherence. *See* causation
confidence interval, 94, 299. *See also* uncertainty range
    breast cancer excess rates, 160–61, 165
    leukemia in Pelham Bay, 248–49
    lung cancer deaths and residential radon, 64, 71, 78, 93–94
    simple illustrative example of, 249–50
    thyroid cancer from nuclear test fallout, 45, 47
Congress (U.S.),
    breast cancer research funding, 153–54
Curie, Irene, 15
Curie, Marie, 13–15
Curie, Pierre, 13

"De Re Metallica," 67
Dickinson, H., 132
DNA. *See also* molecular biology, mutations
    chemical makeup of, 25–26
    duplication during cell division, 173
    parental shares in, 175
    radiation damage of, 25, 56–57
    RNA role in protein synthesis, 173
Doll, Sir Richard, 133
Donora smog episode, 283
dose-response relationship
    arsenic and skin cancer, 310
    childhood leukemia and magnetic fields, 213–14
    importance of, in health studies, 31–33
    proportionality in, 39
    between radiation and cancer, 31
    between smoking and cancer, 32
drinking water contamination. *See also* arsenic
    fecal, in Bangladesh, 303
    in Pelham Bay, 236

in Toms River, 261
in Woburn, 260
dysentery
fecal contamination of drinking
water and, 303

ecological studies
of arsenic in Taiwan water, 307
definition of, in epidemiology, 70
in residential radon studies, 69–70
electric fields
description of, 202, 231
health effect plausibility, 203
electrical appliances
cancer risk, 209–10
cancer risk from electric blankets, 209
cell phones and brain cancer, 201
electricity
direct and alternating current, 230
negative and positive, 230
electromagnetic fields, 201. *See also*
electric fields; magnetic fields
from electric appliances, 9–10
health effects (*see* childhood
leukemia, cancer, breast cancer)
nature of, 230–33
from power lines, 9–10
environment
definitions, 11–12
heredity and, 11
lifestyle and, 12
environmental activism
accomplishments, 196–97, 315
in breast cancer, 138
funding for breast cancer research
and, 151
National Breast Cancer Coalition,
151
need for science, 315
rise of, 20
Silent Spring Institute, 153
Environmental Protection Agency (U.
S.) (EPA), 309
arsenic standards, 308–9
Bangladesh study funding, 308
radon safety standard, 61
TEAM studies of indoor air, 263–66,
287, 291–92, 313–14

environmental science
multidisciplinary character of, 11
epidemiology. *See also* case-control
studies; dose-response
relationship; occupational
studies; rates of diseases; *and
under* specific diseases, rates of
diseases, and risk factors
coherence, testing for, 221–27
causation and, 220–21
description of, 184–85
ecological studies, definition, 70
molecular biology role in, 171–72
nonrandomness of disease
occurrence, 121–26
"Erin Brockovitch," 3, 4, 7
estrogens. *See also* hormones
breast cancer and, 178–79
formation of in body, 179
function, 147
production, 147, 179
promoters in carcinogenesis, 178–79
tamoxifen and estrogen receptors, 179
estrogen receptors, 175–79
and cell proliferation, 175
description of, 175
receptor positive cells, 175
tamoxifen and, 175, 179
exposure assessment
air pollutants, 287
of arsenic in Bangladesh, 309–10
becquerel, 79
becquerel, definition, 96
of chemical hazards in Pelham Bay,
238–39
dose determination in Japan, 29–30
electric blankets, magnetic fields
from, 209
Geographic Information System,
189–90, 192–94
gray (unit of radiation dose), 55
importance in environmental
health studies, 309–10
indoor and outdoor pollutants, 287
joule (energy), 55
magnetic fields, 205–9
old glass, for radon, 72, 93–94
personal monitors of air pollution, 291

exposure assessment (*continued*)
picocurie, 79
picocurie, definition, 96
radiation dose definition, 27–28
radiation dose determination, 55
radiation dose, 27–28
radiation types from atomic bombs
in Japan, 24–25
radon, 79–80
radon and miners, 75–81
relative biological effectiveness
(RBE), 55–56
retrospective, in Pelham Bay, 259–60
sievert, 55
TEAM studies of indoor and
outdoor air, 263–66, 287, 291–92,
313–14
wire code reliability, 211
wire codes and magnetic fields, 206,
208–9
working level month, 80
working level month, definition, 97
working level, 80
working level, definition, 97
X-rays as radiation standard for, 55–
56
extrapolation
air pollution health effects, 284
animals to humans, 221
linear and non-linear, 77–79
linear no-threshold model, 39, 84–
85, 90
occupational studies, 77–78
radiation models compared, 90
reason for, 38–39, 76–77
saturation of radiation damage and,
87–90
threshold for radiation harm, 35,
39, 90

fallout. *See* nuclear accidents, nuclear
weapons tests
false positives and false negatives,
245–46
Farr, William, 219

gamma rays. *See* radiation, types of
Gardner, Martin, 106

gauss. *See* magnetic fields; exposure
assessment
genes. *See also* molecular biology
"expression," 173
BRCA1 and BRCA2 genes in breast
cancer, 176
definition, 172
dominance, 175
p450 gene and cancer, 177
p53 gene in breast cancer, 175
polymorphism, definition, 175
protein synthesis and, 172
radiation and, 56–57
tumor suppressor genes, 175
genetic susceptibilities, 11, 196
in arsenic study in Bangladesh, 311–12
in breast cancer, 172, 175–78
deterrminants of, in asthma, 274
detoxifying enzymes and, 177
in Jewish women, and breast
cancer, 177
p450 gene and cancer, 177
protective effect of breast feeding
and, 177–78
smoking and breast cancer, 177
genetic defects
in bomb survivors, 34
Geographic Information System (GIS),
189–90, 192–94
Greaves, Mel, 148

Hachiya, Michihiko, 17,19
Harvard Center for Risk Analysis
costs of magnetic field remediation,
228–29
Hei, Tom K., 87,88
high energy radiation. *See* radiation
Hippocrates, 281, 292
Hiroshima. *See* atomic bombing
of Japan, Life Span Study (Japan)
hormones. *See also* estrogens
hormonally active agents, 151, 168–
69, 186–88
replacement therapy and breast
cancer, 181–82
and vaginal cancer, 139
xenoestrogen, definition, 155
xenoestrogens, 169, 187–88

hospital emergency room visits
  in asthma epidemics, 276–77
  data from, in Barcelona epidemics,
    277
house dust mite. *See* asthma, triggers
  of; allergens

immune system. *See also* asthma;
  allergy
  development of, 129
  challenges to, 314
Immunoglobulin E (IgE). *See* asthma;
  allergy
incidence. *See* rates of disease
insulation of homes
  asthma and, 297–98
  indoor air pollution and, 297–98
  radon exposure and, 72
ionizing radiation. *See* radiation
isotopes. *See also* radioactive elements
  definition, 99

Kinlen, Leo, 131–33

Leeper, F., 203, 211
leukemia. *See also* childhood
  leukemia
  animal studies of magnetic fields
    and, 221–24
  benzene, 109
  bomb survivors and, 32–34
  delay time after exposure, 234
  medical X-rays and, 36
  nuclear plants and, 103 (*see also*
    Sellafield, *and under* cancer
    clusters}
  Pelham Bay, 235, 238, 250–55
  radiation dose and, 30, 32–34
  radiation, 15
  strontium-90 and, 43–44
Life Span Study (Japan)
  cancer rates, 30–34
  comparison with Bangladesh
    arsenic study, 311–12
  dose determination in, 29–30
  initiation of, 23–24
  as model for environmental health
    studies, 20, 49, 309

paternal irradiation and, 111
  results summarized, 30–34, 48–49
lifestyle and disease
  asthma, 297–98, 300
  breast cancer, 183, 197–98
  distinction from "environment," 12
  modernization, health effects of,
    213–14, 313
linear no-theshold assumption. *See*
  extrapolation, radiation, radon
linear regression, 77
Linet, Martha, 214–15
London smog episode, 282–83
lung cancer
  arsenic from smelters and, 307
  death rates in U. S. and radon, 63–
    64
  radiation dose and, 30–31
  residential radon and, 8, 69–71
  residential radon and, summary,
    94–96
  risk estimates for residential radon,
    91–93
  smoking and asbestos, 82–83
  smoking and radon, 82
  smoking and, 70
  in uranium miners, 67–68
lung function
  of asthmatics, 289
  and exposure to air pollutants, 289

magnetic fields
  animal studies of, 222, 224
  cell studies of, 222–23
  cell signaling and, 224–25
  costs of remediation, 229
  discovery of health risks of, 10, 191
  exposure in homes, 202, 205–9
  frequency of 60 hertz, 203
  gauss, definition, 233
  health risks (*see* childhood
    leukemia; leukemia; cancer)
  ionizing radiation compared, 203
  National Cancer Institute study of,
    209
  ornithine decarboxylase, effects on,
    225
  penetration of body by, 203

magnetic fields (*continued*)
  possible mechanisms for harm by, 202–3
  properties relevant to risk, 212–13
  recommendations on exposure to, 228–29
  static and alternating, 232–33
  tesla, definition, 233
  wire codes as estimate of, 206, 208–9, 211–12
Maimonides, 293
Massachusetts Department of Health
  Cape Cod breast cancer study, 153, 188
  Woburn study, 260–61
melatonin
  magnetic fields and cancer, 223–24
mental retardation
  in bomb survivors, 34
microwaves, 203
miners studies. *See* occupational studies
molecular biology. *See also* carcinogenesis; genes; genetic susceptibilities; DNA; mutations
  alpha particle microbeam studies, 84–91
  arsenic study in Bangladesh, 310–11
  biomarkers for allergy, 294
  biomarkers for arsenic exposure, 311
  of breast cancer, 172–80
  carcinogenesis and radiation, 85–89
  cell division, 57
  cell nucleus, 57
  chromosomes, 57
  environmental health studies and, 11
  exposure assessment using, 268
  p450 gene, 177
  p53 tumor suppressive genes, 311
  pesticides and, 179–80
  radiation damage, 56–57
  role in epidemiology, 171–72
  TGF-alpha and arsenic exposure, 311
mutations
  as biomarkers of exposure, 174–75
  carcinogenesis and, 25–26, 56–57, 85–86, 87–88, 173–75

  causes of, 173
  definition, 173
  effects on protein synthesis, 173–74
  frequency during cell division, 178
  frequency during cell proliferation, 178
  as initiators of carcinogenesis, 178
  microbeam studies, 87–88
  radiation and, 25, 56–57

Nagasaki. *See* atomic bombing of Japan; Life Span Study (Japan)
Nagel, Ernest, 156
National Academy of Sciences (U.S.)
  review of arsenic standard, 308
National Cancer Institute (U.S.)
  agricultural study, 195
  estimate of thyroid cancer from fallout, 45–47
  leukemia and magnetic field study, 209
National Institute of Environmental Health Sciences (U.S.) (NIEHS)
  leukemia and magnetic field report, 218, 227–29
National Heart, Lung and Blood Institute (U.S.)
  asthma social cost estimate, 271
National Institutes of Health (U.S.)
  breast cancer research, 154
  Long Island breast cancer study, 195–96
National Research Council (U.S.)
  Committee on Health Risks of Exposure to Radon, 63–64, 69
  hormonally active agents report, 168
  magnetic fields report, 214, 218, 225–26
nerve damage
  from arsenic, 305
Neutra, R. R., 258
New Jersey Department of Health
  Toms River study, 261–62
New York City Department of Environmental Protection (DEP)
  Pelham Bay landfill remediation, 235–37, 270

New York City Department of Health (DOH)
Pelham Bay cancer study, 237–38
nuclear accidents
Chelyabinsk, 104
Chernobyl, 47, 95–96, 104, 147
Three Mile Island, 20, 104
Windscale, 104–5
nuclear plants. *See also* Sellafield; Windscale
Dounreay and childhood leukemia, 112
health effects (*see* childhood leukemia; leukemia)
nuclear waste
discharge from Sellafield plant, 103
health effects (*see* childhood leukemia)
plutonium recovery from, 101
nuclear weapons tests, 44–47
fallout from, 21–23
health effects (*see* cancer; childhood leukemia; thyroid cancer)
historical background of, 21

Oak Ridge National Laboratory
animal experiments on radiation, 37
occupational studies, 293
agricultural health study, 195–96
asbestos workers, 75
asthma, 293
breast cancer, 180
chemical industry and breast cancer, 180–81
electrical workers and cancer, 211
extrapolation from, to lower exposures, 76
"healthy worker" effect in, 75–76
miners and radon, 79–80
nuns and breast cancer, 139, 159
power of, 74–75
radiologists, 75
smoking adjustment for miners, 81–83
ventilation in mines, 81
watch dial painters, 15

Parker, L., 132
Pelham Bay
cancer in, 240–41
chemical hazards in, 4–6
childhood leukemia cluster in, 235
DOH study conclusions, 255–56
DOH study, 237–38
exposure assessment, retrospective, 259–60
landfill, 235
leukemia in, 235, 239–40, 250–53
pancreatic cancer in, 244–45, 246–47
pesticides, 9, 149–151 (*see also* chemical hazards, hormonally active agents)
breast cancer studies of, 182, 184–87
in breast milk, 151
chemical hazards and breast cancer, 185–86
DDT, 149, 167, 185–87
DDT, DDE and breast cancer, 184–87
estrogenicity of, 168–69
farmers and cancer, 195–96
in fat tissue, 151
health effects (*see* breast cancer)
Seveso accident, 182–83
wildlife, effect on, 149–50
physics, laws of
magnetic field-cancer link, 226–27
plasticizers
breast cancer and, 151
Poisson, S. D., 116
Poisson distribution, 116–20
population mixing. *See* childhood leukemia
power (statistical), 74–75, 251–54
Bangladesh arsenic study, 310
detectability of increased disease rates, 253
leukemia excess in Pelham Bay, 250–53
radiation health studies, 38
sample size and, 74
simple illustrative example of, 253
specificity and, 253–54
power lines. *See* electromagnetic fields, magnetic fields

radiation. *See also* entries under "nuclear" and exposure assessment; radiation, types of; radioactivity; radioactive elements; radon
  atomic bombs, 8
  biological mechanism of harm, 26, 56–57
  discovery of, 13
  DNA damage from, 25, 56–57
  dose, equivalent, 28
  dose, fatal, 28
  dose, sievert as unit, 27–28
  electromagnetic wave energy, 53
  electromagnetic waves, 49–53
  health effects (*see* breast cancer; birth defects; cancer; childhood leukemia; Life Span Study; thyroid cancer)
  ionizing radiation, definition, 49
  medical uses of, 42–43
  microwaves, 53
  mutations and cancer, 56–57
  mutations, 25
  natural background, 25–26, 39–40
  nature of, 49–57
  non-ionizing, 54–55
  occupational exposure, 40
  particle, 54
  photons, 53
  ultraviolet light, 53
radiation sickness, 17, 30, 43
radiation, types of
  alpha particles, 14
  alpha particles, nature of, 24
  beta particles, nature of, 24
  electromagnetic waves, nature of, 24
  gamma rays from atomic bombs, 29
  gamma rays, nature of, 24–25
  medical X-ray exposure studies, 35–36
  neutrons from atomic bombs, 29
  neutrons, nature of, 24–25
  X-rays and animal experiments, 37
  X-rays, discovery of, 13
  X-rays, nature of, 24

radioactive elements. *See also* radon
  ingestion of, 61–63
  iodine-131 and thyroid cancer, 25
  iodine-131 and thyroid gland, 44
  iodine-131 from fallout, 45–47
  iodine-131 in milk, 21, 45–47
  lead, as decay product, 14
  lead-210 in old glass, 72
  penetration of alpha particles from, 62–63
  penetration of beta particles from, 62–63
  polonium in lung tissue, 44, 63
  polonium, 14
  polonium-214, 64–66
  polonium-218, 64–66
  radium and bone cancer, 15
  radium and watch dial painters, 15
  radium, 14
  radon as polonium source, 44
  radon-222, 65–66
  strontium-90 and bones, 43–44
  strontium-90, 62
  uranium, 13–14
  uranium-238, 14, 64–65, 100
radioactivity
  alpha particle emission, 99
  atomic theory of, 97–100
  beta particle emission, 99
  discovery of, 13–14
  electrons and protons, 98
  exposure from, 25
  fission, 100
  half-life, 65, 99
  health effects (*see* cancer, leukemia, lung cancer, thyroid cancer)
  isotopes, 99–100
  neutrons, 99
  nucleus of atom, 98–99
radon. *See also* exposure assessment; radiation; radioactive elements; radioactivity
  alpha particles from, 66
  chemical inertness of, 66
  "daughters," 65–66
  EPA remediation standard, 96
  exposure assessment from old glass, 71–72, 93–94

health effects (*see* lung cancer)
mechanism of harm from, 66
natural background, 67
polonium from, 65–66
progeny, 65–66
in Reading Prong, 60–62
residential levels of, 96–97
residential, 8–9
risk discovered, 59
source of residential, 60
uranium as source, 64–65
Ramazzini, Bernardino 139, 159, 293
random variation. *See also* chance
rates of disease, 72
Seascale cluster and, 126
signals and noise, 72–75
simple illustrative examples of, 115–20, 242–44
small samples, 72
"square root estimate," 74, 84
rates of disease. *See also* asthma rates;
breast cancer rates; cancer
clusters
cancer in Pelham Bay, 240–41
definition, 73, 240
diarrhea in Bangladesh children, 304
incidence defined, 156
infant and child mortality in
Bangladesh, 304
risk factors and, 241
Reading Prong, 60–62
risk estimates. *See also* safety standards
"acceptable risk," 308–9
arsenic and cancer, 309
linear model for radon risk, 89–91
lung cancer and radon, 64, 91–93
medical X-rays, 41–42
of natural background radiation, 42
radiation and cancer, 40–41
"relative risk" definition, 92–93
of thyroid cancer from fallout, 45–47
risk factors. *See also* breast cancer risk
factors
adjustment, reason for, 155–56
cancer in Pelham Bay, 241
for childhood leukemia, 133, 204
definition, 140–41
risk perception, 94–96

safety standards. *See also*
Environmental Protection
Agency, risk estimates
scientific basis for arsenic, 308
arsenic, U.S., 308
arsenic, European, 308
arsenic, World Health Organization,
308
air pollution, 283–84
radon in homes, 61
radiation, 38
Schneider, Konrad, 293
science
activist need for, 315
basis for safety standards, 308
causation, concept of, 221–27
public understanding of, 12
Seascale, town of. *See* cancer clusters,
childhood leukemia
Selikoff, I., 262
Sellafield nuclear plant, 101–2
closure, 134
Shapiro, S., 161
Sierra Club
magnetic field testing, 201
sievert
radiation dose unit, 21, 55–56
Silent Spring, 149
Silent Spring Institute
Cape Cod breast cancer study, 189–90
skin lesions
from arsenic in Bangladesh, 310
from arsenic, 305
smoking
lung cancer in asbestos workers
and, 82–83
lung cancer in miners and, 81–83
lung cancer and, 59, 70
synergism with asbestos exposure,
82–83
synergism with radon exposure, 82–83
Snow, John, 219
soy beans. *See* asthma epidemics
statistical significance. *See also*
confidence interval
controversy in magnetic field study,
216–17
explanation of, 244–49

statistical significance (*continued*)
  misuse of, 254–55, 258–59
  multiple comparisons and, 247–48,
    258
  rationale for 5% criterion, 245–46
  testing for, 245–46
statistics. *See* chance; confidence
    interval; power (statistical);
    statistical significance
Sunyer, J., 278
synergism
  definition, 82–83
  smoking and asbestos, 82–83
  smoking and radon exposure,
    82–83

Taiwan
  arsenic in drinking water, studies of,
    307–8
tamoxifen
  biological mechanism of action, 173
  therapy in breast cancer, 175
TEAM studies of indoor air pollution,
    263–66, 287, 291–92, 313–14
tesla. *See* exposure assessment;
    magnetic fields
"Texas sharpshooter" effect, 122–26,
    259
threshold
  radiation harm, 38, 39
thyroid cancer
  Chernobyl accident and, 47
  nuclear test fallout and, 36–38, 45–
    47
  iodine-131 and, 24, 44
Toms River. *See* cancer clusters
toxic waste dumps. *See also* chemical
    hazards
  Pelham Bay landfill, 4, 235
  breast cancer and, 9, 152
  in Toms River, 6–7, 261–62
  in Woburn, 6, 260
toxicology. *See* animal experiments,
    cell studies
tube wells
  Bangladesh and West Bengal, 303–4

typhoid fever
  fecal contamination of water and, 303

uncertainty range, 49, 93. *See also*
    confidence interval
  of breast cancer excess rates, 160–
    62, 165
  extrapolation in radon studies, 76–78
  of lung cancer deaths from radon, 94
  of residential radon and lung cancer, 71
United Kingdom study of magnetic
    fields
  conclusions, 217
  relevance to U. S. conditions, 217
United Nations Children's Fund
    (UNICEF)
  tube well program in Bangladesh, 304
Utah
  fallout from nuclear tests in, 21–23,
    46

weather
  air pollution and, 284
  inversions, definition, 282
  inversions and London smog, 282
  thunderstorms and asthma, 280–81
  health and, 282, 284, 291
Wertheimer, N., 203, 211
West Bengal (India)
  tube well program, 304
  arsenic contamination discovered
    in, 304–5
Whitman, Christine T., 308
Windscale nuclear plant, 101. *See also*
    Sellafield nuclear plant
  fire at, 104–5
wire codes. *See under* exposure
    assessment
Woburn, Massachusetts. *See under*
    cancer clusters; childhood
    leukemia
Wolff, Mary, 186
World Health Organization (WHO)
  arsenic standard, 308

X-rays. *See* radiation, types of